The book deals briefly with the normal structure, functioning and biochemistry of the esophagus and with the histological and genetic changes accompanying the development of esophageal cancer in humans and animals. Factors implicated in causing esophageal cancer are described in relation to its very dramatic epidemiology. Thus dietary deficiencies and consumption of foods contaminated by *Fusaria* mycotoxins are discussed in connection with the extremely high incidence of the disease in certain sharply demarcated regions in China and South Africa, and alcohol and tobacco use are discussed in relation to the epidemiology in Europe and USA. Other hazards mentioned include opium in Iran, betel nut in Asia and bracken in Japan.

The sole group of chemicals known to be very potent esophageal carcinogens in animal experiments, the nitrosamines, are described especially in terms of the widespread human exposure. The concept is put forward that these chemicals are responsible for initiation of the disease, but that promotion by the secondary risk factors is generally essential for symptomatic cancer to develop. This could explain why the epidemiology reflects exposure to secondary risk factors rather than levels of exposure to nitrosamines. The secondary risk factors increase cell replication but do not initiate cancer. The recent perturbing increase in adenocarcinoma is considered.

T0291731

Cambridge Monographs on Cancer Research

Cancer of the esophagus

Cambridge Monographs on Cancer Research

Books in this Series

Martin R. Osborne and Neil T. Crosby *Benzopyrenes*

Maurice M. Coombs and Tarlochan S. Bhatt
Cyclopenta[a]phenanthrenes

M. S. Newman, B. Tierney and S. Veeraraghavan *The chemistry and biology of benz[a]anthracenes*

Jürgen Jacob *Sulfur analogues of polycyclic aromatic hydrocarbons (thiaarenes)*

R. G. Harvey *Polycyclic aromatic hydrocarbons*

W. Lijinsky *The chemistry and biology of* N-*nitroso compounds*

W. F. Karcher *Dibenzanthracenes and environmental carcinogenesis*

John Higginson, Calum S. Muir and Nubia Muñoz *Human cancer: epidemiology and environmental causes*

Anne R. Kinsella *Colorectal cancer*

Valda M. Craddock *Cancer of the esophagus*

Cancer of the esophagus

Approaches to the etiology

VALDA M. CRADDOCK

Senior Scientist, Medical Research Council
Toxicology Unit

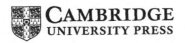

CAMBRIDGE UNIVERSITY PRESS
Cambridge, New York, Melbourne, Madrid, Cape Town, Singapore, São Paulo, Delhi

Cambridge University Press
The Edinburgh Building, Cambridge CB2 8RU, UK

Published in the United States of America by Cambridge University Press, New York

www.cambridge.org
Information on this title: www.cambridge.org/9780521102582

First published 1993
This digitally printed version 2009

A catalogue record for this publication is available from the British Library

Library of Congress Cataloguing in Publication data

Craddock, Valda M.
Cancer of the esophagus: approaches to the etiology / Valda M.
Craddock.
    p.   cm. – (Cambridge monographs on cancer research)
Includes index.
ISBN 0 521 37393 X (hardback)
1. Esophagus – Cancer – Etiology.   I. Title.   II. Series.
[DNLM: 1. Esophageal Neoplasms – etiology.   WI 250 C884c]
RC280.E8C7   1993
616.99'432 – dc20
DNLM/DLC
for library of congress 92-49058 CIP

ISBN 978-0-521-37393-7 hardback
ISBN 978-0-521-10258-2 paperback

Contents

Preface

The surprising discovery that a small simple chemically inert compound, dimethylnitrosamine, was a potent carcinogen, was made by Barnes and Magee in 1956. A few years later I joined them in an attempt to find out how and why, in terms of metabolism of the carcinogen, and reactions with protein, RNA and DNA. From work carried out mainly in Heidelberg and in America, it was very soon found that many of the N-nitroso compounds were carcinogenic, they showed a surprising organospecificity, and that more than half of the 300 tested were carcinogenic for the esophagus. When it became apparent that human exposure to the compounds in the environment was widespread, and that no other chemically identified environmental compounds were potent esophageal carcinogens in animal experiments, the obvious possibility that they were a major cause of esophageal cancer was considered.

The problem in testing this concept was that human exposure was so widespread but difficult to quantify that epidemiological surveys could not associate the disease with exposure to nitrosamines. Instead incidence correlated with other risk factors, especially alcohol consumption and dietary deficiencies. A likely explanation seemed to me to be in the induction of cell replication. I had found that, while continuous feeding of dimethylnitrosamine induced liver cancer, one single injection of the compound was not carcinogenic unless given when the liver cells were dividing in response to partial hepatectomy. The secondary risk factors of alcohol, dietary deficiencies and mycotoxins were shown to stimulate basal cell replication in the esophagus. It therefore seemed highly probable that nitrosamines could initiate malignancy, but that in the esophagus promotion by an increase in cell replication was essential for clinical cancer to appear.

The incidence of esophageal cancer world-wide is one of the highest, in the UK the incidence in women is the highest in Europe, and for men it is second only to France and Switzerland, and ranks among the ten most frequent cancers. The rate of liver cancer in the UK is very low. In spite of this, study of cancer of the liver receives infinitely more support than that of the esophagus. This book was written in the hope that an updated discussion of the problem might stimulate interest and research.

For one person to attempt to write a book considering such broad issues was a formidable prospect, and I have been helped by colleagues with expertise in certain aspects of the subject. The friends I would like to thank especially are the following: Dr Clifford Waters, formerly of Surrey University; Dr J.V. Frei, University of London, Ontario; Dr P. Grasso, formerly of British Industrial Biological Research Association; Dr R. Schoental, formerly of MRC Toxicology Unit; Dr M. Hill, European Cancer Prevention Chairman.

I would like to express my gratitude also to my secretary, Mrs Joan Nicholass, for her hard work and moral support, and to Mr Brian Street, without whose help in enabling me to work after a motor accident the writing of this book would have been very much delayed.

V.M.C.

Abbreviations

NOC   *N*-nitroso compounds

Nitrosamines

NDMA	*N*-nitroso-dimethylamine
NDEA	*N*-nitroso-diethylamine
NDPA	*N*-nitroso-dipropylamine
NDBA	*N*-nitroso-dibutylamine
NMEA	*N*-nitroso-methylethylamine
NMBA	*N*-nitroso-methylbutylamine
NMAA	*N*-nitroso-methylamylamine
NMAlA	*N*-nitroso-methylallylamine
N-SAR	*N*-nitroso-sarcosine
NMBzA	*N*-nitroso-methylbenzylamine
NMPhA	*N*-nitroso-methylphenylamine
N-PIP	*N*-nitroso-piperidine
N-PYR	*N*-nitroso-pyrrolidine

Tobacco-specific nitrosamines

TSN	Tobacco specific nitrosamines
NNN	*N*-nitrosonornicotine
NNK	4(methyl-nitroso-amino)-1-(3 pyridyl)-butanone
NAB	*N*-nitrosoanabasine
NAT	*N*-nitrosoanatbine

Direct-acting nitroso compounds

NMU	Nitrosomethylurea
NEU	Nitrosoethylurea
MNNG	Methylnitronitrosoguanidine

ENNG   Ethylnitronitrosoguanidine
NMUR   Nitrosomethylurethane
NEUR   Nitrosoethylurethane

DNA adducts
7MG   7-methylguanine
O^6MG O^6-methylguanine
3MA   3-methyladenine

Alcohols
EtOH   Ethanol
3Mb   3-methylbutanol
2Mb   2-methylbutanol

Mycotoxins
DS   Deoxyscirpenol

1

Introduction: the problem, incidence, etiology. A working hypothesis

Esophageal cancer is one of the most common cancers world-wide, having a higher global incidence than the much-studied cancer of the liver. When added to oral and pharyngeal cancers, which have a similar etiology, cancers of the upper alimentary tract form the most prevalent cancers world-wide (Parkin *et al.* 1988). The difference in rate between high and low incidence areas around the world is extreme, ranging from 0.4/100000 for women in the state of Utah, USA, to 170/100000 in the Gonbad region of Northern Iran. Even within any country, the geographical distribution of the cancer is often very sharply demarcated, exceptionally high-risk regions neighbouring onto districts with a much lower risk. At the French/Belgian and the Kenya/Uganda borders there is a sharp change in incidence at the political boundaries. Epidemiological studies carried out in these situations have very strongly implicated a variety of risk factors, notably alcohol consumption, deficiencies of certain micronutrients, consumption of food contaminated by mycotoxins, and a low consumption of fresh fruit and vegetables. None of these factors, however, has been shown to cause esophageal cancer in experimental animals.

Thousands of chemicals have been tested for carcinogenicity, but the only compounds found to be potent carcinogens for the esophagus in animal experiments are the nitrosamines. All species tested were found to be susceptible, from amphibia to primates, and there is no apparent reason why man should be excepted. Human exposure to *N*-nitroso compounds, either from intake in food or consumer products, or from *in vivo* formation in the human stomach, is probably ubiquitous. Although other environmental esophageal carcinogens may exist, for example in bracken fern or in opium, they have yet to be identified. At present, the sole contenders for the role of initiators of esophageal cancer in man are the nitrosamines.

It is only in a few instances that a high rate of esophageal cancer associates with a high exposure to nitrosamines. Usually the levels of exposure, while they could be initiating malignant changes in the genetic material of a few basal cells of the esophagus, are apparently too low to cause symptomatic cancer. However, the initiated cells do progress to form tumors when the action of the nitrosamines is promoted by secondary risk factors. Many of these promoters, including alcohols, deficiency of riboflavin or zinc, and mycotoxins, have been shown to increase the rate of replication in the basal cells of the esophagus. A very plausible working hypothesis is therefore that the cancer is initiated by nitrosamines, and promoted by one or more of the secondary risk factors. The epidemiological and animal studies described in this volume give support to this concept.

The fact that esophageal cancer is one of the most unpleasant forms of cancer, and is one with an exceptionally poor prognosis, make a study of the etiology imperative. In spite of this, the proportion of research effort put into study of the esophagus has been exceptionally low in most developed countries. Knowledge of the basic enzymology and ultrastructure is almost non-existent. The reason is obvious: it is far easier in animal experiments to study an organ such as liver than a small tube such as esophagus. As stated nearly 20 years ago (Wynder *et al.* 1975), 'we need to study the biochemistry of epithelial cells in the upper alimentary and upper respiratory tracts – a far more pertinent target of study than the liver cells. We should not act like the drunk who looks for his lost keys under the lantern simply because that is where the light is and look only at the liver cell because it is relatively an easy system to investigate. We believe that an understanding of the biochemical framework of the squamous cell of the upper alimentary tract of an alcoholic and knowledge of why it is more susceptible to tobacco carcinogens will provide major clues to the biochemical parameters controlling the transformation of a squamous cell into a neoplastic cell.' Sadly the majority are still behaving like drunks, even though modern techniques make study of the esophagus more approachable.

The dramatic epidemiology of esophageal cancer shows that the causes lie in the environment, and suggest obvious measures for prevention. It was stated in 1982 (van Rensburg) that we were 'on the threshold of a period that may be dominated by preventive intervention'. At present, owing to the neglect of basic work, we are still only on the threshold.

The few books and reviews considering the etiology of esophageal cancer are now out of date or limited in their scope to one country. It is now ten years since publication of the excellent reviews of Day *et al.*

(1982*a*, *b*), and the book edited by Pfeiffer (1982). Several books entitled *Cancer of the Esophagus* have appeared but they have not discussed the general problem of etiology. The excellent book edited by Huang *et al.* (1984) deals mainly with conditions in China, that by DeMeester *et al.* (1985) is devoted almost entirely to diagnosis, pathology and treatment, and that of Matthews *et al.* (1987) to incidence of cancer in the UK. Recently a brief review (Craddock 1992) has been published.

This book has been written in an attempt to draw attention to the fascinating concepts relating to the etiology of esophageal cancer, and to stimulate work which might lead to a reduction in the high incidence of this tragic, preventable disease.

References

Craddock, V.M. (1992) *Eur. J. Cancer Prev.* **1**, 89–103. Etiology of esophageal cancer: some operative factors.

Day, N.E., Munoz, N. and Ghadirian, P. (1982a) In: *Epidemiology of Cancer of the Digestive Tract* (Correa, P. and Haenszel, W. eds.). Dordrecht: Martinus Nijhoff, pp. 21–57. Epidemiology of esophageal cancer: a review.

Day, N.E. and Munoz, N. (1982b) In: *Cancer Epidemiology and Prevention* (Schottenfeld, D. and Fraumeni, J.F. eds.). Philadelphia: Saunders, pp. 596–623. Esophagus.

DeMeester, T.R. and Levin, B. (1985) *Cancer of the Esophagus.* New York: Grune and Stratton.

Huang, G.I. and K'ai, W. (eds.) (1984) *Carcinoma of the Esophagus and Gastric Cardia.* New York: Springer.

Matthews, H.R., Waterhouse, J.H.A., Powell, J., Robinson, J.E. and McConkey, C.C. (1987) *Clinical Cancer Monographs*, vol. I. London: Macmillan. Cancer of the Oesophagus.

Parkin, D.M., Laara, E. and Muir, C.S. (1988) *Int. J. Cancer* **41**, 184–197. Estimates of the world-wide frequency of sixteen major cancers in 1980.

Pfeiffer, C.J. (ed.) (1982) *Cancer of the Esophagus*, vols. I and II. Boca Raton: CRC Press.

van Rensburg, S.J. (1982) *S. Afr. Cancer Bull.* **26**, 153–159. Nutritional factors in human carcinogenesis.

Wynder, E.L., Hoffmann, D., Chan, P and Reddy, B. (1975) In: *Persons at High Risk of Cancer. An approach to Cancer Etiology and Control* (Fraumeni, J.F. ed.). New York: Academic Press, pp. 485–501. Interdisciplinary and experimental approaches: metabolic epidemiology.

2

Biology of the esophagus

The esophagus is a relatively simple tube which is well adapted to fulfil its function of transporting material from the mouth to the stomach. The elasticity of the mucosa and musculature allows for extension of the lumen during the passage of a bolus of food, and a coordinated nerve plexus and musculature enables peristaltic waves of contraction and relaxation to propel the contents of the lumen to the stomach. On the other hand, the esophagus is one of the first organs to encounter toxic and carcinogenic chemicals in the diet, and the fact that esophageal cancer is one of the cancers with the highest incidence world-wide (Parkin *et al.* 1988) implies that biochemical defence mechanisms are not sufficiently well developed to protect man against this hazard. While the structure and physiology of the esophagus have been studied in some detail, the biochemistry has been almost completely neglected.

Structure of the normal esophagus
The esophagus is comprised of a straight muscular tube running from the pharynx to the stomach. In the neck region it lies dorsal to the larynx and to the anterior end of the trachea, but in the thorax it is slightly to the left of the trachea. After piercing the diaphragm, the esophagus enters the stomach in the middle of the lesser curvature. It therefore lies mainly in the thorax. The length of the esophagus obviously varies very much with the species of animal. In man it is about 25 cm long, in the rat 5 cm.

While an interesting variety of modifications of the esophagus occur in lower animals, in mammals the histological structure follows a common pattern (Figs. 2.1–2.4). The lumen is lined by stratified squamous epithelium, which rests on a corium of connective tissue, the basement membrane. In mammals, the stratified squamous epithelium of the external body surface is continuous with that of the oral cavity, which in turn is continuous with the esophagus. The epithelia differ in their embryonic development, however, as that of the epidermis and oral cavity are ectodermal in origin, while the esophageal epithelium is derived from endoderm.

During embryonic development, the esophagus and stomach are derived from the foregut. During the fifth week of pregnancy in man, the stomach appears as a dilation in the foregut, and during the seventh week the cervical flexure is reduced, the neck forms, and the back straightens. At the same time, the esophagus lengthens. The esophageal epithelial cells proliferate and undergo developmental changes which are unique to the esophagus and are not shared by other stratified squamous epithelia (Johns 1952). The epithelium is at first simple low columnar, and at the ninth week of pregnancy it becomes ciliated. At the eleventh week ciliated cells begin to be replaced by squamous cells. Ciliated cells disappear last from the upper end of the esophagus, although patches of ciliated cells may remain at birth and for a short time after birth. Superficial glands are present at birth, but deep glands are scanty, most of their development being post-natal. In other mammals, no ciliated cells appear in the esophagus during embryonic development.

A complete basal layer of cuboid replicating cells rests on the basement membrane. After replication, one or both of the daughter cells may be displaced away from the underlying connective tissue and move upwards towards the lumen. The cells differentiate as they move towards the surface, forming first larger spinous cells, then polygonal granular cells, and finally becoming flatter and giving rise to squamous cells which may or may not produce keratin (Fig. 2.3) (Leblond *et al.* 1984). Blood vessels do

Fig. 2.1. Diagrammatic representation of transverse section of rat esophagus.

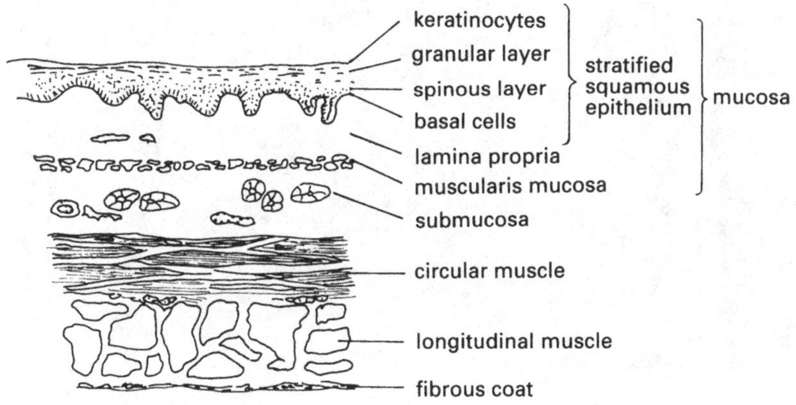

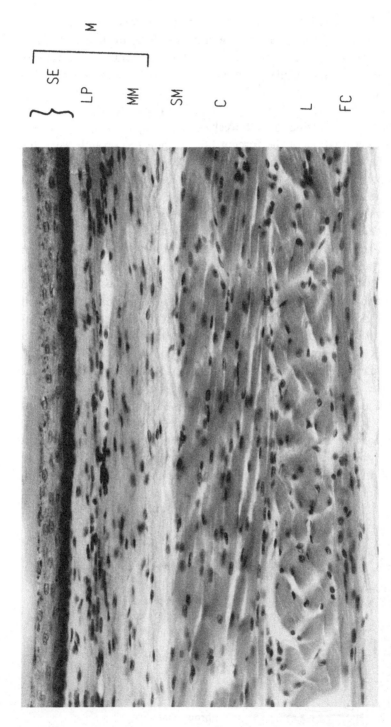

Fig. 2.2. Transverse section of rat esophagus. C, circular muscle; FC, fibrous coat; L, longitudinal muscle; M, mucosa; MM, muscularis mucosa; SE, squamous epithelium; SM, submucosa. H&E, × 200.

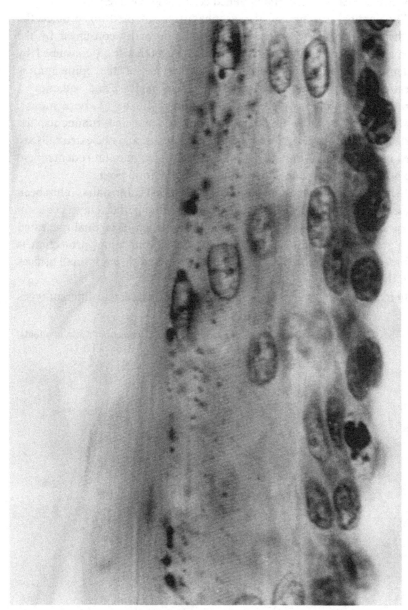

Fig. 2.3. Transverse section of rat esophageal epithelium. B, basal cells; G, granulocytes; K, keratinocytes; S, spinocytes. H&E, ×1000.

not extend into the epithelium, so that the supply of nutrients decreases as the cells move away from the basement membrane. As a result they become less metabolically active, the flattened cells being relatively inert.

The luminal surface of the esophagus is adapted to protect the epithelium, depending on the type of food normally consumed by the animal. For protection against the coarse vegetable food consumed by rodents, ruminants and the horse, the surface of the epithelium is keratinized. In the superficial cells the nuclei regress, and squames of keratin are continuously shed into the lumen. In the newborn mouse, however, and possibly in other newborn rodents and ruminants, the surface cells are not keratinized but produce mucus, and nucleated cells are shed into the lumen (Parakkal 1967). Surprisingly, in adult rodents there are no glands to provide mucus to lubricate the food bolus.

In man, monkeys, cats and dogs, keratinization is rare, unless it has been caused by trauma, although flattened cells in the superficial layers contain a few keratinohyaline granules. Layers of flattened hexagonal nucleated cells are shed from the surface. Instead of keratinization, protection is afforded by production of mucus, which is secreted through small orifices into the lumen.

In man, the mucus glands are of two types, which secrete different types

Fig. 2.4. Transverse section of rat esophagus to show mucosa thrown into folds which allow expansion during passage of food bolus. H&E, × 12.

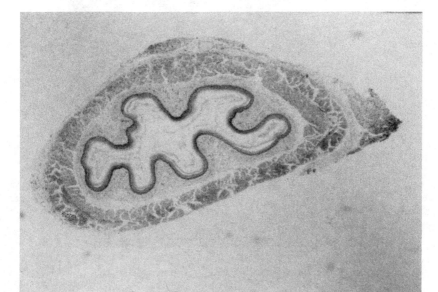

of mucus and differ in their staining properties. The superficial glands occur in the mucosa, and are limited to narrow zones near the two ends of the esophagus. As they resemble the glands in the cardiac end of the stomach, they are sometimes referred to as cardiac glands. The deep glands occur in the submucosa, and are scattered throughout the length of the esophagus, usually predominating in the upper region. The number of glands varies greatly in different individuals.

In the pig, an increasingly popular experimental animal for work on the alimentary canal, the situation is intermediate between that of man and rodents, as keratinization is partial but not complete, and mucus glands are present but are limited to the upper part of the esophagus. The cat is also unusual in being protected neither by mucus glands nor by keratin. These species differences are important to bear in mind when relating the results of experimental work on animals to the situation in man.

In the rat and the mouse, the stratified squamous epithelium of the esophagus continues into the stomach and forms the forestomach. As food passes rapidly down the esophagus and remains in the stomach often for some hours, it has been suggested (Grice 1988) that the forestomach could act as an experimental model for the effect of carcinogens on the esophagus in man. However, although the histological structure of the rodent esophagus and forestomach are very similar, the two organs are susceptible to different carcinogens. In contrast to the situation in rodents, in man there is an abrupt transition from stratified squamous epithelium to simple columnar epithelium at the junction of the esophagus with the cardia of the stomach. Here the white mucus membrane of the esophagus changes abruptly to the pink of the gastric mucosa.

Below the stratified squamous epithelium is a layer of loose connective tissue, the lamina propria. Among the thin collagenous fibres and the network of fine elastic fibres are numerous scattered cells. These cells are mainly lymphocytes, which in man occasionally form small lymphatic nodules, located especially around the ducts of the mucus glands. In addition, plasma cells, macrophages, and eosinophils are present, the numbers rapidly increasing after injury. As mentioned above, in man and certain other species the lamina propria also contains mucus glands.

The lamina propria is separated from the submucosa by the muscularis mucosa. This layer is composed of circular and longitudinal smooth muscle fibres. It is more apparent in lower regions of the alimentary canal, and in view of the fact that it is said to be absent in the mouse (Hummel *et al.* 1966) it may not have an important role in the esophagus.

The submucosa is composed of dense connective tissue, and is fibrous rather than cellular in nature. Broad coarse elastic and collagen fibres are present. The major part of the blood supply to the esophagus reaches the organ at the submucosa, where the arteries branch and pass up to the mucosa and down into the muscle layers. The pink muscle layers are well vascularized to provide oxygen for the repeated contractions involved in peristalsis, while the pale mucosa has a poor blood supply. As a result the mucosa is very sensitive to the nature of material passing down the lumen, and to the gastric juice which is regurgitated from the stomach during reflux. The veins from the mucosa and the muscle anastomose in the submucosa, and leave the esophagus beside the arteries. Lymphatics arise as blind tubes in the mucosa, and anastomose to form larger vessels in the submucosa.

The muscle layers occur below the submucosa. Apparently there is a difference of opinion concerning the nature of the muscle fibres in man and animals. In man, the generally accepted view, expressed by Stinson and Reznik (1982), is that the upper third is composed of striated fibres and the lower third of smooth fibres, while the two types are intermingled in the central region of the esophagus. On the other hand, according to Heading (1984), and as he says contrary to popular belief, only the proximate 3–4 cm of the human esophagus contains striated muscle. For ruminants and rodents, according to Stinson and Reznik (1982), the entire length of the muscle layer is composed of striated muscle, while other publications state that the upper, central, and lower thirds of the esophagus have striated, mixed, and smooth muscle fibres respectively. It is unfortunate that this state of confusion has not been resolved.

The arrangement of the two layers of fibres is similar to that which occurs throughout the alimentary canal. The fibres run in a circular direction round the esophagus in the inner layer, and are longitudinally arranged in the outer layer. However, in neither layer is the organization regular and uniform, and obliquely running fibres are present in both layers.

Contraction of the longitudinal muscle shortens the esophagus, while contraction of circular muscle constricts the lumen, and throws the mucosa into longitudinal folds. As the circular muscle has tonus, the normal state of the mucosa is folded (Fig. 2.4). It is the circular muscle which is thickened at the pharyngeal-esophageal and esophageal-gastric sphincters, and tonus results in the sphincters being closed, except when relaxation occurs as a consequence of swallowing. The ganglionated nerve plexuses which control peristalsis are situated in the muscle layers, the myenteric plexus of Auerbach between the inner and outer muscle layers, and the submucosa plexus of Meissner between the submucosa and the circular muscle.

The outermost coat of the esophagus, the adventitia, is composed of loose connective tissue, and contains blood vessels, lymphatics, and nerves. Elastic fibres attach the adventitia to the trachea and to the diaphragm, and in these regions the connective tissue is stronger and more fibrous than elsewhere. As a result of the elasticity of the esophagus and of its connections with surrounding organs, the functioning of the esophagus is not impeded by respiratory movements. Thus while the histological structure of the esophagus conforms to the basic plan for the alimentary canal from mouth to rectum, it is modified to form an extremely efficient tube for the rapid propulsion of food.

The upper end of the esophagus is closed by the pharyngeal-esophageal sphincter, which prevents the contents from regurgitating into the pharynx, and prevents the passage of air into the esophagus during inspiration. The lower end is closed by the esophageal-gastric sphincter.

Functioning of the esophagus

After solid material has been swallowed, the bolus is seized by a peristaltic wave, and contraction of circular muscle behind the bolus and relaxation of longitudal muscle in front propels the material down the esophagus. The response to swallowing (primary peristalsis) is initiated through afferent reflexes in the pharynx and can occur in the absence of a bolus. The passage of the peristaltic wave down the esophagus (secondary peristalsis) is coordinated by the intramural plexuses in the esophagus, and depends on distension of the lumen, usually caused by the presence of a food bolus.

Under normal resting conditions, the pressure in the esophagus, as in the remainder of the thorax, is below atmospheric pressure, and contraction of the esophageal-gastric sphincter is therefore necessary to prevent reflux of injurious stomach contents into the esophagus. When a food bolus reaches the sphincter, relaxation allows its passage into the stomach. The sphincter then closes immediately. The action of the sphincter is helped by the fact that the esophagus enters the stomach at an oblique angle. In the bat, an animal which spends much of its life upside down, the entrance into the stomach is blocked also by lax folds of the gastric mucosa, which block the aperture, and help to prevent the stomach contents from entering the esophagus by gravity. This factor is operative, but of less importance, in other species.

The fact that the rate of movement of lumen contents is not the same at all levels down to the stomach is important in relation to carcinogenesis, as there has been much discussion concerning differences in the cancer incidence at different levels in men and women. In man, in the cervical region, which is about 6 cm long, the striated muscle is capable of rapid contraction, and solid material passes down rapidly, in approximately 1 second. In this region, peristalsis is controlled by nerve reflexes involving the spinal cord. In the upper thoracic region, 10 cm long, where striated and smooth fibres are intermingled, the transit time is 1.5–2.0 seconds. In the lower thoracic region, where the length is more variable, and the fibres are smooth, the transit time is around 3 seconds. Solid and semisolid food therefore takes 6–7 seconds to pass from the mouth into the stomach. In the lower thoracic region, peristalsis is controlled by the nerve plexus within the muscle layers. The process can, however, be influenced by nerve impulses from outside the esophagus.

In contrast to the effect of swallowing solid material, repeated deglutition of liquids causes an inhibition of peristalsis, and the lower esophageal sphincter remains relaxed. The action of the sphincter is very relevant to esophageal cancer, as the irritant action of gastric juice which occurs if the sphincter is too relaxed, and of stasis in the esophagus which can be caused if the sphincter does not relax, can both cause hyperplasia and so promote carcinogenesis.

The mechanisms involved in the passage of liquids down the esophagus are adapted to differences in anatomy and feeding habits of different species. In the dog, liquid is forcibly squirted into the pharynx and down the esophagus, so that the animal can drink in the head-down position. In birds, including fowl and geese, the passage of liquid as well as of solid is dependent on peristalsis. There is no squirting action from the oral cavity, and the bird must raise its head to drink. These species differences are important in relation to carcinogenesis. For example, it was noticed that in regions in China with higher rates of esophageal cancer the domestic hens often suffer from the disease, and for this reason carcinogenesis produced by giving esophageal carcinogens *per os* has been studied in hens (quoted as unpublished data in Tang *et al.* 1984).

In addition to the voluntary deglutition of food and drink, under normal resting conditions swallowing of saliva is said to occur between one and ten times every fifteen minutes, and less often during sleep. Thus the lumen is continuously washed with saliva and, apart from the brief contact with swallowed material, the lumen is empty. This contrasts with the situation in stomach, where in man the mucosa is exposed to possibly toxic material for several hours after a meal. In the rat, even after 1–2 days' starvation, the stomach is not completely empty. In view of the fact that in certain regions of the world the incidence of esophageal cancer is higher than that of stomach cancer, this implies that duration of contact of carcinogens with the epithelium may not always be relevant in carcinogenesis.

An important factor which may promote carcinogenesis in the esophagus is the upward movement of irritant material, i.e. movement in the abnormal direction. True reverse peristalsis is a rare event, and occurs only in the case of obstruction in the lumen. During vomiting, contraction of the gastric muscles ejects the stomach contents through the esophageal-gastric sphincter and up the esophagus. The muscles of the esophagus, including those of both sphincters, are relaxed. However, ripples of contraction and relaxation often pass upwards. This upward movement is responsible for some of the symptoms of dyspepsia, for example the appearance of 'fur' on the back of the tongue, and also for the upward movements of pockets of air which may have accumulated at the bottom of the esophagus, as occurs during 'belching'. The important issue of gastric reflux is discussed in Chapter 3.

Cell replication and differentiation

As mentioned above, replication normally occurs only in the basal cells of the esophageal epithelium. The process was studied initially by examination of sections of esophagus by autoradiography after injection of the animals with tritiated thymidine (Leblond *et al.* 1964, 1967). These authors showed that, in the rat, the majority of the basal cells divide every three days, mitosis taking place 12 hours after DNA synthesis. Replication is not focal but has a random distribution along the epithelium. The newly replicated cells do not move up immediately into the spinous layer, but the fact that few transitional cell types are seen implies that the transformation of basal into spinous cells must be rapid when it does occur. Migration of the two daughter cells formed from a mitosis does not necessarily occur at the same time, and the factors which determine when migration takes place have not been well defined. It is generally assumed that the state of the microenvironment, i.e. pressure from neighbouring cells, and the supply of nutrients from the circulation, control the process. The 'turnover time', i.e. the time taken by basal cells to replicate, differentiate into spinocytes, granulocytes, keratinocytes, and finally to be shed as squames into the lumen is 4–5 days in the rat (Leblond *et al.* 1964, 1967), and is similar in mice and hamsters (Blenkinsopp 1970). In the normal esophagus, but not during carcinogenesis, the migration of cells from the basal layer precludes further replication and triggers differentiation.

The rate of replication in the basal cells must be adjusted to the rate of loss of cells into the lumen, as the thickness of the epithelium normally remains unchanged. The way in which this steady state is maintained is not understood. One factor known to affect the process is food consumption. Mice tend to eat by night, and as a result a peak of incorporation of tritiated thymidine into the basal cells occurs at around 0400–0600 hours, with a trough at 1600–1800 hours (Burholt *et al.* 1985). Fasting caused a reduction of tritiated thymidine incorporation into the forestomach, but not into the esophagus, although when animals were fed after a 48-hour fast there was an increase in replication to around three times control values in both organs. Presumably a corresponding increase in the rate of cell differentiation and loss of squames must have occurred. Food consumption also influences the replication rate during the recovery period following irradiation (Burholt 1986).

The subcellular events occurring during cell differentiation, i.e. the loss of the rough endoplasmic reticulum, the Golgi apparatus and the mitochondria, the recession of the nucleus, and the appearance of large amounts of keratin in the cells have been studied to a limited extent by histochemical techniques.

Biochemistry and histochemistry of the esophagus

The basic biochemical processes which have been studied in great detail in liver and to variable extents in other organs have been largely neglected in the esophagus. Also, in spite of the fact that in certain regions of the world esophageal cancer is the main form of cancer death, biochemical defense mechanisms and the responses of enzyme systems in the esophagus to toxic compounds and carcinogens have barely been investigated. For example, it has been pointed out (Newberne *et al.* 1989) that 'a major research need is to determine why, under conditions of zinc deficiency, DNA synthesis and cell proliferation in the esophageal epithelium increases, whereas it slows down in all other tissues of the same animal'.

Although different types of stratified squamous epithelia are similar morphologically, their biochemical make-up is characteristic for each tissue. Esophagus, skin and cornified vagina were among the various types of stratified squamous epithelia studied by comparative histochemistry (Maeir *et al.* 1962). Qualitative and quantitative differences were found which did not parallel any morphological characteristic. These are shown in part in Table 2.1. It is striking that, in contrast to the skin and the vagina, no alkaline phosphatase was detected in the esophagus. Also, in the esophagus but not in the other tissues, adenosine monophosphatase (AMPase) was limited to the granular layer. Even now, approximately 30 years later, the explanation of the cellular localization of these enzymes is not known.

One of the few detoxication systems which have been studied in the esophagus is glutathione *S*-transferase. This enzyme catalyses the reaction of glutathione with electrophiles. The system is especially important in relation to carcinogenesis, as the reactive forms of many carcinogens,

Table 2.1. *Comparative enzymatic histochemistry of various stratified epithelia (abbreviated from Maeir et al. 1962)*

	Acid phosphatase			Alkaline phosphatase			Adenosine triphosphatase			Adenosine monophosphatase		
	Esophagus	Skin	Vagina	Esophagus	Skin	Vagina	Esophagus	Skin	Vagina	Esophagus	Skin	Vagina
Cornified layer	+	+	+	−	−	+	−	−	−	−	−	+
Granulocytes	+	+	+	−	+	+	−	−	−	+	+	+
Spinocytes	−	−	−	−	−	+	−	+	+	−	+	−
Basal cells	−	−	−	−	−	−	+	+	+	−	+	−

including nitrosamines carcinogenic for the esophagus, are electrophilic. The level of activity (Sparnins *et al.* 1982) in the esophagus was found to be similar to that in the liver (Neal *et al.* 1987). Feeding certain compounds which occur naturally in food, including certain phenols, lactones, and benzyl isothiocyanate, in the diet to mice, produced an increase in the esophageal glutathione *S*-transferase activity by 68–135 % (Sparnins *et al.* 1982). Benzyl isothiocyanate is a natural component of cruciferous vegetables (Wattenberg 1980), and has been shown to inhibit carcino-genesis induced by tobacco-specific nitrosamines (Morse *et al.* 1989). Obviously similar studies are needed on the effect of other naturally occurring inhibitors of esophageal carcinogens, including ellagic acid (Mandal *et al.* 1986) and diallyl sulfide (Wargovich *et al.* 1988). The activity in the esophagus of other likely protective mechanisms should be studied. These include the mixed function P450 cytochrome systems, antioxidants including glutathione, α-tocopherol and ascorbic acid, radical scavengers, superoxide dismutase, and epoxide hydrolases – to mention a few lines of defense found in other organs.

An interesting event which occurs during cell differentiation in the esophagus is the disappearance of the nucleus, but there is apparently no information concerning the biochemical mechanisms involved or the fate of the DNA. Lysosomes might be expected to contain the proteases and deoxyribonucleases responsible for the disintegration of the nucleus, and these organelles appear in all layers of the esophageal mucosa in man (Hopwood *et al.* 1978). In rodents, however, where regression of the cell nucleus takes place during the conversion of granular cells to form keratinocytes and finally to give the squames which are lost into the lumen, the activity of the hydrolytic enzymes has not been studied.

An aspect of the biochemistry of esophagus which is important in relation to carcinogenesis is the attempt to identify a system which may be useful as an aid for the detection of premalignant lesions. An enzyme which has been studied in this respect is γ-glutamyl-transferase (γGT). This enzyme transfers the γ-glutamyl group from γ-glutamylpeptides to amino acids, and may play a role in the transport of neutral amino acids into cells. In initial work, it was found (Fiala *et al.* 1980) that γGT could not be detected in normal human esophagus, but was present in esophageal carcinoma. However, in a survey of a high-risk population in China, using balloon cytology, γGT was detected in a high proportion of the people not previously suspected of having esophageal cancer (Chen *et al.* 1989). It was suggested that the presence of γGT-positive cells in normal esophageal squamous epithelium might be useful for the detection of suspect subjects.

Another biochemical system which shows encouraging possibilities as a marker for the early stages of malignancy is the composition of the intermediate filaments. These structures were detected first in skeletal muscle, where their characteristic diameter (10 nm) is intermediate between that of the microtubules (25 nm) and myosin filaments (15 nm), and that of actin filaments (6 nm). There are five different groups of intermediate filaments, differing in biochemical composition, the various families occurring in different cell types. In epithelial cells and cells of epithelial origin, the filaments are composed of keratin. The cytokeratins are the 'soft' keratins, as distinct from the 'hard' keratins of hair, wool, nails, and claws. Their importance lies in the fact that the filaments form the cytoskeletal of cells, and appear to have a role in cellular differentiation. Keratinocytes contain bundles of keratin filaments, the keratins accounting for up to 30 % of the cellular protein.

The keratins are composed of families of proteins or polypeptides of molecular weight 40000–65000 in man. The polypeptides can be separated by electrophoresis in denaturing gels, and this technique has shown that different types of epithelia normally synthesize different groups of keratins. In the esophageal epithelium, keratins are synthesized by cells in the lower layers, and become increasingly cross-linked through disulfide bridges as differentiation proceeds. In rodents and ruminants the dead outer layers of the esophagus contain highly cross-linked keratins (Lazarides 1982). In man, high molecular weight keratins are not synthesized. This contrasts to the pattern found in the epidermis, and is consistent with the absence of a granular layer and an anucleate stratum corneum in the esophagus (Banks-Schlegel *et al.* 1983). It was found that human esophageal carcinomas showed consistent alterations in the keratin patterns (Banks-Schlegel *et al.* 1984). A difference in keratin expression between normal esophageal epithelium and squamous cell carcinoma was found also by Grace *et al.* (1985). Although this could be a result of a change in differentiation to give a malignant cell type, it could also be due to a difference in vitamin A levels in the tissue, or to an alteration in the proportion of different cell types in the esophageal epithelium.

The families of keratins from different types of epithelium and from different species have some amino acid sequence homology, but the differences are sufficient to allow the groups to be distinguished immunologically. With reference to carcinogenesis, monoclonal antibodies have been used to detect keratin peptides present in bladder carcinomas which do not occur in the epithelium of normal bladder (Settle *et al.* 1985). These sensitive antibody techniques should be investigated as a means of detecting early signs of esophageal cancer. An autoimmune response to the abnormal keratins in diseased esophagus may also indicate malignancy (Veale *et al.* 1988). Although these changes show much promise as early warning systems for carcinogenesis, it is necessary to bear in mind that changes in keratin expression could result from diseases other than malignancy.

References

Banks-Schlegel, S.P. and Harris, C.C. (1983) *Exp. Cell Res.* **146**, 271–280. Tissue-specific expression of keratin proteins in human esophageal and epidermal epithelium and their cultured keratinocytes.

Banks-Schlegel, S.P. and Harris, C.C. (1984) *Cancer Res.* **44**, 1153–1157. Aberrant expression of keratin proteins and cross-linked envelopes in human esophageal carcinomas.

Blenkinsopp, W.K. (1970) *Cell Tissue Kinet.* **3**, 83–88. Absence of effect of multiple intraperitoneal injections on cell cycle time in epithelium of oesophagus and forestomach in mice, hamsters and rats.

Burholt, D.R., Etzel, S.L., Schenken, L.L. and Kovacs, C.J. (1985) *Cell Tissue Kinet.* **18**, 369–386. Digestive tract cell proliferation and food consumption patterns of Ha/ICR mice.

Burholt, D.R. (1986) *Br. J. Cancer* **53**, Suppl. VII, 7–8. Oesophageal epithelial cell proliferation and food consumption patterns following irradiation.

Chen, Y., Huang, J., Liu, S. and Wang, J. (1989) *Proc. Soc. Exp. Biol. Med.* **190**, 170–173. γ-Glutamyl transpeptidase localization in esophageal exfoliative cytology of a Chinese population at risk for carcinoma.

Fiala, S., Trout, E.C., Teague, C.A. and Fiala, E.S. (1980) *Cancer Detect. Prev.* **3**, 471–485. γ-Glutamyltransferase, a common marker of human epithelial tumors?

Grace, M.P., Kim, H.K., True, L.D. and Fuch, E. (1985) *Cancer Res.* **45**, 841–846. Keratin expression in normal esophageal epithelium and squamous cell carcinoma of the esophagus.

Grice, H.C. (1988) *Food Chem. Toxicol.* **26**, 717–723. Safety evaluation of butylated hydroxyanisole from the perspective of effects on forestomach and esophageal squamous epithelium.

Heading, R.C. (1984) In: *Disorders of the Esophagus* (Watson, A. and Celestin, L.R. eds.). London: Pitman, pp. 3–12. Normal esophageal function.

Hopwood, D., Logan, K.R. and Milne, G. (1978) *Histochem. J.* **10**, 159–170. The light and electron microscopic distribution of acid phosphatase activity in human esophageal epithelium.

Hummel, K.P., Richardson, F.L. and Feketi, E.F. (1966) In: *Biology of the Laboratory Mouse* (Green, E.L. ed.) New York: McGraw-Hill, pp. 247–307. Anatomy.

Johns, B.A.E. (1952) *J. Anat.* **86**, 431–442. Developmental changes in the esophageal epithelium of man.

Lazarides, E. (1982) *Ann. Rev. Biochem.* **51**, 519–550. Intermediate filaments: a chemically homogeneous, developmentally regulated class of proteins.

Leblond, C.P., Greulich, R.C. and Pereira, J.P.M. (1964) In: *Advances in Biology of Skin*, vol. 5, *Wound Healing* (Montagna, W. and Billingham, R.E. eds.). Oxford: Pergamon, pp. 39–67. Relationship of cell formation and cell renewal of stratified squamous epithelia.

Leblond, C.P., Clermont, Y. and Nadler, N.J. (1967) In: Canadian Cancer Conference, Proc. 7th. Canadian Cancer Research Conference, 1966, vol. 7,

References 19

3-30. (Morgan, J.F., Noble, R.L., Rossiter, R.J., Taylor, R.M., Wallace, A.C. and Whitelaw, D.M. eds.). Oxford: Pergamon. The pattern of stem cell renewal in three epithelia, esophagus, intestine and testis.

Maeir, D.M. and Angrist, A.A. (1962) *Lab. Invest.* **11**, 440-451. Comparative enzymatic histochemistry of various stratified squamous epithelia.

Mandal, S., Shivapurkar, N., Superczynski, M. and Stoner, G.D. (1986) *Proc. Am. Assoc. Cancer Res.* Abstract No. 489. Inhibition of nitroso methylbenzylamine-induced esophageal tumors in rats by ellagic acid.

Morse, M.A., Hecht, S.S. and Chung, F.L. (1989) Proceedings of Tenth International Meeting on N-nitroso compounds, mycotoxins and tobacco, IACR, Lyon, p. 94. Chemoprevention of tobacco-specific nitrosamine 4-(methylnitrosoamino)-1-(3-pyridyl)-1-butanone tumorigenesis with aromatic isothiocyanates.

Neal, G.E., Nielsch, U., Judah, D.J., Hulbert, P.B. (1987) *Biochem. Pharmacol.* **36**, 4269-4276. Conjugation of model substrates or microsomally-activated aflatoxin B^1 with reduced glutathione, catalysed by cytosolic glutathione-S-transferases in liver of rats, mice and guinea pigs.

Newberne, P.M., Schrager, T.F. and Conner, M.W. (1989) In: *Nutrition and Cancer Prevention* (Moon, T.E. and Micozzi, M.S. eds.). New York: Marcel Dekker, pp. 33-82. Experimental evidence on the nutritional prevention of cancer.

Parakkal, P.F. (1967) *Am. J. Anat.* **121**, 175-196. An electron microscope study of the esophageal epithelium in the newborn and adult mouse.

Parkin, D.M., Laara, E. and Muir, C.S. (1988) *Int. J. Cancer* **40**, 184-197. Estimates of the world-wide frequency of sixteen major cancers in 1980.

Settle, S.A., Hellstrom, I. and Hellstrom, K.E. (1985) *Exp. Cell Res.* **157**, 293-306. A monoclonal antibody recognizing cytoskeletal keratins of stratified epithelia and bladder carcinomas.

Sparnins, V.L., Chuan, J. and Wattenberg, L.W. (1982) *Cancer Res.* **42**, 1205-1207. Enhancement of glutathione S-transferase activity of the esophagus by phenols, lactones, and benzyl isothiocyanate.

Stinson, S.F. and Reznik, G. (1982) In: *Cancer of the Esophagus*, vol. II (Pfeiffer, C.J. ed.). Boca Raton: CRC Press, pp. 139-168. Comparative pathology of experimental esophageal carcinoma.

Tang, W.C., Lin, P.Z., Frank, N. and Wiessler, M. (1984) *J. Cancer Res. Clin. Oncol.* **108**, 221-226. Metabolism of, and DNA methylation by, N-nitroso-methylbenzylamine in chicken.

Veale, R.B., Thornley, A.L., Scott, E., Antoni, A., Segal, I. (1988) *Br. J. Cancer* **58**, 767-772. Quantitation of autoantibodies to cytokeratins in sera from patients with squamous cell carcinoma of the esophagus.

Wargovich, M.J., Woods, C., Eng, U.W.S., Stephens, L.C. and Gray, K. (1988) *Cancer Res.* **48**, 6872-6875. Chemoprevention of nitroso methylbenzylamine-induced esophageal cancer in rats by the naturally occurring thioether, diallylsulfide.

Wattenberg, L.W. (1980) In: *Naturally Occurring Carcinogens-Mutagens and Modulators of Carcinogenesis* (Miller, E.C., Miller, J.A., Hiromo, I., Sugimura, T. and Takayama, S. eds.). Baltimore: University Park Press, pp. 315-329. Naturally-occurring inhibitors of chemical carcinogens.

3

Esophageal carcinogenesis

High-risk diseases

A number of diseases, not only those directly affecting the esophagus, are associated with an increased risk of esophageal cancer. These diseases (Table 3.1) include chronic esophagitis, stricture, certain motility diseases, reflex esophagitis, Barrett's esophagus, Plummer–Vinson syndrome, celiac diseases, and tylosis. Chronic esophagitis is sometimes considered to be an essential precursor lesion for esophageal cancer in man, and is more conveniently discussed in the following section where the precursor lesions are considered.

High-risk diseases are a useful guide to the etiology of esophageal cancer. These diseases may have the same initial cause as cancer of the esophagus, but develop independently from it and for different reasons. Thus iron deficiency may be a contributing cause to esophageal cancer, as well as causing the anemia associated with Plummer–Vinson syndrome. Alternatively, the high-risk disease may obstruct the flow of food and drink through the esophagus and thus increase its vulnerability to carcinogens, as in the case of achalasia. Finally, a combination of mechanisms may be operative, as when gastro-esophageal reflux develops. In this case, smoking and alcohol consumption together are sufficient to cause esophageal cancer, but in addition they may provoke reflux, and then damage to the esophagus caused by contact with irritant stomach contents enhances the direct action of the carcinogens.

Stricture

Stricture occurs whenever there is damage to esophageal mucosa followed by esophagitis and fibrosis, as after the deliberate or accidental swallowing of corrosive chemicals, especially lye or acid. The esophagitis may be diffuse, and the consequent strictures long and tortuous or, as when

Table 3.1. *High-risk diseases associated with esophageal cancer*

Chronic esophagitis
Stricture
Motility diseases, achalasia
Reflux esophagitis
Barrett's esophagus
Plummer–Vinson syndrome
Celiac disease
Tylosis

for example hold-up of tablets taken without water occurs, the esophageal damage may be more localized (Bennett 1984). Thus aspirin-containing analgesics and antibiotics can have this effect. Certain tablets which have been used to test urine for sugar are strongly alkaline and also produced heat on hydration, so that when lodged in the esophagus they caused ulceration and stricture (Postlethwait 1983). The scarred strictures cause stenosis (a narrowing of the lumen) with a slow insidious onset of dysphagia, a situation which often leads to carcinoma (Lancing *et al.* 1969; Wychulis *et al.* 1971; Hankins *et al.* 1975; Appelquist *et al.* 1980). The long-term effects of accidents of this type cannot be ignored, as the number of people at risk is not insignificant. In the USA, for example, accidental swallowing of lye occurs in approximately 5000 children under 5 years of age each year (Postlethwait 1983). The latent period, however, may be as long as 40 years. Study of the enzymic and ultrastructural characteristics of patients with mid-esophageal stricture suggest that the condition causes metaplastic deviation of the tissue (Berenson *et al.* 1974).

The evidence from clinical studies that stricture is often associated with carcinogenesis is supported by work with experimental animals, but long-term experiments with animals in which the lumen of the esophagus has been narrowed by some means are difficult. In an early experiment, surgically inserted polyethylene cuffs were used to constrict the lumen of the esophagus just above the point of entry into the stomach (Dunham *et al.* 1974). This procedure produced atrophy at the level of the cuff, with proximal dilatation. Benz[*a*]pyrene was then instilled twice weekly. The stasis caused by the treatment might be expected to prolong the contact of the carcinogen with the esophagus, and so to increase its potency. The results of these experiments were inconclusive, but a similar experiment, using the more potent esophageal carcinogen *N*-ethyl-*N*-butyl-nitrosamine, showed that stricture caused an increase in the number of esophageal papillomas which developed in rats (Sons *et al.* 1985).

Very relevant to the human population are experiments in which the effects of dilute acid and of thermal burn injury were studied (Alexandrov *et al.* 1989). Acetic acid 3 %, i.e. the concentration present in vinegar, instilled into the esophagus, caused hyperplasia, and when given before treatment with the carcinogen *N*-nitroso-sarcosin ethyl ester it increased the incidence of benign and malignant esophageal tumors. Thermal burn injury was produced at different locations in the esophagus by use of a heating element in a polyethylene tube 15 days before administering the carcinogen. This treatment resulted in an increase in the multiplicity and incidence of papillomas in the burn zone. In each case the exacerbation of cancer was considered to be due to the co-carcinogenic and promoting effects of hyperplasia.

There are several ways in which stricture can predispose the esophagus to cancer. It was suggested many years ago (Hurst 1939) that stagnating food and saliva in a dilated esophagus can become infected, the products of fermentation and putrification cause esophagitis, and then healing involving epithelial hyperplasia lead to squamous cell carcinoma. An increase in cell replication can have a co-carcinogenic effect when it occurs simultaneously with treatment with the carcinogen, or a promoting action when replication is triggered at later stages in carcinogenesis. In addition, stasis in the esophagus prolongs the time for which any carcinogens present in the food or drink would remain in contact with the esophageal mucosa. Stasis would also increase the time period during which bacteria originating in the mouth could continue to catalyse the reduction of nitrate to nitrite, with the consequent increased possibility of nitrosamine formation either while the swallowed bolus remained in the esophagus, or under acid conditions when it finally reached the stomach.

Several years ago there was an interesting finding of an unusual situation in which a high incidence of esophageal cancer was very probably caused by swallowing lye. This occurred in Alaska where, although the overall incidence of malignant tumors in Eskimos is relatively low, there is a unique predominance of carcinoma of the esophagus in Alaskan Eskimo women (Hurst 1964). This was suggested to be due to the method of making the sealskin mutluks worn by Eskimos on the feet. The sealskin hide is stretched on wooden frames and left outdoors until it is stiff. Wood ashes containing lye are then sprinkled on the hide to act as an abrasive, to help in the scraping and cutting procedures used in the removal of hair. The hides can then be cut to shape, but the edges are made sufficiently soft to enable stitching by being perpetually chewed by the Alaskan women. By the time the women are elderly their teeth have been worn to stumps, and dysphagia leads to the diagnosis of esophageal carcinoma. The continuous swallowing of lye originating in the wood ashes could well be the cause.

Motility diseases, achalasia

Another condition which can cause stasis in the esophagus is achalasia (the Greek for 'without relaxation'), when relaxation of the esophageal-gastric sphincter fails to occur at the critical moment, and the rapid passage of a bolus of food into the stomach cannot take place. In addition, there may be an absence of peristalsis. These conditions can be caused by abnormalities of the fibres of the vagus nerve, of the intramural nervous plexuses in the esophagus, or of the esophageal smooth muscle. The resulting retention of food and fluid causes the esophagus to become dilated and tortuous. The disorder has a world-wide distribution, the incidence ranging from 0.6 to 2 per 100000 per year (Blackwell *et al.* 1984). The incidence of esophageal cancer in patients with achalasia was found to vary from 0 to 20%, depending on the group of cases examined (Just-Vierra *et al.* 1969). The cancer was most often located not in the narrowed cardiac end of the esophagus but in the dilated often inflamed segment preceding it. Other motility disorders, for example the 'nutcracker esophagus' of the 'super-squeezers', may lead to achalasia.

Reflux esophagitis

A further condition under which the contents of the alimentary canal can damage the esophagus is esophageal-gastric reflux. In normal individuals there are usually episodes of asymptomatic gastric reflux, which can be detected only by prolonged pH monitoring of the distal esophagus (DeMeester 1984). The most common cause of more pronounced occasions of reflux is consumption of alcoholic beverages, especially spirits, as discussed in Chapter 6 (in the section 'Effect of ethanol and higher alcohols on basal cell replication'). Dysfunction of the esophageal-gastric sphincter allows regurgitation of the acidic contents of the stomach, with consequent damage to the esophageal mucosa, and then healing associated with hyperplasia. An increase in intra-abdominal pressure, as in obesity, during pregnancy, or after excessive flood or drink, can also cause reflux.

Detailed histological consequences of reflux in man have been described (Ismail-Beigi 1970, 1974), the significant events in relation to carcinogenesis probably being the basal cell hyperplasia and increase in thickness of the layer of basal cells. Study of the incorporation of tritiated thymidine into cultured biopsy specimens from patients with gastric reflux has also shown an increased rate of cell replication (Lipkin *et al.* 1988) which, as mentioned above, can have either a co-carcinogenic or a promoting action. It is therefore not surprising that adenocarcinomas are 'increasingly related in clinical experience to the previous existence of a chronic reflux esophagitis' (Pera *et al.* 1989). The importance of bile in the regurgitated material is as yet uncertain (Gillen *et al.* 1989).

Barrett's esophagus

Prolonged reflux esophagitis can lead to a condition known as Barrett's esophagus. When originally described by Barrett (1957), this lesion was considered to be a congenital disease which resulted in failure of the embryonic lining of the gullet to achieve normal maturity. Barrett's epithelium, however, is almost always associated with esophageal-gastric reflux, even in young patients (Bremner 1984), but severe reflux may be present without the development of Barrett's esophagus (Gillen *et al.* 1990). Reflux is therefore associated with, but may not be the sole cause of, Barrett's disease.

The probable sequence of events is that regurgitation of gastric contents damages the esophagus, and at first the damage is repaired by an increase in the rate of proliferation of basal cells. When this cannot keep pace with the loss of epithelium due to injury, an ulcer develops. Scarring may occur with the formation of fibrous tissue, which may result in stenosis, or alternatively the normal squamous epithelium which has been lost may be replaced by columnar epithelium similar to that lining the stomach. Apparently this can take place by metaplastic conversion (Jass 1981), in which case reflux might result in the appearance of Barrett's columnar cells only when abnormal cells are already present in the esophagus. Alternatively, an upgrowth of columnar cells may invade the esophagus from the cardia.

As a result of the change of cell type, there is secretion of various types of mucus, an increase in the rate of cell replication (Herbst *et al.* 1978), and an increase in the level of the enzyme associated with cell replication: ornithine decarboxylase (Garewall *et al.* 1988). A few oxyntic and parental cells may be present, as well as 'immature' cells (Ozzello *et al.* 1977) and intestinal-like cells. The cellular composition of the affected region of Barrett's esophagus varies in different parts of the lesion and in different patients.

There is convincing evidence that esophageal adenocarcinoma, which is rare in the general population, occurs at high incidence with Barrett's esophagus (Ming 1984). As might be expected from the association between alcohol consumption and reflux, in many series of Barrett's esophagus patients, consumption of tobacco and alcohol was high (Gillen *et al.* 1989). Other case–control studies, however, have suggested that tobacco and alcohol were unlikely to play a major role in the etiology of

Barrett's esophagus (Levi *et al.* 1990). The situation therefore remains uncertain. The condition is important as, while the incidence of gastric cancer has been decreasing for some years in the USA and elsewhere, the proportion of adenocarcinomas in the proximal stomach, which includes the gastric cardia region, is increasing. A considerable proportion of these adenocarcinomas consist of Barrett's adenocarcinomas (Hamilton *et al.* 1988). The explanation of the progression of Barrett's esophagus to malignancy is not clear, but is likely to be associated with the increased rate of cell replication.

Plummer–Vinson syndrome

A condition in which esophageal cancer was associated with sideropenic anemia was previously very common in certain regions of the world, especially among women in rural areas of Sweden, the UK, and the USA. A high incidence of post-cricoid dysphagia was first noticed to occur in patients with hypochromic anemia by Plummer and by Vinson in the USA and by Patterson and by Kelly in the UK around 1920. Cancer of the esophagus associated with sideropenic anemia was documented by Ahlbom (1936) and by Wynder *et al.* (1956), and has since been confirmed by many authors. The disease came to be known as the Plummer–Vinson or Patterson–Kelly syndrome, although the precise list of symptoms used to define the disease has varied from one author to another.

A detailed description of the epithelial changes in the nails, tongue, mouth and skin, and of the relation of the disease to oral and pharyngeal cancer, has been given by Larsson *et al.* (1975). At one time it was thought that iron deficiency caused the anemia and the unusual variety of epithelial lesions. Iron deficiency in tropical countries, however, is not associated with epithelial lesions, and iron deficiency has not been shown to induce these lesions in experimental animals. Other nutritional deficiencies could be involved, and riboflavin deficiency is especially likely to be relevant (see Chapter 10). In the case of the Swedish women, the diet was deficient in the winter months, when fresh vegetables, meat and fish were not available, and malignant changes in the genetic material could ensue. The initiated cells would lie quiescent while the period of poor nutrition lasted, and then be stimulated to develop into cancers in the summer months when the vitamins and minerals necessary for growth were in supply. Intermittent exposure to risk factors has been shown to be important in other types of cancer, for example the higher risk of skin cancer associated with sunbathing in summer in comparison with exposure to sun throughout the year. When there was a general improvement in diet in Sweden, the incidence of sideropenic anemia decreased. In older women, however, there remained a high incidence of esophageal cancer, and it was therefore suggested that the association between the two diseases was merely coincidental. A more likely explanation may be that the improved diet led to a rapid recovery from the hematological changes, while the esophageal cancer, once initiated during the winters of deprivation, was unfortunately irreversible.

Celiac disease

Two diseases which are associated with esophageal cancer and have a genetic component are celiac disease and tylosis. Celiac disease is a malabsorptive disease of the small intestine, and as the upper small intestine is most severely affected, one consequence is a deficiency in the absorption of iron. Patients with a long history of celiac disease have a high incidence of esophageal cancer (Harris 1967; Holmes 1976). This long latent period suggests that the association of the disease with cancer of the esophagus is more likely to be an indirect one caused by nutritional deficiencies rather than the esophageal cancer being a genetically determined disease.

Tylosis

The rare disease tylosis (the Greek for woody) involves hyperkeratosis of the palms of the hands and soles of the feet, and squamous cell carcinoma of the tylotic skin has been reported. Apparently the disease is due to a single dominant autosomal gene. Esophageal cancer has been detected in a high proportion of the patients studied, including families in Liverpool (Harper *et al.* 1970) and in Southern India (Yesudian *et al.* 1980). As the esophagus is an anatomical continuation of the external skin, it is possible that the state of the soles and palms is genetically associated with that of the esophagus. A change in the same dominant gene could therefore predispose both sites towards the development of squamous cell carcinoma. The disease is interesting, as it is the only well-established example of an association between a genetic disease and esophageal cancer, but it accounts for only a minimal proportion of the total incidence.

Overall, study of the diseases associated with esophageal cancer suggests that any condition which damages the esophagus either increases the *in vivo* formation of carcinogens, or exacerbates the effect of preformed carcinogens.

Precursor lesions and histopathology in experimental animals

An understanding of the early stages of esophageal cancer should give a lead to understanding the nature of the initial insult. For example, histological examination should reveal whether superficial or basal cellular layers are first affected, and whether gross injury or specific, possibly genetic, damage is involved. In addition, knowledge of early cellular changes should make possible early diagnosis, and the sooner the disease is detected the greater is the chance of establishing the cause. Also, of course, the greater is the chance of successful treatment.

Study of the early stages of esophageal cancer in man is difficult, as by the time dysphagia has finally led to diagnosis, the disease is already well advanced. However, as the vast majority of human esophageal cancers and of experimental animal cancers are squamous cell carcinomas, experiments with animals should provide a guide for determining which early lesions might be suspect in man.

In the majority of studies, rats have been the preferred experimental animal, and various nitrosamines have been used to initiate cancer. A description of the nitrosamines carcinogenic for the esophagus is given

Fig. 3.1. Esophagus of a rat fed NMBzA dissolved in arachis oil mixed in the diet (16 ppm, 10 weeks), split open longitudinally to show surface view of tumors with papillomas and thickenings which may or may not imply carcinoma. (From Craddock *et al.* 1987, by permission of Oxford University Press.)

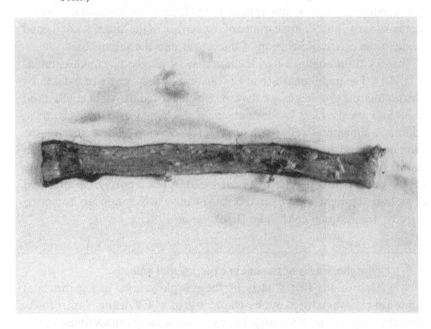

in Chapter 5. Most effort has been directed towards describing the histopathology of the tumors, the animals being killed at a time when the cancers were well established, and far fewer studies have been carried out on the sequential changes preceding the tumors. To some extent the nature of the sequential changes depends on the identity of the nitrosamine used and on the time/dosing techniques employed. With the very potent esophageal carcinogen, *N*-nitroso-*N*-methylbenzylamine (NMBzA), experimental cancer is often initiated by giving a small number of injections of the carcinogen. This regime results in initial necrosis of the esophageal epithelium. The slower acting carcinogen, *N*-nitroso-*N*-diethylamine (NDEA) is generally administered by feeding in the diet, and does not cause the complication of esophageal necrosis. However, NDEA has the disadvantage of being also a hepatocarcinogen, and as liver cancer develops before the esophageal cancer, the animals may need to be killed as a result of liver injury (Reuber 1982).

Whether a potent toxic fast-acting nitrosamine or a slower less toxic carcinogen is employed, a fundamental sequence of events generally takes place. An early response is basal cell hyperplasia, followed by dysplasia, with the appearance of polymorphic nuclei, cellular atypia, replication in more superficial cells in addition to the basal layer, and disorganization of the epithelium. Hyperkeratosis may lead to leukoplakia. The surface of the epithelium may appear 'cobblestone'-like, and the entire surface may be involved, or alternatively a few pedunculated papillomas may appear. Small patches of carcinoma appear as thickenings on the surface, which increase in size, but the appearance of the surface of the lumen is not a good guide to the extent of invasion of the cancer into the submucosa.

Tumors in the squamous epithelium may be papillomas or carcinomas (Fig. 3.1). The papillomas are not invasive, but they may cause death by obstructing the esophagus, or they may be detached by passage of a food bolus and are then lost in the contents of the lumen. Alternatively, or in addition, squamous cell carcinomas may develop. These invade the submucosa and muscle layers, but in animal experiments do not often invade surrounding organs or metastasize. Small 'nests' of carcinoma may appear in the papillomas (Iizuka *et al.* 1982). A few reports have appeared describing 'straight-away' carcinoma, a cancer which appears to spring directly from normal epithelium (Iizuka *et al.* 1982).

Morphogenesis of tumors in experimental animals

One of the first studies of the morphogenesis of experimental tumors in rats was carried out by Napalov *et al.* (1969) using *N*-nitroso-*N*-methyl-phenylamine (NMPhA). The carcinogen was given six times weekly throughout the experiment, groups of animals being killed each month. The experiment lasted for 20 months. NMPhA is not an especially potent esophageal carcinogen, and did not cause necrosis of the esophagus. Leukoplakia was reported, which was followed by thickening of the epithelium, mitoses in superficial cellular layers, and the development of papillomas. Similar sequential morphological changes were described in animals treated with *N*-nitroso-*N*-methyl-*N*-amylamine (Sasajima *et al.* 1982). Treatment with NDEA at 114 ppm in the diet for 26 weeks also induced hyperplasia, the formation of hyperplastic nodules, and then small carcinomas which increased in size and finally killed the animals by blocking the esophagus (Reuber 1977).

While NMBzA has the advantage of being a specific carcinogen for the esophagus (Stinson *et al.* 1978), it also causes frequent ulceration of the epithelium (Stinson *et al.* 1979). However, as two or three injections of NMBzA per week for 2–3 weeks very rapidly produce esophageal tumors, the system has been used for studying the effect of possible promoting or co-carcinogenic agents (Fong *et al.* 1978). The early cellular changes which

Fig. 3.2. Esophagus from a control rat stained using the BUdR–monoclonal antibody technique, showing five nuclei in the basal cell layer which were actively synthesizing DNA during the 1-hour pulse treatment with BUdR, and several others in which the DNA synthesis period partly extended into the beginning or end of the 1-hour pulse labelling. × 80. (From Craddock *et al.* 1987, by permission of Oxford University Press.)

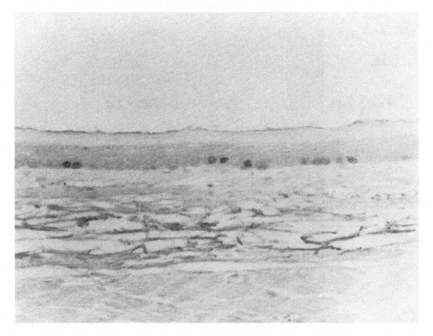

occur using this regime were studied by Craddock *et al.* (1987). NMBzA injected twice weekly for 4 weeks induces papillomas by 4 weeks and carcinomas after 9 weeks. The initial response was an increase in basal cell replication. This was detected by injecting the animals, 1 day after the first injection of NMBzA, with bromodeoxyuridine (BUdR), which became incorporated into newly synthesized DNA in place of thymidine. After 1 hour the animals were killed, and the sites of BUdR incorporation, i.e. the replicating nuclei, were visualized by the BUdR-antibody technique (Figs. 3.2 and 3.3). The increase in replication resulted in thickening of the basal cell layer (cf. Figs. 3.4 and 3.5). Later, extensive destruction of the basal cells occurred, with some injury in the spinous layer (Fig. 3.6). Cell injury lead to a massive influx of mixed inflammatory cells (Fig. 3.7). However, it is surprising that even during the continued treatment with the nitrosamine the basal cell layer was restored, and there was a reduction in the inflammatory cell infiltrate (Fig. 3.8). This suggests that the newly formed basal cells had somehow become resistant to the toxic effects of the NMBzA. It would be of much interest to determine whether this was due

Fig. 3.3. Esophagus from a rat 1 day after a single dose of 2 mg/kg NMBzA, stained using the BUdR–monoclonal antibody technique. There is a marked increase in the number of nuclei synthesizing DNA, but the mitotic cells are still confined to the basal layer. × 80. (From Craddock *et al.* 1987, by permission of Oxford University Press.)

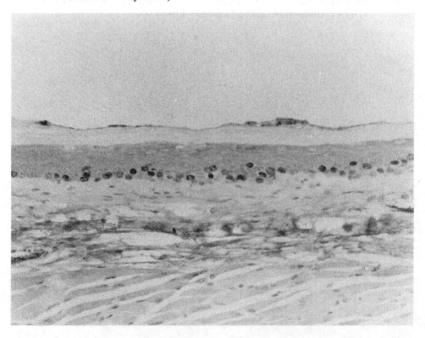

Fig. 3.4. Esophagus from a control rat. H&E, × 80. (From Craddock *et al.* 1987, by permission of Oxford University Press.)

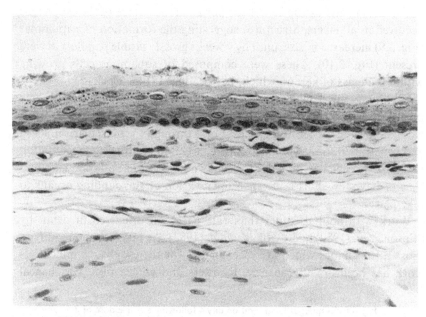

Fig. 3.5. Esophagus from a rat 1 day after a single dose of 2 mg/kg NMBzA. The basal layer is thickened and contains cells in mitosis. H&E, × 80. (From Craddock *et al.* 1987, by permission of Oxford University Press.)

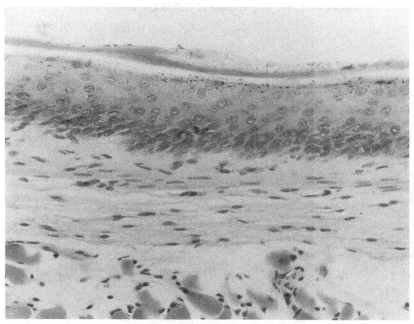

to a loss of the metabolizing enzymes, or to an increase in the activity of a protective mechanism.

Thickening and disruption of the normal architecture of the esophagus occurred in all layers. Structures suggesting the formation of papillomas (Fig. 3.9) increased in size, until by 4 weeks grossly visible papillomas were present (Fig. 3.10). These were composed of squamous cells growing within the mass of keratin which they produced (Fig. 3.11).

Papillomas are benign neoplasms, and have not been shown to become invasive or to metastasize. When the NMBzA treatment results in malignancy, the cancerous basal cells pass through the muscularis mucosa and penetrate into the submucosa (Fig. 3.12). In contrast to the situation in man, experimental animals are usually not kept for a sufficient length of time or have too short a life span for invasion of surrounding organs to take place.

Work with animals other than rats has been discussed in detail by Stinson *et al.* (1982) and by Iizuka *et al.* (1982). As rats respond readily to those nitrosamines which are carcinogenic for the esophagus, much less work has been done with mice, hamsters and guinea pigs. Esophageal

Fig. 3.6. Esophagus from a rat on day 4 following a single dose of 2 mg/kg NMBzA. The basal layer is thickened and markedly dysplastic, still with increased mitosis and some downgrowth. Apoptosis is occurring in the basal and spinous layers. Some hyperkeratosis is already present. H&E, × 80. (From Craddock *et al.* 1987, by permission of Oxford University Press.)

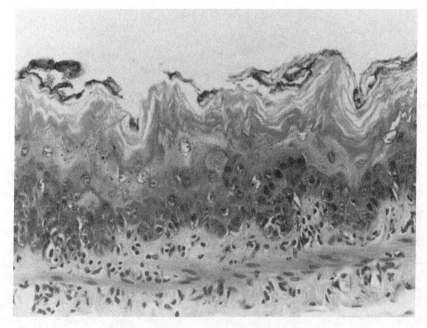

cancer has been induced in these animals by treatment with nitrosamines, but the tumor incidence is much lower than that readily attained in rats. Rabbits, however, appear to be more responsive, and esophageal carcinoma has been induced in rabbits by giving NMBzA and sodium nitrite in the drinking water (Iizuka *et al.* 1977). This technique, in which the active carcinogen is formed in the stomach of the experimental animal, has the advantage of avoiding exposure of personnel to potent carcinogens. The use of larger animals has the advantage of allowing endoscopic and radiographic examination of the esophagus at intervals during the course of carcinogenesis. Roentgenography of rabbits treated with *N*-methyl-*N*-nitroso-*N*-amylamine showed that esophageal tumors could be detected at an early stage and their subsequent enlargement could be followed (Iizuka *et al.* 1982).

A disadvantage of using rodents is the fact that a small proportion of esophageal cancers in man are adenocarcinomas, and the experimental study of this type of tumor has been limited to those animals in which submucosal glands are present, i.e. cat, dog, pig, ruminant, horse and monkey. The cat is unusual in being the only animal so far studied in which a high incidence of so-called spontaneous carcinomas of the esophagus has

Fig. 3.7. Esophagus from a rat on day 7 following two doses of 2 mg/kg NMBzA. The basal layer is disrupted and there is a mixed inflammatory infiltrate in the submucosa extending into the epithelium. H&E, × 80. (From Craddock *et al.* 1987, by permission of Oxford University Press.)

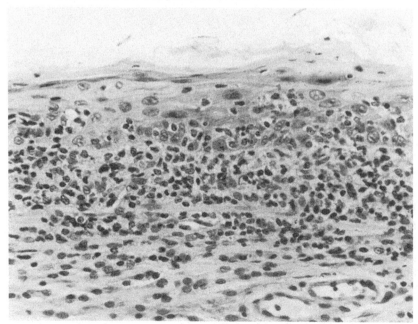

been detected. This is possibly a result of the lack of protection of the mucosa either by mucus secretion or by keratinization (see Chapter 2). There is only one report of the apparently experimental production by NDEA of esophageal papillomas in a cat (Schmahl *et al.* 1978). Esophageal cancer has been induced in dogs by treatment with *N*-ethyl-*N*-nitro-*N*-nitrosoguanidine (Sasajima *et al.* 1977), and in monkeys with 1-nitroso-1-methyl-urea (Adamson *et al.* 1977). Recently, however, an interesting technique was developed by which adenocarcinomas were induced in rat esophagus (Pera *et al.* 1989). Esophago-jejunostomy with gastric preservation was performed, an operation which results in chronic reflux esophagitis. When this procedure was followed by injection of the esophageal carcinogen 2,6-dimethylnitrosomorpholine, a high incidence of adenocarcinomas developed. This experimental model should serve as a basis for studying precursor lesions in man.

Precursor lesions and histopathology in man

By far the most common type of esophageal cancer in man is squamous cell carcinoma, although adenocarcinomas are of increasing

Fig. 3.8. Esophagus from a rat on day 11 after three doses of 2 mg/kg NMBzA. The basal layer is restored, but remained dysplastic. There is a reduction in the inflammatory infiltrate, but acantholysis is prominent in the upper layers of the epithelium and there is marked hyperkeratosis. H&E, × 80. (From Craddock *et al.* 1987, by permission of Oxford University Press.)

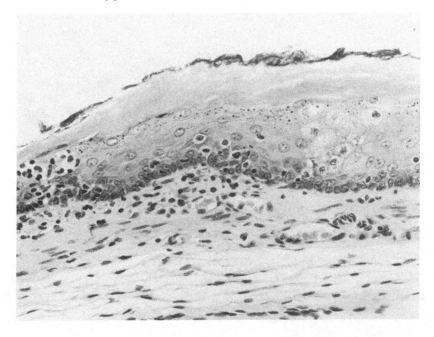

importance. These two diseases differ not only in histological type, but also in global distribution. They occur in different regions of the esophagus, and incidence in relation to sex shows very different male:female ratios. For example, the incidence of squamous cell carcinoma in the USA is 2.6/100000 (male:female ratio 3:1), and of adenocarcinoma is 0.4/100000 (male:female ratio 7:1) (Yang *et al*. 1988). These factors suggest different etiologies. Squamous cell carcinoma occurs with the highest frequency in China and Iran, and is associated with low living standards and poor diet. The highest incidence of adenocarcinoma on the other hand occurs in more affluent countries. Thus the rate is increasing in the UK (Powell *et al*. 1987) and in the USA (Yang *et al*. 1988), where the rate of adenocarcinoma in white men increased by 74% between 1973 and 1982. The majority of the studies on the sequence of changes which occur in the esophagus during carcinogenesis have been carried out in China, where work was stimulated by the urgent need to establish methods for the early detection of the disease, and for scanning populations in areas of especially high incidence.

Fig. 3.9. Esophagus from a rat on day 20 following eight injections of 2 mg/kg NMBzA, showing the early stage of papilloma formation. H&E, × 80. (From Craddock *et al*. 1987, by permission of Oxford University Press.)

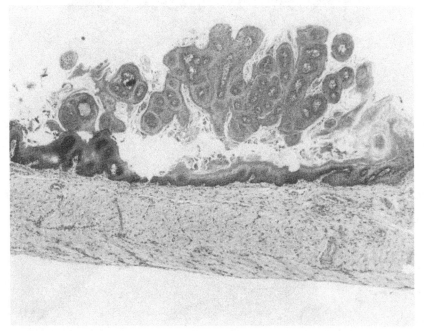

Region of esophagus affected

At one time it was suggested that in women cancers occurred more often at the top end of the esophagus, while in men the higher incidence

Fig. 3.10. Squamous papilloma of the oesophagus in a rat at 30 days following eight injections of 2 mg/kg NMBzA. The papilloma consists of nests of keratin-producing squamous cells with a fibro-insular stalk. H&E, × 20. (From Craddock *et al.* 1987, by permission of Oxford University Press.)

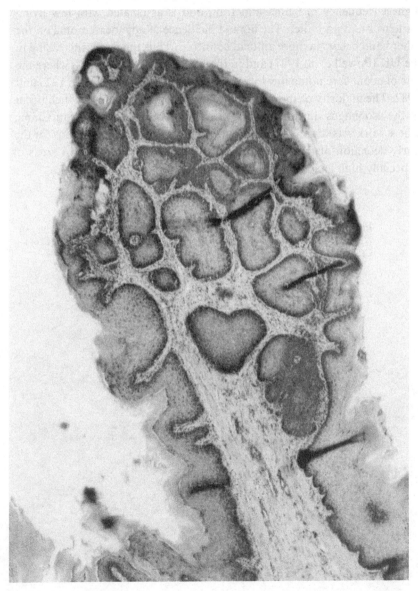

Fig. 3.11. A region of the papilloma in Fig. 3.10, showing squamous cells in bed of keratin. H&E, × 120. (From Craddock *et al.* 1987, by permission of Oxford University Press.)

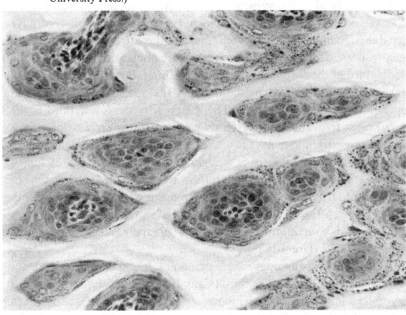

Fig. 3.12. Esophagus of a rat fed NMBzA in the diet (16 ppm, 10 weeks), showing invasion of the submucosa by malignant basal cells. H&E, × 40. (From Craddock *et al.* 1987, by permission of Oxford University Press.)

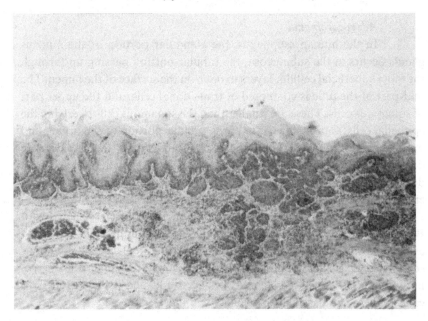

occurred nearer to the stomach. The cause was thought to be the consumption of hot strong tea by women and of alcohol, with consequent gastro-esophageal reflux, by men. The high rate of esophageal cancer in the upper region of the esophagus in women, however, is more likely to have been due to Plummer–Vinson syndrome, and this attractive simplification has now been abandoned. Squamous cell carcinomas occur mainly in the middle third of the esophagus. A survey in China showed the distribution in the cases studied to be middle third 58.3%, lower third 38.9%, and upper third 2.8% (Yang 1980). The reason why the lower third is the second most frequent site may be that, even with full relaxation of the esophageal-gastric sphincter, the diameter of the lumen is less than that of the esophagus, so that there is a slight delay in the passage of lumen contents at this site. This slowing results in an increase in exposure time of the mucosa to irritant compounds or carcinogens which may be present in the diet (Hurst 1939). Another common site of squamous cell carcinomas is at the level of bifurcation of the trachea, where there is a slight narrowing of the esophagus (Hurst 1939).

In contrast to squamous cell carcinomas, the majority of adeno-carcinomas occur in the lower third (Yang 1988) as a result of the fact that they are mainly Barrett's carcinomas caused by reflux of the stomach contents. A proportion of the adenocarcinomas found in China may be outgrowths from the gastric cardia, as tumors of this site are also common in the same region of China.

Adenocarcinoma

In the human esophagus, the glandular portion of the mucous glands occurs in the submucosa, the tubular portion passing up through the more superficial cellular layers to open on the surface of the lumen. The mid-part of the tube is composed of transitional cells, and the upper part of squamous cells. These are smaller than the squamous cells overlying the epithelial cells. Carcinomas arise in the tubular portion of the organ, and may be transitional or squamous. The cells lining the tubules are desquamated and pass with the mucus to the surface, where they can be detected at biopsy. Pre-cancerous cells were found to be dysplastic, with enlarged nuclei and prominent nucleoli (Shen *et al.* 1982).

The more frequent type of adenocarcinomas are those associated with Barrett's disease (see previous section). The squamous cells lining the esophagus which are destroyed by reflux may be replaced by columnar cells. These cells may resemble gastric or intestinal columnar cells in type, but in either case they secrete mucins (Jass 1981), and if they give rise to cancers these are classified as adenocarcinomas.

Squamous cell carcinoma

By the time dysphagia has led to diagnosis of squamous cell carcinoma, the disease is already at a late stage. In one survey, by the time of diagnosis more than 50 % of the cancers had metastasized to the lymph nodes (Shen *et al.* 1982). The consequences of metastases and invasion by esophageal cancers are especially tragic, as several vital organs, including the trachea, lungs and aorta, are adjacent to the esophagus, and are affected either directly or via lymphatic involvement. The result is a very short survival time after diagnosis. This has stimulated attempts to develop screening methods which might be applied to high-risk populations, if not to the general public.

Screening techniques

The two most popular screening methods have been endoscopy and biopsy, and interesting information concerning sequential changes during carcinogenesis has been produced during the course of this work. Specimens for biopsy may be obtained by direct abrasion with Nylon brushes, a procedure which may be performed either blindly, or with the brush inserted into an endoscopy tube (Cabre-Fiol 1982). Alternatively the specimen may be obtained by suction. In this case a double-lumen tube with an inflatable balloon covered by a Nylon mesh net attached to one end is swallowed, the balloon passing into the stomach. Air is injected through one tube into the balloon, which then contracts as the air is sucked out. As the balloon is withdrawn up the esophagus, cells are collected onto the mesh net, and smears can be made for cytological examination (Shen *et al.* 1982). Use of this technique has led to the detection of early lesions which had been missed by endoscopy and by radiographic examination (Yang 1980).

Sequence of histological changes in man

Normal esophagus, when studied by microscopic examination of biopsy specimens, showed large flat squamous epithelial cells, with small, often pycnotic, nuclei. The nuclear chromatin was homogeneous, with no evidence of a nucleolus. Only superficial cells and a few intermediate (granular) cells, but not basal cells, are collected from normal esophagi by the usual techniques.

Unfortunately no specific identifying characteristics have been detected in premalignant or malignant cells. In general the nuclei were found to be larger, and irregular in outline, the chromatin was more intense and irregularly distributed, and mitoses were sometimes abnormal. Multinucleate cells, and keratinized tadpole-shaped cells were occasionally present. Degenerate cells, inflammatory cells, and red cells, which are absent in the early stages, may occur in samples from late carcinomas (Shen *et al.* 1982). With carcinoma *in situ*, biopsy techniques remove not only superficial cells but, in addition, material from the tumor.

For the detection of chronic esophagitis, endoscopy is a suitable technique. There is reddening and swelling of the mucosa as a result of the increase in temperature caused by dilatation of blood vessels in the submucosa. Necrosis, erosion, and ulceration can also be detected.

As expected, surveys carried out in China, Iran, and in Europe have revealed differences in the precursor lesions in different countries (Munoz *et al.* 1983). In China and Iran high-risk populations showed a high incidence of chronic esophagitis, characterized by an irregular friable mucosa, edema, hyperemia, and leukoplakia. In Europe, where the cancer incidence is much lower, esophagitis is less prevalent. Erosions and ulcerations in the pericardium region, caused by reflux, were more often detected.

On the basis of surveys carried out on high-risk populations, two sequences of changes, which may not be incompatible, have been suggested (Fig. 3.13).

Mass surveys of high- and low-risk populations have been carried out in China since 1970 (Li *et al.* 1980). Nearly all surveys where it has been looked for have found a high incidence of hyperplasia in high-risk populations. Many surveys have found chronic esophagitis and atrophy, but not all have detected dysplasia.

Hyperplasia

As with animal experiments, hyperplasia is likely to be an important event at some stage in carcinogenesis. In one survey, pathological examinations of cancerous lesions showed a zone of hyperplasia to be present near to the cancer in all cases; 82 % showed marked hyperplasia,

Fig. 3.13. Two suggested sequences of changes producing esophageal cancer.

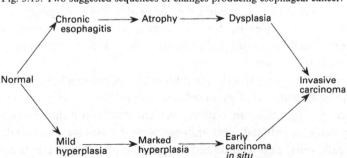

and in 18 % of the cases it was less extensive (Li *et al.* 1980). In early cancerous lesions, background hyperplasia was present in 90 % of the cases (Munoz *et al.* 1985). While cell replication normally occurs only in the basal cell layer, proliferation in the upper layers was found to occur more commonly in a high-risk group than in a low-risk population (Munoz *et al.* 1985). An expansion of the basal layer of proliferating cells in high-risk populations was confirmed by Yang *et al.* (1987). These two latter groups of authors stressed the value of studying replication by measuring tritiated thymidine incorporation into biopsy specimens of esophagus.

During the progression from normal through mild hyperplasia to marked hyperplasia, the epithelium becomes thickened until there are on average 35 cell layers. The nuclei may be spindle-shaped or oval, the presence of enlarged nuclei suggesting delayed maturation. The cells may assume irregular shapes, and cytoplasm may be scanty. The spinous cells may also increase in number, and parakeratosis may be present (Li *et al.* 1980). Detailed studies of mass surveys have been presented by many authors (Pfeiffer 1982).

Chronic esophagitis

While the occurrence of hyperplasia at some stage during the course of carcinogenesis was fairly rapidly established, the generality of chronic esophagitis as a precursor lesion in high-risk populations was more debatable. One of the earliest reports of a high incidence of chronic esophagitis was from the high-cancer population in Northern Iran (Kmet *et al.* 1972). In this population chronic esophagitis occurred frequently even in the young age groups (15–24 years old), and therefore was probably due to widespread damage to the esophagus which occurred from an early age. The esophagitis thus differs from that seen in lower-incidence areas in Europe and the USA, where it is usually a result of reflux. The chronic esophagitis in Iran occurred in 80 % of the individuals examined, and was accompanied by proliferation and dilatation of submucosal blood vessels (Crespi *et al.* 1979). These lesions occurred most frequently in the middle and lower thirds of the esophagus, the sites most commonly affected by esophageal cancer; in contrast to the situation in the USA and UK, the precardial region was almost always normal. Chronic esophagitis and dysplasia were frequently found also in the high-risk area in North West China (Munoz *et al.* 1982). In the USA, where the incidence of esophageal cancer is low, there is a lower frequency of dysplasia (Postlethwait *et al.* 1974).

In order to assess further the precancerous nature of certain lesions, a comparison of their prevalence was carried out between a region of China with a low cancer incidence (Jiaoxian), one with a high incidence (Linxian), and Iran (Crespi *et al.* 1984). Very much lower levels of chronic esophagitis, esophagitis with atrophy, and of dysplasia were measured in the low-compared with the high-incidence areas, data which suggest that the lesions are in fact precancerous. Hyperkeratosis, parakeratosis and acanthosis have been stressed by Shen (1984). Studies of young people are important, as it is in young age groups that the early precursor lesions might be detected. To select a suitable high-risk population, young people 15–26 years old were compared on the basis of whether esophageal cancer had or had not occurred in a first-degree relative (Wahrendorf *et al.* 1989). Although chronic esophagitis was known to be present in more than 50% of the high-risk adult population, it was significant to find that 36–44% of the high-risk young population also showed histological signs of chronic esophagitis.

Detailed descriptions of the stages of carcinogenesis and of the pathology of esophageal carcinomas have been given by Shen (1984) and by Liu *et al.* (1984).

The problems preventing the early detection of cancer are the absence of any cancer-specific change, and the variability of the endoscopic and histological appearance of precancerous changes. Early cancers were classified on the basis of their endoscopic appearance by Li *et al.* (1980) into four types:

1. Surreptitious, in which lesions are thin and flat, and difficult to locate by the naked eye.
2. Erosion type, in which the mucosa is dark and depressed.
3. Plaque type, in which slightly elevated greyish plaques appear on the surface.
4. Papillomatous type, in which raised papillomas are attached to the mucosa by a thick peduncle.

When the tumors become malignant they may invade the submucosa and the surrounding organs, and many spread through the esophagus. However, multiple tumors in a single esophagus may not be the result of invasive spread but may have a multifocal origin. Separate cancers may also enlarge and coalesce to form a single large tumor mass (Li *et al.* 1980).

The biochemical changes associated with esophageal carcinogenesis, and the possibility of viral involvement, are discussed in Chapter 11. At present the extent of understanding of the mechanisms involved in carcinogenesis – for example, the genetic changes, activation of proto-oncogenes, changes in the response to epidermal growth factors, production of ectopic keratins – is very limited (see Chapter 11). However, it is very probable that increasing knowledge of these processes will shed light on the etiology of cancer, i.e. on how external factors can initiate the process or affect its development. Also, further information should lead to simple, more specific tests for carcinogenesis, and allow earlier detection of the disease.

References

Adamson, R.H., Krolikowski, F.J., Correa, P., Sieber, S.M. and Dalgard, D.W. (1977) *J. Natl. Cancer Inst.* **59**, 414–422. Carcinogenicity of 1-methyl-1-nitrosourea in nonhuman primates.

Ahlborn, H.E. (1936) *Br. Med. J.* **ii**, 331–333. Simple achlorhydric anaemia, Plummer–Vinson Syndrome and carcinoma of the mouth, pharynx, and esophagus in women.

Alexandrov, V.A., Novikov, A.I., Zabezhinsky, M.A., Stolyarov, V.I. and Petrov, A.S. (1989) *Cancer Lett.* **47**, 179–185. The stimulating effect of acetic acid, alcohol and thermal burn injury on esophagus and forestomach carcinogenesis induced by N-nitrososarcosin ethyl ester in rats.

Appelquist, P. and Salmo, M. (1980) *Cancer* **45**, 2655–2658. Lye corrosion carcinoma of the esophagus.

Barrett, N.R. (1957) *Surgery* **41**, 881–894. The lower esophagus lined by columnar epithelium.

Bennett, J.R. (1984) In: *Disorders of the Esophagus* (Watson, A. and Celestin, L.R. eds.). London: Pitman, pp. 129–136. Benign esophageal strictures.

Berenson, M.M., Herbst, J.J. and Freston, J.W. (1974) *Dig. Dis. Sci.* **19**, 895–907. Enzyme and ultrastructural characteristics of esophageal columnar epithelium.

Blackwell, J.N. and Castell, D.O. (1984) In: *Disorders of the Esophagus* (Watson, A. and Celestin, L.R., eds.). London: Pitman, pp. 37–52. Motor disorders of the esophagus and their medical management.

Bremner, C.G. (1984) In: *Disorders of the Oesophagus* (Watson, A. and Celestin, L.R., eds.). London: Pitman, pp. 94–104. Barrett's oesophagus.

Cabre-Fiol, V. and Vilardell, F. (1982) In: *Cancer of the Esophagus*, vol. II, (Pfeiffer, C.J., ed.). Boca Raton: CRC Press, pp. 17–27. Exfoliative cytology of the esophagus.

Craddock, V.M. and Driver, H.E. (1987) *Carcinogenesis* **8**, 1129–1132. Sequential studies of rat esophagus during the rapid initiation of cancer by repeated injection of N-methyl-N-benzylnitrosamine.

Crespi, M., Munoz, N., Grassi, A., Aramesh, B., Amiri, G., Mojtabai, A. and Casale, V. (1979) *Lancet* **ii**, 217–221. Esophageal lesions in northern Iran: a premalignant condition?

Crespi, M., Munoz, N., Grassi, A., Qiong, S., Jing, W.K. and Jien, L.J. (1984) *Int. J. Cancer* **34**, 599–602. Precursor lesions of esophageal cancer in low-risk population in China: comparison with high-risk populations.

DeMeester, T.R. (1984) In: *Disorders of the Esophagus* (Watson, A. and Celestin, L.R., eds.). London: Pitman, pp. 73–93. Pathophysiology of gastro-esophageal reflux.

Dunham, L.J. and Sheets, R.H. (1974) *J. Natl. Cancer Inst.* **53**, 875–881. Effects of esophageal constriction of benzo[*a*]pyrene carcinogenesis in hamster esophagus and forestomach.

Fong, L.Y.Y., Sivak, A. and Newberne, P.M. (1978) *J. Natl. Cancer Inst.* **61**, 145–150. Zinc deficiency and methylbenzylnitrosamine-induced esophageal cancer in rats.

Garewal, H.S., Gerner, E.W., Sampliner, R.E. and Roe, D. (1988) *Cancer Res.* **48**, 3288–3291. Ornithine decarboxylase and polyamine levels in columnar upper gastrointestinal mucosae in patients with Barrett's esophagus.

Gillen, P. and Hennessy, T.P.J. (1989) In: *Reflux Oesophagitis* (Hennessy, T.P.J., Cuschieri, A. and Bennett, J.R. eds.). London: Butterworth, pp. 87–191. Barrett's oesophagus.

Hamilton, S.R., Smith, R.R.L. and Cameron, J.L. (1988) *Hum. Pathol.* **19**, 942–948. Prevalence and characteristics of Barrett's esophagus in patients with adenocarcinoma of the esophagus or esophagogastric junction.

Hankins, J.R. and McLaughlin, J.S. (1975) *J. Thorac. Cardiovasc. Surg.* **69**, 355–360. The association of carcinoma of the esophagus with achalasia.

Harper, P.S., Harper, R.M.J. and Howel-Evans, A.W. (1970) *Q. J. Med.* **155**, 317–333. Carcinoma of the esophagus with tylosis.

Harris, O.D., Cooke, W.T., Thompson, H. and Waterhouse, J.A.H. (1967) *Am. J. Med.* **42**, 899–912. Malignancy in adult coeliac disease and idiopathic steatorrhoea.

Herbst, J.J., Berenson, M.M., McCloskey, D.W. and Wiser, W.C. (1978) *Gastroenterology* **75**, 683–687. Cell proliferation in esophageal columnar epithelium (Barrett's esophagus).

Holmes, G.K.T., Stokes, P.L., Sorahan, T.M., Prior, P., Waterhouse, J.A.H. and Cooke, W.T. (1976) *Gut* **17**, 612–619. Coeliac disease, gluten-free diet, and malignancy.

Hurst, A. (1939) *Lancet* **i**, 621–626. Cancer of the alimentary tract. II. Carcinoma of the esophagus.

Hurst, E.E. (1964) *Cancer* **17**, 1187–1196. Malignant tumors in Alaskan Eskimos: unique predominance of carcinoma of the esophagus in Alaskan Eskimo women.

Iizuka, T., Ichimura, S. and Kawachi, T. (1977) *Gan No Rinsho*, **68**, 829–835. Carcinoma of the esophagus in rabbits induced with *N*-methyl-*N*-benzylamine and sodium nitrite.

Iizuka, T., Kato, H, Ichimura, S. and Kawachi, T. (1982) In: *Cancer of the Esophagus*, vol. II (Pfeiffer, C.J. ed.). Boca Raton: CRC Press, pp. 185–197. Experimental esophageal carcinoma in rats, rabbits, dogs and other species.

Ismail-Beigi, F., Horton, P.F. and Pope, C.E. (1970) *Gastroenterology* **58**, 163–174. Histological consequences of gastroesophageal reflux in man.

Ismail-Beigi, F. and Pope, C.E. (1974) *Gastroenterology* **66**, 1109–1113. Distribution of the histological changes of gastroesophageal reflux in the distal esophagus of man.

Jass, J.R. (1981) *J. Clin. Pathol.* **34**, 866–870. Mucin histochemistry of the columnar epithelium of the esophagus: a retrospective study.

Just-Viera, J.O. and Haight, C. (1969) *Surg. Gynecol. Obstet.* **128**, 1081–1095. Achalasia and carcinoma of the esophagus.

Kmet, J. and Mahboubi, E. (1972) *Science* **175**, 846–853. Esophageal cancer in the Caspian littoral of Iran: initial studies.

Lansing, P.B., Ferrante, W.A. and Ochsner, J.L. (1969) *Am. J. Surg.* **118**, 108–111. Carcinoma of the esophagus at the site of lye stricture.

Larsson, L.-G., Sandstrom, A. and Westling, P. (1975) *Cancer Res.* **35**, 3308–3316. Relationship of Plummer–Vinson disease to cancer of the upper alimentary tract in Sweden.

Levi, F., Ollyo, J.-B., La Vecchia, C., Boyle, P., Monnier, P. and Savary, M. (1990) *Int. J. Cancer* **45**, 852–854. The consumption of tobacco, alcohol and the risk of adenocarcinoma in Barrett's oesophagus.

Li, M., Li, P. and Li, B. (1980) *Adv. Cancer Res.* **33**, 173–249. Recent progress in research on esophageal cancer in China.

Lipkin, M. (1988) *Cancer Res.* **48**, 235–245. Biomarkers of increased susceptibility to gastrointestinal cancer: new application to studies of cancer prevention in human subjects.

Liu, F.S. and Zhou, C.N. (1984) In: *Carcinoma of the Esophagus and Gastric Cardia* (Huang, G.J. and K'ai, W.Y. eds.). Berlin: Springer, pp. 77–116. Pathology of carcinoma of the esophagus.

Ming, S.-C. (1984) In: *Precancerous States* (Carter, R.L. ed.). Oxford: Oxford University Press, pp. 185–229. Precancerous states of the esophagus and stomach.

Munoz, N., Crespi, M., Grassi, A., Qing, W.G., Quiong, S. and Cai, L.Z. (1982) *Lancet* i, 876–879. Precursor lesions of esophageal cancer in high-risk populations in Iran and China.

Munoz, N. and Crespi, M. (1983) In: *Precancerous Lesions of the Gastrointestinal Tract* (Sherlock, P., Morson, B.C., Barbara, L. and Veronesi, V. eds.). New York: Raven Press, pp. 53–63. High-risk conditions and precancerous lesions of the esophagus.

Munoz, N., Lipkin, M., Crespi, M., Wahrendorf, J., Grassi, A. and Shih-Hsien, L. (1985) *Int. J. Cancer* **36**, 187–189. Proliferative abnormalities of the esophageal epithelium of Chinese populations at high and low risk for esophageal cancer.

Napalkov, N.P. and Pozharisski, K.M. (1969) *J. Natl. Cancer Inst.* **42**, 927–940. Morphogenesis of experimental tumors of the esophagus.

Ozzello, L., Savary, M. and Roethlisberger, B. (1977) *Pathol. Ann.* **12**, 41–86. Columnar mucosa of the distal esophagus in patients with gastroesophageal reflux.

Pera, M., Cardesa, A., Bombi, J.A., Ernst, H., Pera, C. and Mohr, V. (1989) *Cancer Res.* **49**, 6803–6808. Influence of esophago-jejunostomy on the induction of adenocarcinoma of the distal esophagus in Sprague–Dawley rats by subcutaneous injection of 2,6-dimethylnitrosomorpholine.

Pfeiffer, C.J. (ed.) (1982) *Cancer of the Esophagus.* Boca Raton: CRC Press. Vol. I, chapters 7, 8, 9; vol. II, chapters 1, 2, 3, 4.

Postlethwait, R.W. and Musser, A.W. (1974) *J. Thorac Cardiovasc. Surg.* **68**, 953–956. Changes in the esophagus in 1000 autopsy specimens.

Postlethwait, R.W. (1983) *Surg. Clin. North Am.* **63**, 915–924. Chemical burns of the esophagus.

Powell, J., Robertson, J.E. and McConkey, C.C. (1987) *Br. J. Cancer* **55**, 346–347. Increasing incidence of esophageal cancer: in which sites and which histological types?

Reuber, M.D. (1977) *J. Natl. Cancer Inst.* **58**, 313–321. Histopathology of preneoplastic and neoplastic lesions of the esophagus in BUF rats ingesting diethylnitrosamine.

Reuber, M.D. (1982) In: *Cancer of the Esophagus*, vol. II (Pfeiffer, C.J. ed.). Boca Raton: CRC Press, pp. 169–183. Experimental neoplasms of the esophagus in Buffalo strain rats.

Sasajima, K., Kawachi, T., San, T., Sugimura, T., Shimosato, Y. and Shirota, A. (1977) *J. Natl. Cancer Inst.* **58**, 1789–1794. Esophageal and gastric cancers in metastases induced in dogs by *N*-ethyl-*N*-nitro-*N*-nitrosoguanidine.

Sasajima, K., Taniguchi, Y., Okazaki, S., Morino, K., Takubo, K., Yamashita, K. and Shirota, A. (1982) *Eur. J. Cancer Clin. Oncol.* **18**, 559–564. Sequential morphological studies of the esophageal carcinoma of rats induced by *N*-methyl-*N*-amyl-nitrosamine.

Schmahl, D., Habs, M. and Ivankovic, S. (1978) *Int. J. Cancer* **22**, 552–557. Carcinogenesis of *N*-nitrosodiethylamine in chickens and domestic cats.

Shen, C. and Shu, Y.-J. (1982) In: *Cancer of the Esophagus*, vol. II (Pfeiffer, C.J. ed.). Boca Raton: CRC Press, pp. 3–15. Cytology as a screening method for esophageal carcinoma in the People's Republic of China.

Shen, Q. (1984) In: *Carcinoma of the Esophagus and Gastric Cardia* (Huang, G.J. and K'ai, W.Y., eds.). Berlin: Springer, pp. 115–190. Diagnostic cytology and early detection.

Sons, H.U., Borchard, F., Muller-Jah, K. and Sandmann, H. (1985) *Cancer* **56**, 2617–2621. Accelerated tumor induction by distal esophageal constriction in the rat under the influence of *N*-ethyl-*N*-butylnitrosamine.

Stinson, S.F., Squire, R.A. and Sporn, M.B. (1978) *J. Natl. Cancer Inst.* **61**, 1471–1475. Pathology of esophageal neoplasms and associated proliferative lesions induced in rats by *N*-methyl-*N*-benzylnitrosamine.

Stinson, S.F. (1979) *Am. J. Pathol.* **96**, 871–874. Animal model of human disease: Esophageal carcinoma in the rat induced with methyl-alkyl-nitrosamines.

Stinson, S.F. and Reznik, G. (1982) In: *Cancer of the Esophagus*, vol. II (Pfeiffer, C.J. ed.). Boca Raton: CRC Press, pp. 139–168. Comparative pathology of experimental esophageal carcinoma.

Wahrendorf, J., Change-Claude, J., Liang, Q.S., Rei, Y.G., Munoz, N., Crespi, M., Raedsch, R., Thurnham, D. and Correa, P. (1989) *Lancet* iv, 1239–1241. Precursor lesions of oesophageal cancer in young people of a high-risk population in China.

Wychulus, A.R., Woolam, G.L., Anderson, H.A. and Elles, F.H. (1971) *J. Am. Med. Assoc.* **215**, 1638–1641. Achalasia and carcinoma of the esophagus.

Wynder, E.L. and Fryer, J.H. (1956) *Ann. Intern. Med.* **49**, 1106–1128. Etiologic considerations of Plummer–Vinson (Patterson–Kelly) syndrome.

Yang, C.S. (1980) *Cancer Res.* **40**, 2633–2644. Research on esophageal cancer: a review.

Yang, G.-C., Lipkin, M., Yang, K., Wang, G.-Q., Li, J.-Y., Yang, C.S., Winawer, S., Newmark, H., Blot, N.J. and Fraumeni, J.F. (1987) *J. Natl. Cancer Inst.* **79**, 1241–1246. Proliferation of esophageal epithelial cells among residents of Linxian, People's Republic of China.

Yang, P.C. and Davis, S. (1988) *Cancer* **61**, 612–617. Incidence of cancer of the esophagus in the USA by histologic type.

Yesudian, P., Premalatha, S. and Thambiah, A.S. (1980) *Br. J. Dermatol.* **102**, 597–600. Genetic tylosis with malignancy: a study of a South Indian pedigree.

4

Epidemiology

Introduction

The geographical distribution of cancer of the esophagus is the most dramatic of any type of cancer (Day *et al.* 1982). There are large differences in incidence from one country to another, and also from one area to another within any country. In several regions the high- and low-incidence areas are very sharply demarcated.

The global incidence of cancer of the esophagus is one of the highest of all cancers (Parkin *et al.* 1988; Table 4.1). Combined with cancers of the mouth and pharynx, which often have a similar etiology, the incidence of these upper digestive tract cancers is the highest of any form of cancer. The rate ranges from $0.4/100000$ women in the state of Utah, USA, to $174/100000$ for women in the Gonbad region of Iran (Kmet *et al.* 1972). Especially high incidence regions are the notorious 'cancer belt', stretching from Iran to China, certain regions in South Africa, and the Normandy district of France (Sales *et al.* 1985; Fig. 4.1). The astonishingly wide variations in incidence between neighbouring areas have been studied most often in China, where the rate in the Taihang mountains is more than $80/100000$ in the Linxian region, and less than $20/100000$ in the neighbouring Fanxian county (Cai 1982).

This dramatic epidemiology led to the hope that the causes of the cancer would be relatively easy to identify, but in spite of extensive surveys no single predominating cause has been detected. It is probable that several risk factors are involved, exceptionally high rates of cancer occurring where several risk factors co-exist. The nations fall very roughly into three groups. In group 1 the cancer rate is very high, as in the Iran to China cancer belt, and here the predominating causes are very probably related to diet, including micronutrient deficiencies, low levels of the protective factors which occur in fresh fruit and vegetables, and consumption of food

Table 4.1. *Annual numbers of cancers world-wide (after Parkin* et al.
1988)

Stomach	669 000
Lung	660 000
Breast	572 000
Colon/rectum	572 000
Cervix uteri	460 000
Mouth/pharynx	379 000
Esophagus	310 000
Liver	251 000
Lymphoma	238 000
Prostate	236 000

containing mycotoxins and high levels of initiating carcinogens, i.e.
nitrosamines. In group 2 countries, including most of Europe and the
USA, the cancer rate is relatively low, and the major cause is excessive
consumption of alcoholic beverages, a condition which is often ac-

Fig. 4.1. Geographical distribution of cancer on the esophagus (after Sales *et al.*
1985). Black area, very high incidence; hatched area, high incidence; white area,
moderate to low incidence.

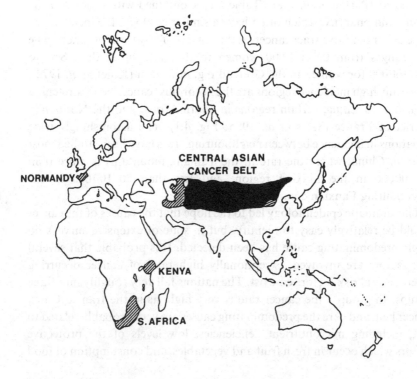

companied by dietary deficiencies. Group 3 countries such as Japan and South Africa have, overall, intermediate cancer rates. Several causes are important, including alcohol, which is not relevant in the Moslem countries of group 1. Dietary deficiencies, and in Japan consumption of very hot tea gruel, and of toxic plants, for example bracken, may be the leading causes in different areas, while in South Africa certain unusual procedures practised during pipe smoking seem to be important. Thus the position of a country on the global league table depends mainly on environmental factors, and no race or religion has been shown to be especially vulnerable.

The survival time after diagnosis is tragically short, usually as a result of late diagnosis. The average survival time in the USA after diagnosis was found to be about six months, with a 5-year survival rate of only 3% for white males and 1% for black males (Axtell *et al.* 1976). The 5-year survival rate was 7% in 1981 for men in England and Wales overall (CRC Annual Report 1990), and 5% for the Midlands (Matthews *et al.* 1987). As a result of the short survival time, mortality rates closely reflect incidence rates (Haas *et al.* 1978).

The age-standardized mortality rates for a number of countries are shown in Table 4.2 (Day *et al.* 1982). Although the incidence in Europe is often said to be low, the rates for Switzerland, Scotland, Ireland, and England and Wales are considerable. Obviously the range for men, as well as for women as mentioned previously, is very large; from 31.7/100000 for males in China to 1.9/100000 in Rumania. The rates for females range from nine times lower than those for males in Switzerland, to the situation in Iceland which apparently is unique in that the female rate is higher than the male rate.

The range for Europe in more detail, for periods between 1985 and 1988, is shown in Fig. 4.2 (La Vecchia *et al.* 1991*a*). While the rate per 100000 males for Switzerland fell from 7.2 in 1976 to 5.6 in 1985–8, the incidence in Scotland increased from 7.1 to 9.2. The rates in Ireland, England and Wales have also risen during this period. The incidence in the former USSR has recently been assessed and added to the data shown in Fig. 4.2 (La Vecchia *et al.* 1991*b*). As with other cancers of the upper alimentary tract in the former USSR, the rate for esophagus is high, and in men is exceeded in Europe only by the rates in France and in Scotland (men 8.4/100000; women 2.3/100000).

Epidemiology at the global level

The geography of a region is very often a major factor in determining incidence of esophageal cancer, as the terrain and climate determine the types of agriculture which are possible, and this in turn

Table 4.2. *Cancer of the esophagus 1976 (China 1981): mortality rates per 100000 (after Day* et al. *1982b)*

Country	Males	Females
China	31.7	15.9
Singapore	14.4	2.3
Puerto Rico	13.6	5.2
Chile	9.8	5.0
Switzerland	7.2	0.8
Japan	7.1	1.6
Scotland	7.1	3.7
Ireland	5.8	3.8
England and Wales	5.5	2.9
Costa Rica	5.3	2.0
Paraguay	5.3	1.4
New Zealand	5.2	2.0
Australia	4.4	1.8
USA	4.3	1.1
Belgium	3.9	0.8
Federal Republic of Germany	3.8	0.7
Austria	3.8	0.5
Iceland	3.7	4.1
The Netherlands	3.2	1.2
Sweden	3.1	0.8
Denmark	3.0	1.1
German Democratic Republic	2.8	0.5
Greece	2.0	0.7
Rumania	1.9	0.5

determines the foods which are available, and the occupations, life-styles, and socioeconomic status of the population. High-incidence regions exist where cereals form the staple diet, and where there is a low consumption of fruit, vegetables, and animal food. The rates can be high in remote regions with limited availability of fresh food, and this may occur especially in the winter months as a result of transport problems. For example, esophageal cancer in women in Europe at one time was highest in remote regions of Sweden (Wynder *et al.* 1957) but, with the improvements in the diet imposed by the Swedish government there was a fall in incidence, and Scottish women now head the league table (La Vecchia *et al.* 1991a).

Urban/rural distribution

Differences have been detected between urban and rural districts. Thus, in South Africa, when coloured men moved to the towns for work, the increase in salary allowed an increase in the use of alcohol and tobacco, and the result was an increase in the esophageal cancer rate in the towns.

Poverty does not necessarily lead to esophageal cancer on account of an inability to purchase healthy food, but is linked to cancer by the fact that low socioeconomic groups often have a higher consumption of alcohol and tobacco.

The higher incidence rates in towns with a high population density than in regions less densely populated was demonstrated also many years ago in the State of Connecticut, USA, and again it was suggested that alcohol consumption, tobacco use, and nutritional deficiencies were the explanation (Mason *et al.* 1964). A similar higher incidence in the towns of other regions of the USA, especially for male whites, has been detected (Haas *et al.* 1978). Occupation was not considered to be a determining factor in Connecticut. The only occupations found to be associated with esophageal cancer are those of the alcohol-associated trades, i.e. brewers, barmen and waiters. Where poor diet is apparently the major cause, a higher incidence is found in rural areas, as in China (Liu *et al.* 1984), Japan (Haas *et al.* 1978) and in women in Sweden (Wynder *et al.* 1957) and Scotland (Kemp *et al.* 1985).

A higher incidence in towns has been detected in certain countries in Europe. Thus in Denmark the increase in squamous cell carcinoma from

Fig. 4.2. Incidence of esophageal cancer in Europe (after La Vecchia *et al.* 1991*a*).

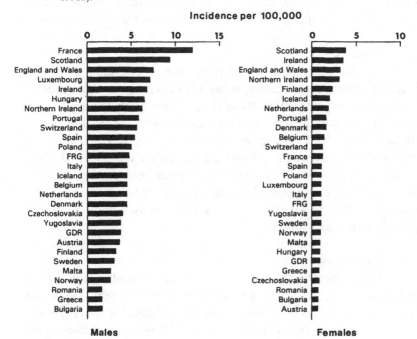

1978 to 1987 was higher in Copenhagen than elsewhere, a fact which correlates with an increase in alcohol consumption over this period (Moller *et al.* 1992). Studying rural areas of Austria in comparison with Vienna, it was found that the urban/rural ratio for men was 0.72, but that for women the incidence was much higher in Vienna (ratio 4.3). The fact that the urban/rural ratio for females for lung cancer was 1.9 suggests that a higher tobacco consumption in the town was partly responsible, but that a higher alcohol consumption was more important (Swoboda *et al.* 1991).

Sex ratios

The esophageal cancer rate in males is on average about twice that in females, but extreme ratios exist at both ends of the scale. The record is in the Normandy region of France, where the male/female ratio is 20/1, but in France overall, Spain and Switzerland the ratios are relatively high at 11.9/1.0, 6.7/1.0 and 5.6/1.0 respectively (La Vecchia *et al.* 1991*a*). At the lower end of the scale, the ratio is 0.85/1 in the Gonbad region of Iran (Kmet *et al.* 1972), while in Iceland, where the dietary nitrosamines are suspect, the rate is also higher in women than in men (3.7/4.4) (Day *et al.* 1982). These data obviously suggest that, as might be expected, the ratio is high where alcohol consumption is the major cause, but that women are more severely affected by a poor diet. There is no evidence to suggest that esophageal cancer is sex-linked, although sex differences have been detected in animal experiments in the rate of metabolism of nitrosamines.

Genetics

Genetic inheritance is not important in determining the epidemiology of esophageal cancer, either with reference to high-incidence countries or to regions within the countries. Very rarely there is a direct genetic link, as with the uncommon disease of tylosis, or the link may be indirect as a result of association with high-risk diseases which may be partly under genetic control, including Barrett's esophagus and celiac disease. The explanation of the fact that the black population of the USA has a higher rate of esophageal cancer than the white is not genetic, but occurs on account of a poorer diet and a higher consumption of alcohol, especially spirits, and tobacco.

Time trends

Where dietary deficiencies are a main cause of a high rate of esophageal cancer, and where these are a result of inclement climate and terrain, the high incidence is likely to have existed since antiquity. Thus in high-incidence regions in China, the infertile arid soil is responsible for the poor socioeconomic conditions, and ancient Chinese scrolls depict people clutching their throats and apparently suffering from esophageal cancer. Cancer registration and mortality reports show that the mortality rate in China did not change between 1959 and 1978 (Liu *et al*. 1984). By contrast, where alcohol and tobacco are the major hazards, the cancer rate can increase dramatically in a short time. In South Africa, for example, there is no evidence that esophageal cancer was common before 1930, but between 1949 and 1958 the incidence increased threefold in the coloured population, with a smaller increase in the whites (Oettle 1964). A more rapid increase followed, so that now it is the most common cancer in men in certain regions (Cook *et al*. 1971).

In Switzerland a decrease in esophageal cancer rate was found to correlate with a decrease in alcohol consumption, with a 20–30 year interval. Thus alcohol consumption decreased 1920–1940, and cohort studies showed a decrease in cancer rate 1951–1984 in the groups born 1880–1910 (Levi *et al*. 1988). The decrease was a result also of improvements in diet, especially in consumption of fresh fruit and vegetables.

Each country has its own unique pattern of changes in esophageal cancer incidence over the years. In Sweden the rate in women decreased with improvements in diet and in men with a reduction in alcohol consumption, while in the UK the rate has increased since around 1950, probably owing to the increase in alcohol consumption which began around 1930. In the USA, while the incidence of squamous cell carcinoma in white men has been relatively stable for some years, that in blacks has been gradually increasing. An interesting temporal change occurred in The Netherlands, where a sudden rise in rate of esophageal cancer correlated with an increase in tea consumption. When inexpensive coffee became available from the Dutch East Indies, and this replaced tea as the most popular drink, the incidence of cancer of the esophagus decreased.

Adenocarcinoma

The frequency of esophageal adenocarcinomas had been considered to be low, around 5 %, but it was noticed by Wang *et al*. (1986) that much higher percentages had been reported. This could have been the result of misclassification, as the frequency of adenocarcinoma depends largely on the method used to classify the lesion. At one time, all adenocarcinomas in the lower esophagus with involvement of the esophageal-gastric junction were thought to be of gastric origin. However, it was found by Wang *et al*. that 11 of 12 of their adenocarcinomas had Barrett's epithelium, a fact which strongly suggests an esophageal origin for the tumors. Thirty-four per cent of all esophageal cancers received at the Beth Israel Hospital in Boston, Massachusetts, between 1975 and 1982 were found to be adenocarcinomas.

A further report from the USA showed that the rate of adenocarcinoma in white men increased 74% over the period 1972–1982, an observation which led to the suggestion that these two major types of esophageal cancer may have different causes (Yang *et al.* 1988). A more detailed report from nine areas of the USA showed that a similar change in pattern was occurring elsewhere (Blot *et al.* 1991). From 1976 to 1987 the rate of increase of adenocarcinoma in men exceeded that of any other type of cancer, and by the mid-1980s it accounted for about a third of all esophageal cancers.

One of the first reports of an important change in the situation with reference to esophageal cancer in Europe appeared in studies carried out in the Western Midlands of the UK (Powell *et al.* 1990). While, in common with the general trend throughout the world, the rate of gastric cancer had been decreasing over the period 1962 to 1981, the incidence of adeno-carcinoma of the esophagus and cardia had increased. In contrast to squamous cell carcinoma, the increase in adenocarcinoma was relatively higher in the higher socioeconomic groups. As, at least in the UK, it was the professional classes who were the first to reduce smoking, it seems that tobacco is not a major factor. It has been suggested that alcohol consumption, especially of spirits, or dietary habits, might be involved.

A meeting of the European Cancer Prevention Organization convened in 1991 to discover whether this change in trend was occurring elsewhere in Europe (Reed 1991). Data from the West Midlands Cancer Registry showed that in 1986 adenocarcinoma accounted for 23.4% of esophageal cancers, compared with 6.6% in 1962. Similar changes were reported from Denmark, Belgium, France, and Switzerland. In Australia also an increase in esophageal adenocarcinoma has been observed (Watson 1991).

While the incidence of squamous cell carcinoma could be reduced in the Third World by improved nutrition and in the West by a reduction in alcohol and tobacco use, there is no certain knowledge on which to base recommendations for preventing the disquieting increase in adeno-carcinoma. A disease which predisposes to adenocarcinoma of the esophagus is Barrett's esophagus, but the incidence of the disease, and the factors which determine whether or not it progresses to malignancy, are unknown. Investigations into the etiology of adenocarcinoma are urgently needed.

Epidemiology at the national level

Only a very brief mention of the geographical distribution and possible causes of esophageal cancer in various countries is given in this section, as each country is discussed in more detail in the chapter where the factors most likely to be relevant are assessed. Thus China is discussed in Chapter 10 (nutrient deficiencies) and Chapter 9 (mycotoxins), and France in Chapter 6 (alcohol).

China

Esophageal cancer has been an obvious well-recognized cause of widespread distress in China since antiquity. 'Ge Shi Ging', the 'hard of swallowing' disease, with blockage of the gullet and vomiting after eating,

Fig. 4.3. Incidence of esophageal cancer in areas of the Taihang mountains, China (after Liu *et al.* 1984).

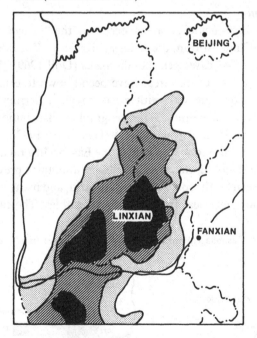

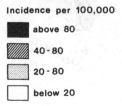

Incidence per 100,000

above 80

40 - 80

20 - 80

below 20

is described in China's earliest surviving scroll, written in 300 BC. Unfortunately, Houwang Miao, the 'Throat God Temple' was destroyed by fire in the war of 1927 (Yang 1980). It is tragic that even now, after many surveys and several intervention experiments, it is still not possible to pin-point the causes of the disease. However, in addition to praying to the Throat God, a general improvement in diet and in living conditions in rural communities should reduce the cancer incidence.

It is in China that the most dramatic examples of neighbouring regions with very different rates of esophageal cancer are found. The geographical distribution of the disease in Linxian and Faxian in the Henan province is shown in Fig. 4.3 (Liu *et al.* 1984). Attempts to find explanations for the sharply demarcated regions of exceptionally high incidence are discussed in Chapters 9 and 10. The problem has been the subject of several reviews (Li 1980; Yang 1980; Liu *et al.* 1984).

USSR and Iran

Exceptionally high-incidence areas occur in the 'cancer belt' region extending from China to Iran, the Ghurjev district of Kazakhstan recording an astonishing 547 cases per 100000 males (Doll 1969). As in China, regions with very high cancer areas have been known to exist for many years, and these correlate well with areas having a terrain and climate unfavourable for agriculture. The geographic distribution of esophageal cancer in Iran is shown in Fig. 4.4 (Day *et al.* 1982b). The highest incidence occurs in the Gonbad region in the Eastern littoral of the Caspian Sea, where the shielding effect of the Elburz mountains prevents clouds from reaching the area, the soil is alkaline and arid, and many of the semi-nomadic population never eat fresh fruit or vegetables. The cancer

Fig. 4.4. Incidence of esophageal cancer in the Caspian littoral of Iran (after Day *et al.* 1982b).

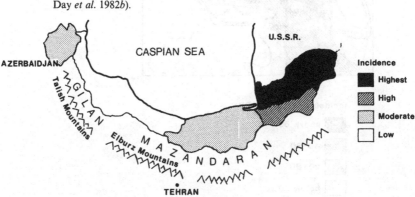

rate falls on passing east, and in the lowest incidence regions there is an abundant rainfall, and consequently an abundant supply of fresh plant food. The etiology of cancer in Iran is discussed in Chapter 10.

South Africa
In contrast to the situation in Iran, high-incidence areas in South Africa do not strictly follow any geographical boundaries. At one time esophageal cancer was unknown in Africa, but it began to appear with more extensive use of alcohol, and when maize was introduced into the country from America. At first the cause was thought to be the associated deficiency in nicotinamide, which occurs when maize forms the staple diet, but later it was found to follow not the consumption of maize but of moldy maize, occurring especially where the cereal was contaminated with *Fusaria* mycotoxins (Chapter 9). The very rapid more recent increase in incidence is likely to be due to importation of alcohol and tobacco.

Saudi Arabia
Esophageal cancer is the most common form of cancer in men in Saudi Arabia after non-Hodgkin's lymphomas, and in women after cancers of the breast and thyroid, and non-Hodgkin's lymphomas (El-Akkad *et al.* 1986). An abnormal clustering of cases was found at Gassim, where a high consumption of thermally very hot food was reported. A low male/female ratio supported the evidence that diet is an important factor.

United States
In women in the USA the incidence of esophageal cancer is low, and regional variations are slight. The cancer rates in men are higher, especially in certain regions, including the north-east, and the incidence throughout America is much higher among blacks than in white men (Schoenberg *et al.* 1971; Tollefson 1985). It has been shown repeatedly that high alcohol consumption is the main cause and that alcoholic beverages are the only factor clearly associated independently with cancer of the esophagus, mouth and pharynx (Keller 1980). Many detailed surveys, such as those carried out in Puerto Rico (Martinez 1969), Washington, DC (Pottern *et al.* 1981; Ziegler *et al.* 1981), South Carolina (Brown *et al.* 1988), and Los Angeles (Yu *et al.* 1988), have shown that spirits are the most hazardous type of drink. The poor diet which often accompanies high alcohol consumption is also responsible (Ziegler 1986; Pottern *et al.* 1988;

58   *Epidemiology*

Ziegler *et al.* 1988; Yu *et al.* 1988). Involvement in manufacturing industries was not a significant factor (Fraumeni *et al.* 1977).

Japan

A variety of causes apparently explain the relatively high incidence of esophageal cancer in Japan. Alcohol has been shown to play a role, spirits being the more hazardous type of beverage (Chapter 6). Hot tea gruel, a gruel made of rice and tea, has also been implicated, and bracken consumption may cause esophageal and stomach cancer (Chapter 8). The popular diet of fish and vegetables is apparently widespread and should be protective.

Europe

By far the highest incidence of esophageal cancer in men in Europe occurs in France, where it is exceptionally high in the north-west in the region of Calvados (Fig. 4.5; Picheral 1986). The cause was not difficult to identify as the high consumption of apple brandy. The high cancer rate in Switzerland is also due to spirit consumption. Italy apparently avoids a rate which might be commensurable with the amount of ethanol consumed, as this country is the second in Europe as regards litres of alcohol consumed *per capita* per year, but is sixth in the mortality rate for esophageal cancer in men (Table 6.1). The highest rate occurs in the north-east of Italy (Fig. 4.6; Cislaghi *et al.* 1978, quoted in Day 1984). A detailed survey has shown that alcohol and tobacco use are the major cause, and in

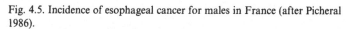

Fig. 4.5. Incidence of esophageal cancer for males in France (after Picheral 1986).

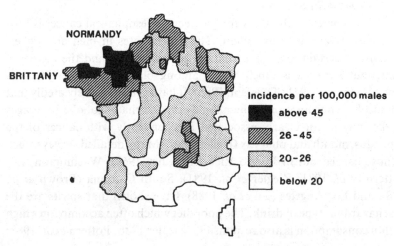

Italy wine is a greater hazard than spirit consumption (Barra *et al.* 1990). It was suggested that the most hazardous type of drink in each region, based on the cancer incidence and total amount of ethanol consumed in that type of beverage, is the most favoured drink for the region.

Although the major cause of esophageal cancer in men is alcohol consumption, even in the affluent society of Northern France, where there are no obvious dietary deficiencies, case–control studies have shown an effect of diet (Tuyns *et al.* 1987). Animal proteins, fresh meat, and polyunsaturated fats were protective and, while vitamin A in the form of retinol in butter increased risk, β-carotene in vegetables decreased the risk.

The geographical distribution of the disease for women in Europe is very different from that for men. Even in the Calvados region of France the rate for women is low, the male/female ratio being around 20/1. As described in detail elsewhere, the incidence for women was highest in remote regions in Sweden, but after improvements in diet Scotland now is at the head of the league table.

Fig. 4.6. Incidence of esophageal cancer in Italy (after Cislaghi *et al.* 1978).

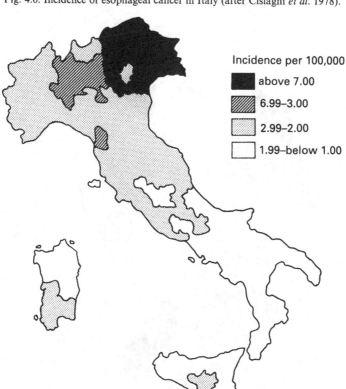

The geographical distribution of cancer of the esophagus for women in Scotland is shown in Fig. 4.7 (Kemp *et al.* 1985). The highest rates occur mainly in the more remote regions, in the Hebrides and Caithness. Owing to the mountainous terrain, the inclement weather, and the cost of transporting perishable food over the mountains, especially in winter, it is very probable that the cause is dietary deficiencies. There is no obvious explanation for the high rate in Nithsdale and Annandale. The high-incidence regions for men are strikingly different from those for women

Fig. 4.7. Incidence of esophageal cancer for women in Scotland (after Kemp *et al.* 1985).

Incidence per 100,000 females

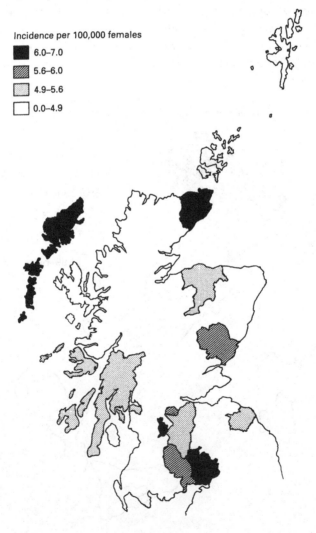

(Fig. 4.8; Kemp *et al.* 1985). While the Spey Valley in the north is well known for its whisky distilleries, there is also a high incidence in Nithsdale and Annandale, as is the case for women. The high-incidence area on the east coast, the Angus district, is the location of many of the smokeries which produce smoked Scotch salmon and there could well be a high local consumption of this delicacy. Smoked fish and meat are the foods most likely to contain high concentrations of carcinogenic nitrosamines.

As with Scotland, the high-incidence regions for women in England and

Fig. 4.8. Incidence of esophageal cancer for men in Scotland (after Kemp *et al.* 1985).

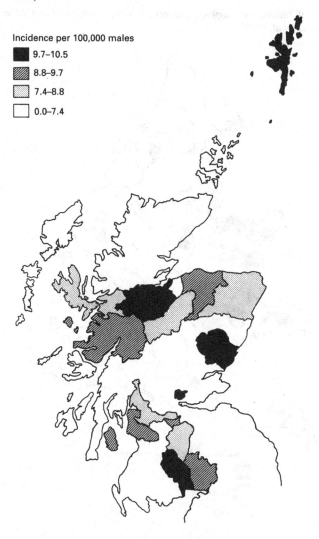

Incidence per 100,000 males

- 9.7–10.5
- 8.8–9.7
- 7.4–8.8
- 0.0–7.4

Wales are mainly in the more remote regions in the west (Fig. 4.9; Gardner *et al.* 1983). In winter the fresh fruit and vegetables consumed in the UK are mainly imported from Spain and other countries with warmer climates. As the food is imported mainly into ports on the south-east coast, the cost of distribution increases the price in the more remote districts. Thus seasonal dietary deficiencies are a possible explanation. Fresh fruit and vegetables are the food items which show the greatest regional variations in consumption in the UK. For men the geographical distribution of high-incidence regions is very scattered (Fig. 4.10). As the cause of esophageal cancer in men is likely to be alcohol consumption, and this is not known to

Fig. 4.9. Incidence of esophageal cancer for women in England and Wales (after Gardner *et al.* 1983).

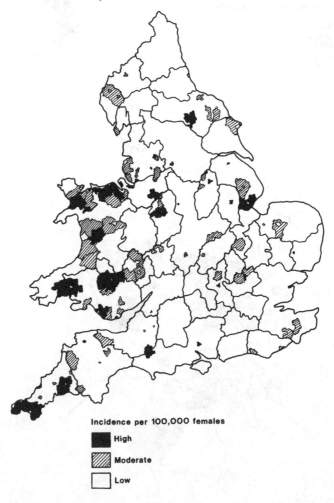

Incidence per 100,000 females

High

Moderate

Low

vary significantly over England and Wales, an ill-defined epidemiology would be the result. Studies of the etiology of esophageal cancer in men and women in the UK, especially in relation to the amount and type of alcoholic beverages consumed, are urgently needed. Esophageal cancer is one of the ten most frequent cancers for men in the UK, the incidence is increasing, the survival time after diagnosis is tragically short, and yet study of this disease in the UK has been neglected.

Germany is fortunate in having a relatively low incidence of esophageal cancer. In men, the rate of the most frequent neoplasms decreased over the period 1952–1981, but esophageal cancer was one of the exceptions

Fig. 4.10. Incidence of esophageal cancer for men in England and Wales (after Gardner *et al.* 1983).

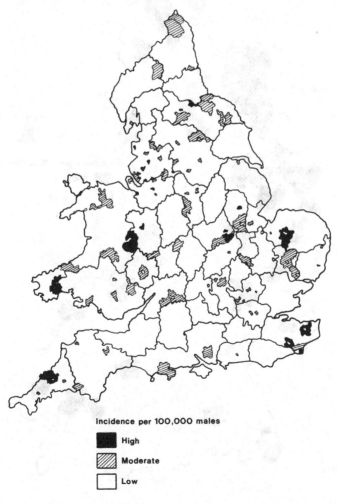

(Becker *et al.* 1984). There was a large increase in the incidence of lung tumors, which have now supplanted stomach cancer as the most frequent cancer. As this was due to an increase in tobacco use, a factor which also acts synergistically with alcohol in causing esophageal cancer, the increase in smoking was probably the cause of the increase in esophageal cancer also. In contrast, the incidence in women decreased over this period. The regional distribution shows that the 'hot spots' for women are mainly on

Fig. 4.11. Incidence of esophageal cancer for women in Germany (after Becker *et al.* 1984).

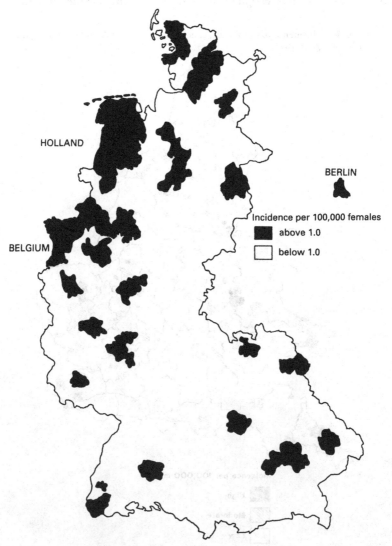

the borders with Holland and Belgium (Fig. 4.11; Becker *et al.* 1984), while those for men are more scattered (Fig. 4.12). There are no convincing explanations for these differences.

Although the cause of the high incidence of esophageal cancer in men in the West is alcohol and tobacco consumption, and in both sexes around the world dietary factors are partly responsible, it has not yet been possible to introduce effective preventive measures. More research is needed into

Fig. 4.12. Incidence of esophageal cancer for men in Germany (after Becker *et al.* 1984).

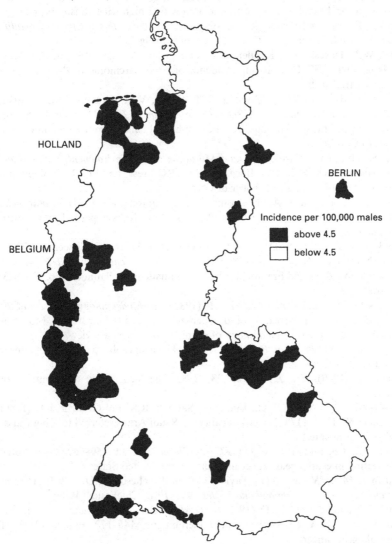

the mechanism by which these factors cause cancer. As esophageal cancer is one of the most obviously environmentally dependent cancers, it should then be possible to introduce acceptable preventive measures.

References

Axtell, L.M., Asire, A.J. and Myers, M.H. (1976) Cancer Patient Survival. U.S. DHEW Public Health Service Publication No. 5 (NIH), pp. 64–69. Washington DC.: U.S. Govt. Printing Office.

Barra, S., Franceschi, S., Negri, E., Talamini, R. and La Vecchia, C. (1990) *Int. J. Cancer* **56**, 1017–1020. Type of alcoholic beverage and cancer of the oral cavity, pharynx and esophagus in an Italian area with a high wine consumption.

Becker, N., Frentzel-Beyme, R. and Wagner, G. (1984) *Atlas of Cancer Mortality in the Federal Republic of Germany*. Berlin: Springer.

Blot, W.J., Devesa, S.S., Kneller, R.W. and Fraumeni, J.F. (1991) *J. Am. Med. Assoc.* **265**, 1287–1289. Rising incidence of adenocarcinoma of the esophagus and gastric cardia.

Brown, L.M., Blot, W.J., Schuman, S.H., Smith, V.M., Ershow, A.G., Marks, R.D. and Fraumeni, J.F. (1988) *J. Natl. Cancer Inst.* **80**, 1620–1625. Environmental factors and high risk of esophageal cancer among men in coastal South Carolina.

Cai, H. (1982) In: *Carcinogens and Mutagens in the Environment*, vol. I, *Food Products* (Stich, H.F. ed.). Boca Raton: CRC Press, pp. 39–52. Etiology and prevention of esophageal cancer in China.

Cislaghi, C., De Carli, A., Morosini, P. and Puntoni, R. (1978) *Atlante della mortalita per tumori in Italia 1970–72*. Rome: Lega Italiana per la Lotta Contro i Tumori.

Cook, P.A. and Burkitt, D.P. (1971) *Br. Med. Bull.* **27**, 14–20. Cancer in Africa.

Day, N.E. and Munoz, N. (1982a) In: *Cancer Epidemiology and Prevention* (Schottenfeld, D. and Fraumeni, J.F. eds.). Philadelphia: Saunders, pp. 596–623. Esophagus.

Day, N.E., Munoz, N. and Ghadirian, P. (1982b) In: *Epidemiology of Cancer of the Digestive Tract* (Correa, P. and Haenszel, W. eds.). Dordrecht: Martinus Nijhoff, pp. 21–57. Epidemiology of esophageal cancer: a review.

Day, N.E. (1984) *Br. Med. Bull.* **40**, 329–334. The geographic pathology of cancer of the esophagus.

Doll, R. (1969) *Br. J. Cancer* **28**, 1–8. The geographic distribution of cancer.

El-Akkad, S.M., Amer, M.H., Lin, G.S., Sabbah, R.S. and Godwin, J.T. (1986) *Cancer* **58**, 1172–1178. Pattern of cancer in Saudi Arabs referred to King Faisal Specialist hospital.

Fraumeni, J.F. and Blot, W.J. (1977) *J. Chron. Dis.* **30**, 759–767. Geographic variation in esophageal cancer mortality in the United States.

Gardner, M.J., Winter, P.D., Taylor, C.P. and Acheson, E.D. (1983) *Atlas of cancer mortality in England and Wales 1968–1978*. Chichester: Wiley.

Haas, J.F. and Scottenfeld, D. (1978) In: *Gastrointestinal Tract Cancer* (Lipkin, M. and Good, R.A. eds.). New York: Plenum, pp. 145–172. Epidemiology of esophageal cancer.

Keller, A.Z. (1980) *Prev. Med.* **9**, 607–612. The epidemiology of esophageal cancer in the West.

Kemp, I., Boyle, P., Smans, M. and Muir, C. (1985) IACR Scientific Publ. No. 72. Atlas of Cancer in Scotland, 1975–1980.

Kmet, J. and Mahboubi, E. (1972) *Science* **175**, 846–853. Esophageal cancer in the Caspian littoral of Iran: initial studies.

La Vecchia, C., Boyle, P., Franceschi, S., Levi, F., Maisonneuve, P., Negri, E., Lucchini, F. and Smans, M. (1991a) *Eur. J. Cancer* **27**, 94–101. Smoking and cancer with emphasis on Europe.

La Vecchia, C., Levi, F., Lucchini, F., Evstieeva, T. and Boyle, P. (1991b) *Int. J. Cancer* **49**, 678–683. Cancer mortality in the USSR, 1986–1988.

Levi, E., De Carli, A. and La Vecchia, C. (1988) *Rev. Epidemiol. Sante Publique* **36**, 15–25. Trends in cancer mortality in Switzerland, 1951–1984.

Li, M., Li, P. and Li, B. (1980) *Adv. Cancer Res.* **33**, 173–249. Recent progress in research on esophageal cancer in China.

Liu, Q. and Bing, Li. (1984) In: *Carcinoma of the Esophagus and Gastric Cardia* (Huang, G.J. and K'ai, W.Y. eds.). Berlin: Springer, pp. 1–24. Epidemiology of carcinoma of the esophagus in China.

Martinez, I. (1969) *J. Natl. Cancer Inst.* **42**, 1069–1094. Factors associated with cancers of the esophagus, mouth and pharynx in Puerto Rico.

Mason, M.J., Bailar, J.C. and Eisenberg, H. (1964) *J. Chron. Dis.* **17**, 667–676. Geographic variation in the incidence of esophageal cancer.

Matthews, H.R., Waterhouse, J.H.A., Powell, J., Robinson, J.E. and McConkey, C.C. (1987) *Clinical Cancer Monographs*, vol. 1. London: Macmillan. Cancer of the oesophagus.

Moller, H., Boyle, P., Maisonneuve, P., La Vecchia, C. and Jensen, O.M. (1992) *Eur. J. Cancer Prev.* 159–164. Incidence of cancer of the esophagus, cardia and stomach in Denmark.

Oettle, A.G. (1964) *J. Natl. Cancer Inst.* **33**, 383–439. Cancer in Africa, especially in regions south of the Sahara.

Parkin, D.M., Laara, E. and Muir, C.S. (1988) *Int. J. Cancer* **41**, 184–197. Estimates of the worldwide frequency of sixteen major cancers in 1980.

Picheral, H. (1986) In: *Global Geocancerology: A world geography of human cancers* (Howe, G.M. ed.). Edinburgh: Churchill Livingstone, pp. 144–153. France.

Pottern, L.M., Morris, L.E., Blot, W.J., Ziegler, R.G. and Fraumeni, J.F. (1981) *J. Natl. Cancer Inst.* **67**, 777–783. Esophageal cancer among black men in Washington DC. I. Alcohol, tobacco and other risk factors.

Powell, J. and McConkey, C.C. (1990) *Br. J. Cancer* **62**, 440–443. Increasing incidence of adenocarcinoma of the gastric cardia and adjacent sites.

Reed, P.I. (1991) *Lancet* **338**, 178–179. Changing pattern of oesophageal cancer.

Sales, D. and Levin, B. (1985) In: *Cancer of the Esophagus* (DeMeister, T.R. and Levin, B. eds.). New York: Grune and Stratton, 1–19. Incidence, epidemiology and predisposing factors.

Schoenberg, B.S., Bailar, J. and Fraumeni, J.F. (1971) *J. Natl. Cancer Inst.* 63–73. Certain mortality patterns of esophageal cancer in the United States 1930–67.

Schottenfeld, D. (1984) *Semin. Oncol.* **11**, 92–100. Epidemiology of cancer of the esophagus.

Swoboda, H. and Friedl, H.P. (1989) *Eur. J. Cancer* **27**, 83–85. Incidence of cancer of the respiratory and upper digestive tract in urban and rural Eastern Austria.

Tollefson, L. (1985) *Reg. Toxicol. Pharmacol.* **5**, 255–275. Use of epidemiology, scientific data, and regulatory authority to determine risk factors in cancer of some organs of the digestive system. 2. Esophageal cancer.

Tuyns, A.J., Riboli, E., Doornbos, G. and Pequignot, G. (1987) *Nutr. Cancer* **9**, 81–92. Diet and esophageal cancer in Calvados, France.

Wang, H.H., Antonioli, D.A. and Goldman, H. (1986) *Hum. Pathol.* **17**, 482–487. Comparative features of esophageal and gastric adenocarcinomas: recent changes in type and frequency.

Watson, A. (1991) *Lancet* **338**, 819–820. Oesophageal cancer.

Wynder, E.L., Hultberg, S., Jacobsson, F. and Bross, E.J. (1957) *Cancer* **10**, 470–487. Environmental factors in cancer of the upper alimentary tract: Swedish study with special reference to Plummer–Vinson (Paterson–Kelly) syndrome.

Yang, C.S. (1980) *Cancer Res.* **40**, 2633–2644. Research on esophageal cancer in China: a review.

Yang, P.C. and Davis, S. (1988) *Cancer* **61**, 612–617. Incidence of cancer on the esophagus in the USA by histologic type.

Yu, M.C., Garabrant, D.H., Peters, J.M. and Mack, T.M. (1988) *Cancer Res.* **48**, 3843–3848. Tobacco, alcohol, diet, occupation and carcinoma of the esophagus.

Ziegler, R.G., Morris, L.E., Blot, W.J., Pottern, L.M., Hoover, R. and Fraumeni, J.F. (1981) *J. Natl. Cancer Inst.* **67**, 1199–1206. Esophageal cancer among black men in Washington DC. II. Role of nutrition.

Ziegler, R.G. (1986) In: *Essential Nutrients in Carcinogenesis* (Poirier, L.A., Newberne, P.M. and Pariza, M.W. eds.). New York: Plenum Press, pp. 11–26. Epidemiologic studies of vitamins and cancer of the lung, esophagus and cervix.

5

Chemicals carcinogenic for the esophagus: the nitrosamines

Experimental studies: *N*-nitroso compounds

Introduction

The esophagus is an organ which might not be expected to be especially sensitive to chemical carcinogens. After ingestion, food and drink remain for a short period in the mouth, for a much longer time in the stomach, but pass rapidly through the lumen of the esophagus. Exposure of the oral and gastric mucosa is of very much longer duration than that of the esophageal epithelium, so that direct-acting chemicals, i.e. those which do not require metabolic activation to be effective carcinogens, are more likely to cause oral or gastric cancer. Chemicals which remain inert until activated by metabolism can be absorbed into the circulation and reach the esophagus by this route. However, the chemicals which do require metabolic activation before they become effective are more likely to be carcinogenic for the more metabolically active organs, i.e. liver and kidney, than for organs with lower metabolic activity, and lower cytochrome P450 levels, such as muscle, nerve and esophagus.

In general, this concept appears to be justified, as of all the huge number of chemicals which have been tested for carcinogenicity, very few are carcinogenic for the esophagus. The outstanding exception is a large group of compounds which are very potent esophageal carcinogens: the *N*-nitrosamines. Whether given by oral, intraperitoneal, intravenous or subcutaneous routes, many *N*-nitrosamines are carcinogenic for the esophagus, and for a number of *N*-nitrosamines the esophagus is the sole target organ. Over 300 *N*-nitrosamines have been tested for carcinogenicity, and more than half of these are carcinogenic for the esophagus in the rat. Many *N*-nitrosamines are widespread in the environment, and are present in food, drink, and in widely used industrial products. In

Table 5.1. *Chemical induction of esophageal cancer in rats by dietary treatment*

Chemical	Dose in diet (ppm)	Duration of treatment	Incidence of carcinomas	Reference
Dihydrosafrole	2500	2 years	0/20	Hagen *et al.*
	10 000	2 years	10/20	(1965)
8-Nitroquinoline	2500	1 year	0/11 (1/11 papillomas)	Takahasi *et al.* (1978)
Acetone[4-(5-nitro-2-furyl)-2-thiazolyl] hydrazone	1000	1 year	1/20	Morris *et al.* (1969)
N-nitroso-N-methylbenzylamine (NMBzA)	1	1 year	20/20	Druckrey *et al.* (1967)
	16	12 weeks	5/10	

addition, *N*-nitroso compounds are possibly unique among potent chemical carcinogens in being formed from widely consumed innocuous precursors in the human stomach. Therefore human exposure is very probably ubiquitous. The global incidence of esophageal cancer is high, and some factor(s) widespread in the environment must be responsible.

The potency of the small number of chemicals which are not *N*-nitroso compounds is contrasted with the potency of NMBzA in Table 1. Dihydrosafrole, 8-nitroquinoline, and a nitrofuran derivative, induce a low incidence of carcinomas or papillomas in the esophagus of rats when fed at several thousand parts per million for a year or more, while NMBzA induces 100 % malignancy at much lower dose levels after a much shorter time. The non-nitroso carcinogens do not occur in the environment, and therefore human exposure is very limited. Benzo[*a*]pyrene, given at 30 ppm by forced drinking in 70 % ethanol solution for more than 1½ years, induced one esophageal carcinoma in 63 mice (Horie *et al.* 1965). As the authors state that no esophageal tumors were induced when the benzo[*a*]pyrene was given in olive oil, the presence of the 70 % ethanol was apparently essential. This implies that the usual conditions for human exposure to benzo[*a*]pyrene are unlikely to cause cancer of the esophagus.

In view of its widespread consumption, the possibility that the antioxidant, butylated hydroxyanisole, is an esophageal carcinogen is important (for review, see Grice 1988). This commonly used food preservative induces squamous cell tumors in the forestomach of rats, and when fed in the diet to pregnant pigs it induced proliferative and parakeratotic changes in the esophagus (Wurtzen *et al.* 1986). As the stratified squamous esophageal epithelium of rodents and ruminants is keratinized, while that of pigs and primates is not, the pig could well be a more relevant test animal. The keratin layer, which protects the epithelium from the effects of hard dry food, could also prevent absorption of carcinogens. Obviously, chronic experiments with butylated hydroxyanisole in pigs and primates are urgently needed.

It may well be that as yet unidentified esophageal carcinogens exist in certain items associated with esophageal cancer, for example in opium or in bracken, as discussed in Chapter 8. At present, however, *N*-nitrosamines are the most suspect initiating carcinogens for the esophagus.

Carcinogenicity of *N*-nitroso compounds

For most populations, the levels of exposure to *N*-nitrosamines is low; although cancer may be initiated in a few cells, the exposure may be too low for cancer to become apparent unless the initiated cells are stimulated to progress to malignancy by secondary risk factors. Carcinogenicity of the nitrosamines may be enhanced by associated risk factors such as consumption of alcoholic beverages, dietary deficiencies, or exposure to mycotoxins. As with, for example, stomach cancer, a combination of initiating carcinogen and promoting risk factors is the most plausible etiological concept.

The human toxicity of nitrosamines was discovered on account of an industrial poisoning tragedy (Freund 1937). Two chemists who were developing a method for preparing *N*-nitroso-dimethylamine (NDMA) for use in the prevention of corrosion, were exposed by inhalation. A detailed study was made of the course of the illness which developed; one victim died with centrilobular necrosis of the liver one month after mopping up a spillage. Reports of a similar illness in workers in an automobile factory led to the request that the UK Medical Research Council Toxicology Unit should study the toxicity of NDMA. The effects seen in experimental animals were similar to those recorded in man. In addition, NDMA fed in the diet induced liver cancer (Magee *et al.* 1956), and a single injection produced kidney tumors (Magee *et al.* 1959).

The discovery that a simple chemically inert compound could be a potent carcinogen was surprising at that time, and rapidly led to the extensive investigation of other *N*-nitrosamines (Druckrey *et al.* 1967). Many of these chemicals were found to be potent carcinogens. Most nitrosamines showed a striking organ specificity, the esophagus very often being affected. Although the liver, esophagus and kidney were perhaps the most frequent target sites, almost all organs of the body were susceptible in either rats, mice, guinea pigs or hamsters (Magee *et al.* 1976; Preussmann *et al.* 1984*a*).

There are two main groups of *N*-nitroso compounds (NOC), and the distinction between them is important as it determines the site of their carcinogenicity (Fig. 5.1). The *N*-nitrosamines are chemically inert, and metabolic activation is essential prior to carcinogenicity. The site of their

Fig. 5.1. Carcinogenic *N*-nitroso compounds.

N-nitrosamines
e.g. dimethylnitrosamine

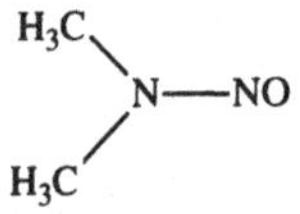

$$H_3C$$
$$\diagdown$$
$$N\text{---}NO$$
$$\diagup$$
$$H_3C$$

N-nitrosamides
e.g. nitrosomethylacetamide

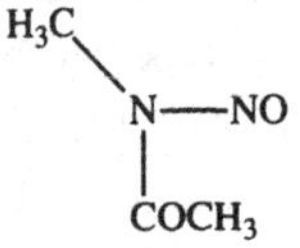

$$H_3C$$
$$\diagdown$$
$$N\text{---}NO$$
$$|$$
$$COCH_3$$

N-nitrosoureas
e.g. nitrosomethylurea

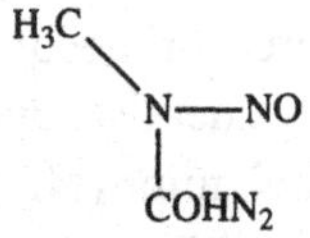

$$H_3C$$
$$\diagdown$$
$$N\text{---}NO$$
$$|$$
$$COHN_2$$

N-nitrosoguanidines
e.g. *N*-methyl-*N*-nitroso-*N'*-nitroguanidine

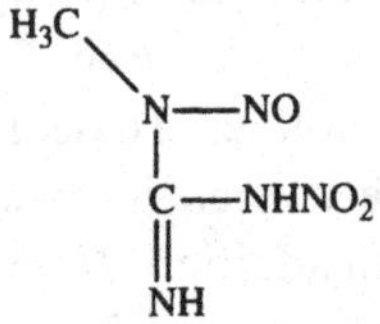

$$H_3C$$
$$\diagdown$$
$$N\text{---}NO$$
$$|$$
$$C\text{---}NHNO_2$$
$$||$$
$$NH$$

N-nitrosourethanes
(*N*-nitroso-*N*-alkylcarbamic acid ethyl esters)
e.g. *N*-nitroso-*N*-methylurethane

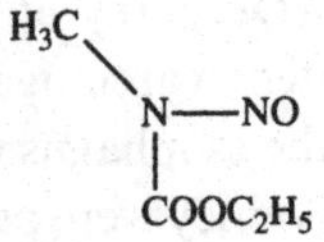

$$H_3C$$
$$\diagdown$$
$$N\text{---}NO$$
$$|$$
$$COOC_2H_5$$

action is therefore dependent not so much on the route of administration as on the ability of different organs to metabolize these compounds. In general *N*-nitrosamines are not metabolized by the brain or in the fetus, and therefore are not carcinogenic for brain or transplacentally. By contrast, the *N*-nitrosamides, *N*-nitroso-ureas, *N*-nitroso-guanidines and *N*-nitroso-urethanes are chemically reactive, and the identity of the main target organ depends largely on the route of administration, and on which organ is exposed to the highest dose. Therefore, while the *N*-nitrosamines which are carcinogenic for esophagus are effective by any route of administration, for the other *N*-nitroso compounds, unless given orally, esophagus is not a major target organ. Thus *N*-nitroso-*N*-methylurea (NMU) induces esophageal cancer in monkeys when given orally, and in Syrian golden hamsters when given by intratracheal installation, possibly as a result of spill-over into the esophagus. After oral treatment esophageal carcinogenicity was shown for *N*-nitroso-*N*-methylurethane (NMUR) for the rat (Schoental *et al.* 1962) and Syrian hamster (Herrold 1966), *N*-nitroso-*N*-ethylurethane (NEUR) for the rat (Hirose *et al.* 1979; Makawa *et al.* 1989), and *N*-nitroso-*N*-ethyl-*N'*-nitroguanidine (NENG) for the mouse (Nakamura *et al.* 1974).

Nitrosamines carcinogenic for the esophagus

As seen from the extensive tables compiled by Preussmann *et al.* (1984*a*), the nature of the nitrosamines which are carcinogenic for the esophagus varies with the species of animal being considered. A high proportion of the nitrosamines tested are esophageal carcinogens in the rat. In the hamster, the esophagus is susceptible to those *N*-nitroso compounds which do not require metabolic activation, but the *N*-nitrosamines have not been found to be carcinogenic for the esophagus.

As shown in Tables 5.2 and 5.3(*a*)–(*c*), *N*-nitrosamines may be dialkyl compounds, symmetric or asymmetric, cyclic, aromatic, or heterocyclic. While NDEA is a potent esophageal carcinogen, NDMA, even when fed to different animal species at varying dose levels for long periods, did not induce a single esophageal tumor (Peto *et al.* 1984). There is evidence that *N*-nitroso-*N*-diethylamine (NDEA) induced esophageal cancer in the F1 progeny when given transplacentally to mice with congenital mega-esophagus (Ghaisas *et al.* 1989). It was necessary to feed tobacco post-natally, to act as a promoter.

A list showing the range and variety of *N*-nitrosamines which are carcinogenic for the esophagus shows that minor changes in structure can dramatically alter the target organ for a nitrosamine – a feature which

Table 5.2. *N-nitrosamines carcinogenic for the esophagus in the rat*

Symmetric	*Cyclic*
N-nitroso-	N-nitroso-methylcyclohexylamine
diethylamine	
dipropylamine	*Aromatic*
dibutylamine	N-nitroso-
	methylphenylamine
Asymmetric	methylbenzylamine
N-nitroso-	
methylbutylamine	*Heterocyclic*
methylamylamine	N-nitroso-
methylvinylamine	piperidine
methylallylamine	hexamethylenemine
ethylbutylamine	
ethylisopropylamine	*Tobacco-specific*
ethylvinylamine	N-nitroso-
sarcosine	nornicotine
	anabasine

For references and an extensive list see Preussmann *et al.* (1984*a*).

Table 5.3(*a*). *Carcinogenicity of N-nitrosamines in rats: symmetric and asymmetric*

Type	Nitrosamine	Esophagus	Liver	Other sites
Symmetric	Dimethyl	−	+	Kidney
	Diethyl	+	+	Lung
	Dipropyl	+	+	
	Dibutyl	+	+	Bladder
	Diamyl	−	+	
Asymmetric	Me-ethyl	+	+	
	Me-*n*-propyl	+	−	Forestomach
	Me-*n*-butyl	+	+	Forestomach, nasal cavity
	Me-*n*-amyl	+		
	Me-vinyl	+	−	Pharynx, tongue
	Me-allyl	+	−	Nasal cavity, kidney
	Me-sarcosine	+	−	−

reveals the high specificity of the enzymes responsible for their metabolism. As shown in Table 5.3, there is a critical minimum length of the alkyl chain and of the size of the heterocyclic ring for the nitrosamine to be carcinogenic for esophagus.

With reference to aromatic nitrosamines, both nitroso-methylphenylamine (NMPhA) and methylbenzylnitrosamine are esophageal carcinogens, although under the conditions of treatment which have been

Table 5.3(*b*). *Carcinogenicity of N-nitrosamines in rats: cyclic and aromatic*

Cyclic and aromatic	Formula	Esophagus	Other sites
Me-cyclohexyl		+	Pharynx, lung
Me-phenyl		+	Forestomach
Me-benzyl		+	—
Me-(2-phenylethyl)		+	—

used, NMPhA is less potent. The carcinogenicity of this compound is surprising, in view of the fact (discussed later) that the carcinogenic metabolic site for nitrosamines is generally an α-carbon hydroxylation, and there is no α-carbon susceptible to hydroxylation in this case. As far as it is possible to generalize, asymmetric nitrosamines, especially those which are more lipophilic, are more likely to be carcinogenic for the esophagus. This feature has been demonstrated repeatedly during studies of structure/activity relationships, and presumably results from the specificity of esophageal P450 isozymes. For example, while *N*-nitroso-diallylamine was not found to be carcinogenic, all the asymmetric nitrosamines containing an allyl group were carcinogenic for esophagus (Lijinsky *et al.* 1984). The esophageal carcinogenicity of nitroso-sarcosine (N-SAR) is of special interest, owing to its widespread occurrence in food. The nitrosamines most often used to study the course of carcinogenesis in the esophagus have been NMBzA and *N*-nitroso-*N*-methylamylamine (NMAA). The sequence of pathological changes following treatment with these nitrosamines is discussed in Chapter 3.

With reference to the mutagenicity of nitrosamines, after initial problems concerning techniques, it was found that in general the carcinogenic nitrosamines were mutagenic when incubated with *Salmonella typhimurium*

Table 5.3(c). Carcinogenicity of N-nitrosamines in rats: heterocyclic

Heterocyclic	Formula	Esophagus	Liver
Azetidine	N—NO	−	+
Pyrrolidine	N—NO	−	+
Piperidine	N—NO	+	+
Hexamethylene-imine	$(CH_2)_6$ N—NO	+	+
Heptamethylene-imine	$(CH_2)_7$ N—NO	+	−

in a liquid system containing the customary activating cytosol fraction from rat liver. NMPhA was an exception. As this nitrosamine is carcinogenic for esophagus but not for liver, an obvious possibility was that it would be activated by esophageal but not by liver P450 systems. However, it was found that NMPhA was not mutagenic in the *Salmonella* assay when the S9 mix was isolated from rat esophagus, unless the co-mutagen norharman was added (Anderson *et al.* 1985).

Mechanism of carcinogenicity of N-nitrosamine
A general consensus at present is that, for many of the nitros-amines which have been studied, the initiation of cancer is comprised of three essential steps:

1. Metabolic activation of the nitrosamine with the formation of an alkylating intermediate.
2. Alkylation of DNA at a relevant site in the molecule, i.e. the oxygen atom of guanine or thymine.

3. Replication of the alkylated DNA before repair mechanisms in the cell have removed the relevant adduct.

Reviews discussing the metabolic activation of nitrosamines (Archer *et al.* 1985), the alkylation and repair of DNA (Saffhill *et al.* 1985), and the significance of DNA replication (Rajewsky 1972; Craddock 1976) have been published.

Metabolism of nitrosamines and alkylation of DNA

When given to rats by the oral route, simple aliphatic nitrosamines disappear rapidly from the blood, and treatment with ^{14}C-labelled nitrosamines results in the appearance of [^{14}C]carbon dioxide in the exposed air and the labelling of urinary metabolites and of normal metabolic intermediates (Heath *et al.* 1958). It was discovered that many nitrosamines are metabolized in the endoplasmic reticulum by enzymes belonging to the cytochrome P450 system responsible for the metabolism

Fig. 5.2. Metabolism of NDMA.

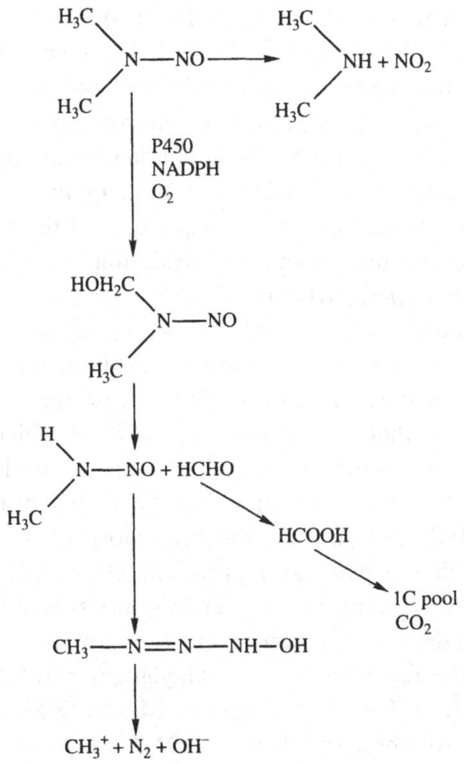

of many xenobiotics. As the P450 isozymes have broad overlapping specificities, different isozymes probably each metabolize a range of nitrosamines, some more effectively than others. The distribution of isozymes in different organs must at least in part explain the organ specificity of nitrosamines.

In vitro experiments carried out in the presence of a trapping agent, for example semicarbazide, showed that on metabolism several nitrosamines gave rise to the corresponding aldehydes, NDMA forming formaldehyde, NDEA producing acetaldehyde. This was the result of initial hydroxylation of the carbon atom in the α-positions adjacent to the nitroso amino group. Substitution of the hydrogen atom at this position with alkyl, aryl or deuterium altered but did not abolish carcinogenicity. Liberation of the aldehyde resulted in the formation of the unstable monoalkylnitrosamine, which on decomposition gave an electrophilic alkylating agent, the ultimate carcinogen, and nitrogen (Fig. 5.2). However, even with aliphatic nitrosamines, this simple scheme is far from the complete story. The binding spectra with P450 are atypical, and the P450 isozymes and are unusual in their response to inducing agents and to inhibitors. The NMBzA demethylase is unusual in being inhibited by zinc, and activity increases on a zinc-deficient diet (Barch *et al.* 1987). According to the scheme shown in Fig. 5.2, the amount of nitrogen liberated would be expected to be equivalent to the nitrosamine metabolized, but experiments with ^{15}N-labelled nitrosamines have not confirmed this prediction. There is evidence that additional reactions occur, including denitrosation, trans-nitrosation, and the formation of hydrazines (Preussmann *et al.* 1984a). With long chain alkyl nitrosamines, oxidation can occur at the terminal oxygen, as with N-nitroso-di-n-butylamine, or β-oxidation can take place, as in the case of N-nitroso-di-n-propylamine.

The electrophilic alkylating agents formed react with proteins and with nucleic acids and the levels of the reaction products have been widely used to study the *in vivo* metabolism of nitrosamines. Now that there is compelling evidence to show that it is the alkylation of DNA which is the relevant reaction for carcinogenesis by many compounds, the level of DNA alkylation is of most interest. The major alkylated base to be formed is 7-methylguanine (7-MG), and this base has been most often studied. However, the base which mis-pairs at replication, O^6-methylguanine (O^6MG), is more likely to be implicated in carcinogenesis. In addition, while 7-MG is lost from DNA by slow non-enzymic depurination, O^6MG is actively removed by the repair enzyme, O^6-alkylguanine–DNA-alkyl transferase (see next section). The initial ratio of 7-MG to O^6MG is 0.1. Therefore, determination of these two bases in DNA can give a good measure of the initial level of alkylation and of the rate of repair of the 'carcinogenic' base. O^4-ethylthymine is another mispairing base which is formed after treatment with NDEA, and as it is not subject to repair in mammalian systems it can accumulate during chronic treatment until it becomes the predominant alkylated base in DNA (Dyroff *et al.* 1986). On account of difficulties in measuring the small amounts formed after a single dose of nitrosamine, O^4-ethylthymine has not often been measured.

Metabolism of nitrosamines in the esophagus has been studied to a limited extent in the intact animal, by determining the level of labelling of esophageal DNA after treatment with labelled nitrosamines. Using whole-body autoradiography and [^{14}C]methyl or [^{14}C]benzyl NMBzA, the highest levels of labelling were found for the nasal cavity, esophagus and lung (Kraft *et al.* 1980*a*). The nitrosamine disappeared rapidly from the circulation, and the evidence was that both methylated and benzylated macromolecules were formed (Kraft *et al.* 1980*b*). Methylation of DNA was highest in the target organ, the esophagus, followed by liver, lung and forestomach (Hodgson *et al.* 1980). In mice, however, the levels of alkylation of DNA did not explain the organotrophy of NMBzA (Kleihues *et al.* 1981). Similar experiments with another potent esophageal carcinogen, NMAA, labelled in the methyl group, showed the methylation of DNA to be highest in the esophagus, followed by nasal epithelium, liver, trachea and lung (Koenigsmann *et al.* 1988). The authors concluded that there is preferential metabolism by the upper respiratory and gastrointestinal tracts. With the tobacco-specific nitrosamines (TSN), N'-nitrosonornicotine (NNN) is carcinogenic for the esophagus, and for the nasal cavity. After injection of [^{14}C]NNN in the mouse, while initially the levels of radioactivity were highest in the liver and kidney, by 24 hours ^{14}C was present only in the nasal epithelium, bronchi, esophagus and salivary gland – a finding which suggests that esophagus among other organs is capable of metabolizing NNN (Waddell *et al.* 1980).

Using a very sensitive peroxidase immunohistochemical method to visualize O^6-alkylguanine in DNA in individual cells, it was found that a single injection of NMBzA gave rise to O^6MG only in the sensitive cells of the target organ, the esophageal basal cells, and not in liver (Scherer *et al.* 1989). NDEA, carcinogenic for both esophagus and liver, formed O^6EG in DNA in both organs, while NDMA, carcinogenic only for liver, formed O^6MG in liver and not in esophagus. Radioimmune assays have been used also to test for O^6MG in DNA isolated from inhabitants of regions in China which have a high incidence of esophageal cancer (Umbenhauer *et al.* 1985). These pioneering experiments suggest that it may be possible to relate alkylation of DNA to esophageal cancer in human populations. The ability to metabolize nitrosamines is maintained in the papillomas which develop during continuous treatment with NMBzA and NMAA, suggesting that additional mutations are acquired during chronic treatment (Dirsch et al. 1990).

Studies on the microsomal metabolism of NMBzA were initiated by Labuc et al. (1982). In esophageal microsomes, oxidation occurred almost exclusively at the methylene carbon, with the formation of benzaldehyde and a methylating intermediate, while in the liver methylating and benzylating intermediates were formed. NMBzA was metabolized to benzaldehyde by esophageal microsomes of the rat, but not by those of Syrian hamster or the mouse, although the reaction occurred with liver and lung microsomes from all three species (Mehta et al. 1984a). In agreement with this finding, acute toxicity studies showed that cellular damage occurred in the esophagus in the rat, but not in hamsters or mice. Metabolism was not induced by pre-treatment of the rats with phenobarbital or with 3-methylcholanthrene (Mehta et al. 1984b). Esophageal microsomes from the rat metabolized also NDEA and N-nitrosodibutylamine (NDBA), but while with liver it was possible to give an average rate of metabolism, with esophagus the variation between different batches of animals was so great that it was possible to give only a range of values (Bertram et al. 1985). Metabolism of NDMA was almost undetectable. When slices or pieces of esophageal tissue were incubated with NMAA, metabolism of the amyl group occurred, with the formation of 2-, 3-, and 4-hydroxyamylmethyl and 4-oxoamylmethyl nitrosamines (Mirvish et al. 1985, 1988).

Studies with cultured rat epithelial cells showed a selective toxicity of different N-nitrosamines for the esophagus, and implied that this system was appropriate for mechanistic studies (Zucker et al. 1991). However, in view of the species differences in carcinogenicity of nitrosamines for the esophagus, studies with cultures of human material are of special interest. NMBzA was metabolized more extensively than NDMA or NDEA and, as with the rat esophagus, oxidation occurred mainly at the methylene group rather than at the methyl group, with the production of benzaldehyde and a methylating intermediate (Autrup et al. 1982). Metabolism in human esophagus, however, was approximately 100 times slower than in the rat. With cultured fetal esophageal explants, NDEA was bound to DNA more extensively than was NMBzA (Autrup et al. 1984).

The metabolism of tobacco-specific nitrosamines is of special interest. NNN, carcinogenic for the esophagus, and 4(methyl-nitroso-amino)-1-(3 pyridyl)-butanone (NNK), not yet shown to be an esophageal carcinogen, were both metabolized in the esophagus, but the level of metabolism of

NNK was less than that occurring in the other organs studied (Castonguay *et al.* 1983). After treatment of intact rats with NNN, however, O^6MG was detected in DNA of nasal mucosa, lung and liver, but not in that isolated from esophagus (Foiles *et al.* 1985). Experiments with tritiated NNN and NNK showed that cultured rat esophagus metabolized NNN to a greater extent than NNK to a reactive species which pyridloxobutylates DNA (Murphy *et al.* 1990). This may be important in determining the carcinogenicity of NNN.

Differences found in the results of whole animal and *in vitro* systems, and also large individual variations in the rates of metabolism of nitrosamines found on using cultures derived from different human individuals, may well be explained by dietary factors. Pretreatment of animals with various dietary constituents which have been suggested to be protective against cancer, including phenols, cinnamic acid, coumarins, indoles and iso-thiocyanates, was found to reduce metabolism of NNN in cultured rat esophagus (Chung *et al.* 1984). The plant phenol ellagic acid, which reduced NMBzA-induced esophageal cancer (Mandal *et al.* 1986, 1990; Daniel *et al.* 1991), inhibited the metabolism of NMBzA in cultured rat esophagus (Mandal *et al.* 1988), and reduced the metabolism of NMBzA by esophageal but not liver microsomes (Barch *et al.* 1989). Diallylsulphide, a thioether present in garlic, also inhibited esophageal carcinogenicity of NMBzA, but surprisingly pretreatment of animals with diallylsulphide reduced the metabolism of NMBzA in liver but not in esophageal microsomes (Wargovich *et al.* 1988). Other workers, however, found that incubation with diallylsulphide had little effect on liver microsomal metabolism of NMBzA (Brady *et al.* 1988).

Another example of a protection from cancer by inhibition of met-abolism of nitrosamine is given by the thiocyanates. Phenethyl iso-thiocyanate, a product of the thioglycosylase-catalysed hydrolysis of gluconasturtin, is a naturally occurring compound found in certain cruciferous vegetables. Rats fed a diet containing the isothiocyanate developed 99–100 % fewer tumors in the esophagus when treated with NMBzA than did the control group. The compound also reduced the metabolism of NMBzA by esophageal tissues (Stoner *et al.* 1991). As well as explaining apparently incongruous results which were in fact caused by consumption of differing diets, inhibition of nitrosamine metabolism may well explain the protective effect against esophageal cancer in man of certain chemicals which occur in various commonly consumed plant foods.

Studies of nitrosamine metabolism by the esophagus in the intact animal and in microsomal systems and cultures of explants indicate that, where the nitrosamine is carcinogenic for the esophagus, it is metabolized by esophageal microsomes, and methylation of DNA ensues. At present there is no sound evidence for the formation of benzyl adducts after treatment with NMBzA, or that NMPhA gives rise to phenyl adducts in DNA, although diazo coupling may occur (Koepke *et al.* 1984). Whether the large number of nitrosamines carcinogenic for the esophagus are metabolized by the identical P450 isozyme, or by a number of isozymes with overlapping specificities, is unknown. There is also no evidence for the induction of nitrosamine-metabolizing enzymes in the esophagus, and no information on their relationship with nitrosamine-metabolizing enzymes in other organs.

Repair of DNA

A landmark in understanding how genetic damage causes cancer was reached around 1966, when evidence began to accumulate to show that DNA damage could be repaired by error-correcting mechanisms in the cell. Three important adducts formed in DNA by metabolites of many nitrosamines are N^7-alkylguanine, O^6-alkylguanine, and 4-alkylthymine. Information on repair of these lesions is mainly limited to the methyl and ethyl adducts. 7-MG is lost slowly from DNA by non-enzymic depurination, and by a very slow repair mechanism in rat liver. O^6MG is repaired by an O^6-alkylguanine–DNA-alkyl transferase, in a reaction whereby the methyl group is transferred to the sulfhydyl group of a cysteine residue in the repair protein (Lindahl 1982). As the reaction is stoichiometric rather than catalytic, the protein involved is not a genuine enzyme, and would more appropriately be called the alkyl acceptor protein. The repair protein is 'consumed' during the reaction, and when the store of this specific protein in the cell is exhausted, repair of DNA cannot proceed until further biosynthesis has occurred. The rate of repair of O^6-alkyl adducts is therefore determined by the amount of repair protein in the cell nucleus. There is a large variation in the level between different organs. In the rat, the liver contains by far the highest concentration. Kidney contains less, and the repair ability of brain and of esophagus is very low (Craddock *et al.* 1986). The disappearance of receptor protein from esophagus is dose-dependent after treatment of rats with NMBzA or with NDEA, and several days may be needed for it to be restored. NMPhA does not affect the level of transferase, a fact suggesting that NMPhA is not metabolized to form an alkylating agent (Craddock *et al.* 1986).

O^4-methylthymine is another base which mis-pairs at replication, and therefore could be important in carcinogenesis. At present the consensus of opinion is that it is not actively repaired by mammalian cells (Brent *et al.* 1988), but the species and cell types which have been studied are very limited.

As repair of O^6-MG in DNA involves simple removal of the methyl group, the DNA is returned to its previous condition, and repair is error-free. Removal of 3-methyladenine (3-MA) involves a very different process, as a glycosylase catalyses the breakage of the purine–deoxyribose bond, with the release of 3-MA and the formation of depurinated DNA. Evidence for the existence of 'insertases' which could 'fill the gap' with a normal base is now known to have been mistaken, and instead the depurinated DNA is subject to further degradation by nucleases. The level of 3-MA glycosylases in different organs varies less than does that of O^6MG–DNA-alkyl transferase (Craddock *et al.* 1982), but the level in esophagus has apparently not been determined. 3-MA, however, is probably responsible for the toxicity rather than for the carcinogenicity of the nitrosamines.

The importance of repair of DNA lesions lies in the fact that, for the lesion to be effective, replication of the DNA must occur before the alkylated adduct has been removed. This is discussed in the next section.

Replication of DNA

The alkylated bases in DNA responsible for initiating cancer act by mis-pairing during DNA replication, thereby introducing a change in base sequence in the daughter strand. For malignancy to ensue, it is therefore essential that replication should take place before the alkylated base has been removed from the DNA. Malignancy thus depends on the initial level of DNA alkylation, the rate of removal of the relevant base, and on the rate of DNA replication. In liver, rapid metabolism of many nitrosamines results in high levels of alkylation of DNA, but repair is rapid and the rate of cell replication normally slow. In esophagus, however, there is rapid metabolism of certain nitrosamines and consequent alkylation of DNA, repair is slow and, as discussed in Chapter 2, replication is comparatively rapid. Esophagus is therefore much more vulnerable than liver to certain nitrosamines. In discussing alkylation of DNA in relation to carcinogenesis in different organs, it is essential to consider all three factors, i.e. the initial level of alkylation, repair, and replication. In the past attempts have been made to relate carcinogenicity simply to the level of alkylation of DNA, and misleading and unjustified conclusions have been made.

Although the level of replication in the basal cells of the esophagus is relatively high, in order to replace cells lost from the surface of the lumen, various factors can increase the rate of replication, either by causing damage and restorative hyperplasia, or by direct mitotic stimulation. The dose schedule often used to initiate cancer in esophagus with NMBzA causes extensive damage, and restorative hyperplasia occurs (Craddock et al. 1987). Risk factors for esophageal cancer very probably act by increasing vulnerability to nitrosamines by stimulating cell replication. Thus alcoholic beverages (Chapter 6), mycotoxins (Chapter 9) and riboflavin and zinc deficiencies (Chapter 10) may act in this way.

Exposure to N-nitroso compounds and risk assessment

Formation of N-nitroso compounds in the environment

It was first suggested by Druckrey et al. (1962) that N-nitrosamines might be formed in tobacco smoke. Evidence for the environmental occurrences of nitrosamines was presented by Enders et al. (1964), who showed that the toxic factor in nitrite-preserved fishmeal responsible for a sheep-poisoning episode in Norway was NDMA. Following this disconcerting discovery of a potent carcinogen in animal feed, surveys were carried out elsewhere, and low levels of a variety of N-nitrosamines were found in human food, drink, manufactured products, and normal human urine. However, it was not until specific sensitive analytical methods were developed, which involved separation by gas–liquid chromatography and thermal energy analysis by detection of chemiluminescence, with mass spectrometry for confirmation of identity (Fine et al. 1974, 1975) that the data was unequivocal.

N-nitrosamines are formed whenever amines and nitrite come together at an appropriate pH. Thus secondary amines react with nitrite to form the corresponding nitrosamine:

$$\begin{array}{c} R_1 \\ \diagdown \\ \diagup NH + NO_2 \longrightarrow \\ R_2 \end{array} \qquad \begin{array}{c} R_1 \\ \diagdown \\ \diagup N\text{---}NO + OH^- \\ R_2 \end{array}$$

As the amine reacts in the un-ionized form, nitrosation occurs more readily with weakly basic amines, such as methylbenzylamine, than with strongly basic amines, for example dimethylamine, which ionize more readily. The rate of nitrosation of secondary amines is proportional to the square of the nitrite concentration. In addition to nitrosation of secondary amines, N-nitrosamines can be formed by unexpected routes. Thus the amine gramine, found in barley malt, reacts with nitrite not only by nitrosation at the tertiary nitrogen atom, but also by nitrosative dealkylation, with the secondary formation of NDMA (Ahmed *et al.* 1985):

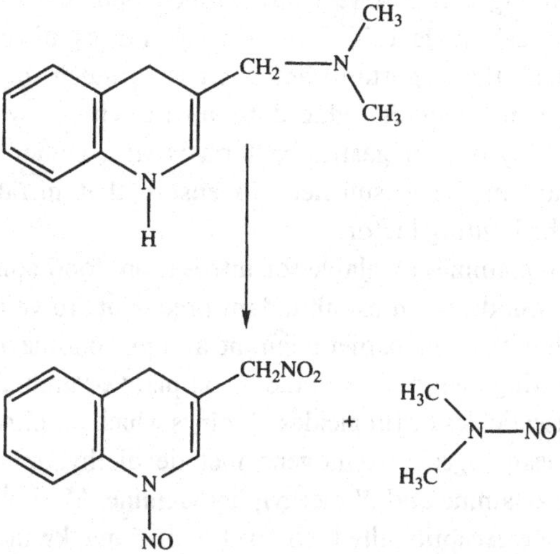

An example of a situation in which nitrosamines carcinogenic for the esophagus are formed is in the smoking of fish and meat. This process converts creatine, present at high concentrations in muscle, into sarcosine, which can be nitrosated by nitrogen oxides in the smoke to form N-nitrososarcosine, an esophageal carcinogen:

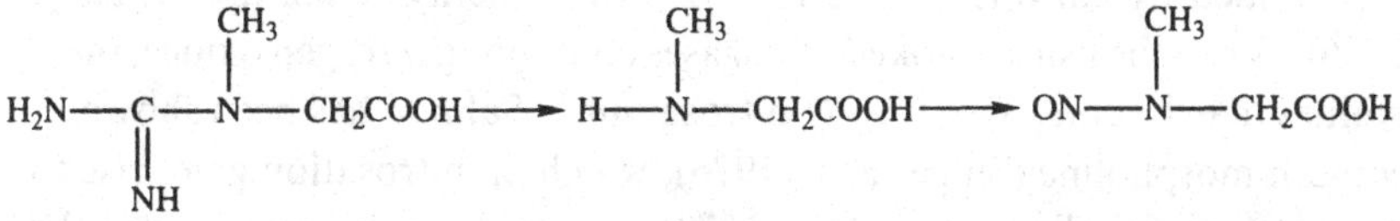

| Creatine | Sarcosine | *N*-nitrososarcosine |

Unexpected routes of nitrosamine formation and the unpredictability of the occurrence of nitrosamines in food and its packaging emphasize the need for careful surveys.

A major source of the nitrite which participates in nitrosation is that added to food in preserving mixtures. The highest levels occur in cured meats, where at present the addition of nitrite is necessary to prevent the growth of *Clostridium botulinum*. Nitrite is also formed from nitrate by bacterial reduction during storage of food. Here nitrite levels depend on the concentration of nitrate and on the duration of storage. The main dietary sources of nitrate are certain vegetables, the levels in different vegetables being very variable. Thus spinach and beets can contain more than 2640 mg nitrate/kg, while tomatoes and cucumbers contain only a few milligrams per kilogram. In contrast, nitrite levels in fresh vegetables are low, but the content in fresh spinach, approximately 30 mg nitrite/kg, increased to 3550 mg/kg after storage for 4 days (Shank 1981). High nitrate levels in drinking water have caused much debate concerning possible hazards for carcinogenesis. However, as far as nitrosamine formation is concerned, the important factor is not so much the nitrate level but how readily it becomes reduced to nitrite, either by microorganisms *in vitro*, or by oral or gastric bacteria *in vivo*. Under normal conditions, the nitrate intake is sufficient to ensure that nitrate concentrations are not the limiting factor.

With reference to the amines available for nitrosation, food contains a variety of these compounds, the most abundant precursors to volatile *N*-nitrosamines being dimethylamine, diethylamine and pyrrolidine. Certain amines are formed during metabolism in the living plant or animal, while others originate in insecticides or fungicides. Amines which on nitrosation give rise to potent esophageal carcinogens include diethylamine, piperidine, *N*-methylbenzylamine and *N*-methylphenylamine. Methylbenzylamine was found at the exceptionally high level of 16.5 mg/kg in carrots (Neurath *et al.* 1977), and methylphenylamine occurs in tea (Maga 1978). The amines may be present in fresh food, but also they are formed by bacterial action during storage. For example, the end product of nitrogen metabolism in fish is trimethylamine oxide, which on storage is converted by bacteria into trimethylamine. Even when stored frozen, trimethylamine is degraded by enzymes in the fish to form dimethylamine (Zeisel *et al.* 1986). When the fish is smoked with gases containing nitrogen oxides, these amines may be converted into *N*-nitrosamines. Salmon has been shown to contain morpholine (Singer *et al.* 1976), which on nitrosation gives rise to *N*-nitrosomorpholine (Haas *et al.* 1973), an esophageal carcinogen in the hamster (Preussmann *et al.* 1984*a*). The presence of these nitrosamines could well account for the high incidence of certain cancers among populations that consume large quantities of preserved fish (see later). Another route by which bacteria can form amines is by decarboxylation of amino acids. Thus lysine gives rise to piperidine, a readily nitrosatable amine, which on nitrosation forms a potent esophageal carcinogen.

Especially hazardous are the amines formed by fungi. Certain fungi can convert primary amines into secondary amines by direct methylation (Ji *et al.* 1986). The secondary amines arising from these reactions are therefore asymmetric, and on nitrosation form nitrosamines which are especially likely to be potent carcinogens for the esophagus. Thus *Fusarium moniliforme* can methylate isoamylamine, which on nitrosation yields *N*-nitroso-*N*-methylisoamylamine, a potent esophageal carcinogen.

Microorganisms increase the levels of nitrosamines not only by catalyzing the formation of amines and of nitrite, but also by their ability to carry out enzyme-mediated nitrosation reactions (Camels *et al.* 1985). Bacteria could be important in forming nitrosamines in fermented foods, for example soya sauce, yoghurts and cheese. Heating food at temperatures used for cooking also leads to the formation of nitrosamines by a variety of routes. The occurrence of NDMA and *N*-nitroso-pyrrolidine (N-PYR) in cooked bacon is the most notorious example of this (Preussmann *et al.* 1984*b*). Oxides of nitrogen are a common product of combustion, being formed during gas cooking, and relatively high concentrations of nitrite are generally present in cured meat. The nitrite reacts with proline in the bacon to form *N*-nitrosoproline, and subsequent heat-induced decarboxylation yields N-PYR.

The nitrosamines formed in these reactions are chemically stable and inert, and remain in food and drink unless they are lost on account of their volatility or are destroyed by sunlight. The direct-acting *N*-nitroso compounds, on the other hand, for example *N*-nitrosoureas and *N*-nitrosamides, react readily with major components of the food. These compounds are therefore generally not consumed in the diet, although their formation from precursors in the stomach may well be important. They would be more likely, therefore, to react with gastric mucosa than with esophageal epithelium.

Occurrence of *N*-nitroso compounds and relation to incidence of esophageal cancer
Occurrence in food

Significant amounts of volatile and non-volatile nitrosamines, including several which are carcinogenic for the esophagus, have been found and assayed in a variety of foods. The concentrations found vary very widely even for the same food item purchased from the same area, but in general the highest levels have been found in foods to which nitrite has been added, or which have been smoked using gases containing nitrogen oxides. Therefore cured meats, salted or smoked fish, and cheese are especially suspect (Table 5.4). High levels may occur in 'fresh' fish as a result of the bacterial action described above, the concentrations depending on the degree of 'freshness'. As seen from Table 5.4, nitrosamines carcinogenic for the esophagus – NDEA, NDBA, N-PIP and N-SAR – occur in common food items. An attempt to assess the percentage contribution of different types of food to total nitrosamine exposure has been carried out for NDMA for males in former West Germany (Preussmann *et al.* 1984*b*). Here beer (see next section) accounted for 64 %

Table 5.4. *N-nitrosamine content of foods*

N-nitrosamine	Food	Content (μg/kg)
N-nitroso-dimethylamine (NDMA)	Cured meats	0–84
	Salted fish	1–35
	Fresh fish	0.2–18
	Cheese	1–15
N-nitroso-N-diethylamine (NDEA)	Cured meats	3–91
	Cheese	2–20
	Fish	4–14
N-nitroso-dibutylamine (NDBA)	Cured meats	0–3.9
N-nitroso-pyrrolidine (N-PyR)	Cured meats	0.6–139
	Cheese	1.4–3.4
N-nitroso-piperidine (N-PIP)	Cured meats	0–60
	Cheese	2–11
N-nitroso-sarcosine (N-SAR)	Icelandic smoked mutton	200–410[a]
	Corned beef	0–30[a]
	Bacon, raw	0–11.5[a]
	Bacon, fried	0–15.5[a]

From Rogers (1982) and [a] Tricker *et al.* (1984).

of the total, preserved or fermented foods being the other major contributors (Table 5). In most western countries, the concentrations of these nitrosamines are usually on the lower side of the range, but in the East the methods of food preparation more often favour the formation of nitrosamines.

To study the relevance of the nitrosamine content of food for human cancer, the diets of populations living in high-incidence areas for certain cancers have been studied. Esophageal, gastric and nasopharyngeal cancers have received most attention. The causes of these three types of cancer may each be related to N-nitroso compounds, although the highest incidence areas for each cancer are not identical, i.e. esophageal cancer is especially high in North Central China, nasopharyngeal cancer in South China and Greenland, and gastric cancer in Japan and Iceland. In each case, with the possible exception of Japan, there is a high consumption of preserved fish, meat or vegetables, i.e. food items known to be especially likely to contain high levels of nitrosamines.

The local diet consumed in the North Central region of China, in the Henan province, Linxian county, has been studied in detail. Water supplies were often inadequate, and the water as collected from the wells contained high levels of nitrate and nitrite. Often water was stored in earthenware jars for considerable periods, during which time bacterial reduction of nitrate to nitrite took place. The diet was severely restricted, being comprised mainly of gruel and pickled vegetables, and it was the latter item which has been most suspect. The vegetables, mainly turnips and sweet potato leaves, were fermented in water, without the addition of salt or vinegar. The pickles were consumed throughout the winter, and were often stored for more than a year. During the storage period, nitrite formed by bacteria from nitrate in the water or in the vegetables can react with amines in the plant material to form nitrosamines. In addition, molds grew on the surface of the pickles, and the fungi produced not only mycotoxins but also reduced nitrate to nitrite and methylated primary amines to form asymmetric secondary amines, as mentioned previously. In addition, the previously unknown nitrosamine, *N*-3-methyl-*n*-butyl-*N*-1-methyl-acetonylnitrosamine (NMAMBA) was found in corn bread which had been inoculated with *F. moniliforme* and incubated with a low concentration of nitrite (Li *et al.* 1986). Similarly, *N*-2-methyl-*n*-propyl-*N*-methylacetonylnitrosamine was detected in millet and wheat flour which had been treated in the same way. NMAMBA induced tumors in the forestomach, an organ often regarded as an extension of the esophagus, in rats and mice.

The first food items from Linxian to be analysed by reliable techniques did not show especially high levels of volatile nitrosamines (Singer *et al.* 1986). However, the foods studied – millet flour, turnip chips, steamed corn cakes and persimmon bran meal – were not especially suspect. Later, items with a reputation for containing high levels of nitrosamines were studied, and pickled and salt vegetables were found to contain up to 15.0 μg/kg NDMA and 25.5 μg/kg N-PYR, dried and salted fish up to 24.4 μg/kg NDMA, and shrimp products up to 131.5 μg/kg NDMA (Song *et al.* 1988). A previously unknown compound, Roussin red methyl ester, was isolated from pickled vegetables (Liu *et al.* 1989). This chemical is a nitroso-iron complex, and is thought to be derived in part from the metal jars used for storage:

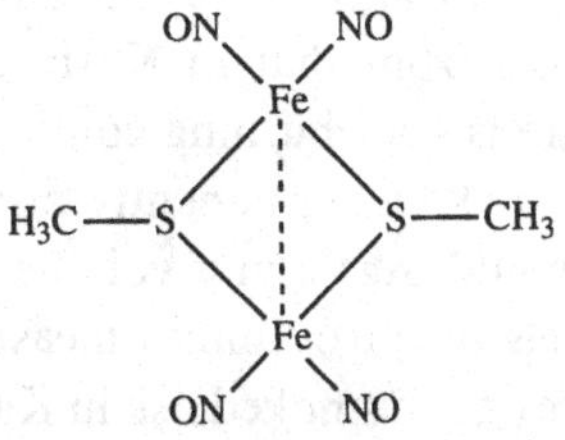

The fact that chronic administration of Roussin red to rats and mice induced papillomas in the forestomach implies that this compound could be carcinogenic for esophagus. In addition, Roussin red can react with benzylamine to form NMBzA, a potent esophageal carcinogen.

Another high-risk area for esophageal cancer in which the diet has been examined for its nitrosamine content is the Kashmir region of India (Siddiqi *et al*. 1989). Factors commonly associated with esophageal cancer, for example consumption of alcohol, tobacco smoking, use of betel quid, dietary deficiencies, and a low intake of fruit, vegetables, meat and fish do not apply to Kashmir. However, on account of the climate and distinct cultural traditions, the Kashmiris have a unique diet, which differs from that of the surrounding areas where there is a lower incidence of esophageal cancer. The long severe winters in Kashmir necessitate the storage of food, which is often kept for more than two years. Plant foods are sun-dried or pickled, and fish is sun-dried or smoked. As with similar food items in North Central China, fungi and bacteria have the opportunity to convert nitrate to nitrite, which then reacts with amines in the food to form nitrosamines. Another local speciality is strong salted tea. Bicarbonate is added to the tea at the time of brewing, and then boiling may be continued for up to two hours. The tea is kept hot in samovars, and sodium chloride is added before consumption. The per capita daily consumption is 6–10 cups per day. Another suspect food item is the mixed spice cake which is used as a source of spices for most Kashmiri foods.

Each of these commonly consumed food items was found to be widely contaminated by *N*-nitroso compounds (Siddiqi *et al*. 1988). Of special relevance for esophageal cancer was the high level of N-sar in pickled vegetables (36.0 μg/kg) and in spice cake (5.0 μg/kg). Other very high levels were of N-PRO (320 μg/kg) in spice cake and *N*-nitrosothiazolidine-4-carboxylic acid (82.0 μg/kg) in smoked fish. Although the levels of *N*-nitroso compounds detected in the dried vegetable *Brassica oleracea* were lower, this food item is consumed in large amounts throughout the year (Kumar *et al*. 1990).

In another region of Northern India, Nagaland, the incidence of nasopharyngeal cancer is exceptionally high, and here again there is a high consumption of smoked fish and meat (Sakar *et al*. 1989). The route of exposure to nitrosamines, however, differs from that in Kashmir. The Naga tribes live in single-room huts, a fire is kept burning continuously, and there is no ventilation. Meat and fish are kept permanently suspended above the fire, so that the inhabitants would inhale any volatile nitrosamines liberated from the food. The levels of nitrosamines measured in the smoked meat were higher than those found in smoked fish in Kashmir, and included the esophageal carcinogen NDEA. A plausible concept is that inhalation of nitrosamines released from smoking food causes nasopharyngeal cancer, while consumption of the food induces esophageal cancer.

Other regions with a high incidence of nasopharyngeal cancer are South China, Tunisia and Greenland, and here again there was found to be a high consumption of dried fish and mutton widely contaminated by nitrosamines (Poirier *et al.* 1987). An important factor may be that in South-East Asia these foods are given to babies when less than two years old. Thus the age of exposure and whether the nitrosamines are inhaled or swallowed is likely to determine the target organ.

It is often in semi-arid regions around the world, such as those near the Caspian Sea, and in Linxian, that there is a high incidence of esophageal cancer. A plant which is widely used as a folk medicine and health tea in semi-arid areas, *Ephedra altissima*, was shown to contain *N*-methylbenzylamine, which on nitrosation would give rise to NMBzA, an especially potent esophageal carcinogen (Tricker *et al.* 1987*a*), and another asymmetric nitrosamine (Tricker *et al.* 1987*b*). In Western countries the incidence of esophageal cancer in men is determined mainly by consumption of alcohol and tobacco, but in women diet can play a more important role. High rates of esophageal cancer in women occur in Iceland, where there is a high consumption of smoke-cured mutton. This has been shown to contain very high levels of N-SAR, as well as other *N*-nitroso compounds (Tricker *et al.* 1984). Recently the potent esophageal carcinogen *N*-nitroso-*N*-methylaniline (i.e. *N*-nitroso-*N*-methylphenylamine, NMPhA), was detected in smoked mutton in Iceland (Sen *et al.* 1990; Sen 1991). The formation of NMPhA was associated with the use of sheep dung as a source of smoke. This was the first time that this particular nitrosamine had been detected in food, and its presence illustrates the fact that because a nitrosamine has not been previously detected in food it should not be assumed that it need not be considered.

In Europe, the highest incidence of esophageal cancer in women occurs in Britain, North Wales having an especially high rate. Here the population was found to have a higher intake of nitrite than in other regions studied, this being due mainly to a high consumption of bacon (Knight *et al.* 1987), a food item notorious for its high nitrosamine content.

This brief survey suggests that high rates of esophageal cancer are associated with consumption of food containing high levels of nitrosamines. Other items, including alcoholic beverages and tobacco, add to the total intake of nitrosamines, and an important factor is the formation of *N*-nitroso compounds in the stomach. The importance of nitrosamines as a cause of esophageal cancer is discussed later in relation to the total intake from different sources.

Occurrence in alcoholic beverages

In view of the fact that consumption of alcoholic drinks is associated with esophageal cancer, and that the amount of ethanol consumed does not explain the epidemiology of the disease (Doll 1967), the question of the nitrosamine content of different beverages is obviously of great interest. Pioneering experiments (McGlashan *et al.* 1968) reported high levels of certain nitrosamines in home-made spirits consumed in regions in Zambia with high rates of esophageal cancer. At that time, however, the analytical techniques used, i.e. polarography, were not sufficiently specific for measuring low concentrations of nitrosamines. In later work, where gas chromatography and mass spectrometry were employed, no nitrosamines were detected in distilled alcoholic beverages from high or low cancer incidence areas in Kenya or Uganda (Collins *et al.* 1971).

In Europe, however, careful surveys of different types of beer from various countries showed surprisingly high levels of NDMA in a high proportion of the samples studied (Preussmann *et al.* 1984*b*). The mean concentration was 2.5 ppb, and the maximum value observed was 68 ppb. Although NDMA was the major nitrosamine to be found in beer, more relevant to the question of esophageal cancer was the detection of NDEA in a small number of samples, and of N-SAR at 7–20 ppb in 5 of 13 samples.

There have been wide variations in the data presented on the nitrosamine content of the same beverage from different localities, and in the content of different types of beverage. Thus Goff *et al.* (1979) detected nitrosamines in beer and Scotch whisky, but not in wines, sherries, liqueurs, brandies, gins, vodkas or rums. When drinks consumed in areas with a high incidence of esophageal cancer were analysed, however, high levels of certain nitrosamines were found (Walker *et al.* 1979*b*). For example, there is an exceptionally high consumption of cider and apple brandy in northern France, the region in Europe which has by far the highest incidence of esophageal cancer for men, and here cider was found to contain up to 18 μg/litre NDMA, farm apple brandy contained up to 10 μg/litre, and industrially produced apple brandy 3.6 μg/litre. NDMA was present at lower levels in beer, whisky, wine and kirsch. The esophageal carcinogen NDEA occurred in cider, apple brandy, wine, whisky and kirsch, but the highest level, 4.8 μg/litre, was detected in the liqueur mirabelle. Another esophageal carcinogen, nitroso-dipropylamine (NDPA), occurred in industrial apple brandy at 2.6 μg/litre. More recent surveys have confirmed the observation that the highest levels of NDEA and of NDPA occur in apple-based alcoholic drinks, i.e. cider and cider distillate (IARC 1988).

While in northern France cider and apple brandy are the most popular alcoholic drinks, in Germany beer accounted for 64% of the total intake of NDMA (Preussmann *et al.* 1984*b*). Elsewhere beer could account for an even higher proportion of the NDMA consumed, as there was found to be a wide variation in the NDMA content of beers of different European countries. The levels ranged from 0.3 μg/litre in Swedish beer to 3.0 μg/litre in Austrian, with German at 0.6 μg/litre. Since the discovery by Preussmann that the NDMA was formed during the malting process, it has been possible to implement changes in the procedures used in brewing which have resulted in dramatic reductions in the NDMA content, at least for German beer. Measures are also being taken to reduce the content in Scotch whisky.

It is improbable that the nitrosamine content of alcoholic beverages plays an important role in their association with esophageal cancer. In general, the highest levels of nitrosamines were found in beer, while spirits present a much greater risk for esophageal cancer, followed by wine, and beer presents a low risk for this particular cancer. In addition, NDMA is the main nitrosamine present in beer, but this potent liver carcinogen is not carcinogenic for esophagus, at least in rats. Also it is significant that the high concentrations of various alcohols present in the drinks would inhibit the metabolism of the very much lower concentrations of nitrosamines when these were consumed in the same item. However, the reason for the high levels of certain nitrosamines in apple-based alcoholic drinks is apparently unknown, and this should be investigated. Another cause for concern is the fact that the identified volatile nitrosamines account for only a small proportion of the *N*-nitroso compounds occurring in beer (MAFF 1987). At present, however, it is probable that the effect on cell replication in the esophagus of contact with high concentrations of ethanol, and also with the fusel alcohols found in spirits, is the key factor in explaining the association of alcoholic drink consumption with esophageal cancer (see Chapter 6).

Occurrence in tobacco

Tobacco and tobacco smoke represent the major source of exposure of man to nitrosamines. While the nitrosamine content of food is expressed in micrograms per kilogram, that of tobacco products is measured in milligrams per kilogram, and is often two orders of magnitude higher than that in any other consumer product. Different types of tobacco, i.e. smoking tobacco, fine-cut chewing tobacco, and the finely ground tobacco used in snuff, all contain high levels of certain nitrosamines. While the US government has limited the total nitrosamine content of food to 10 μg/kg, a sample of snuff was shown to contain 10000 times this concentration (Joyce 1986). The nitrosamines present in tobacco include those which occur elsewhere in the environment, and also others which are specific for tobacco – the tobacco-specific nitrosamines (TSN). Although carcinogenicity depends on the route of exposure and on the species under consideration, as described previously, nitrosamines which are carcinogenic for the esophagus are present in tobacco products.

The formation and occurrence of nitrosamines in different types of tobacco and in tobacco smoke have been studied extensively by Hoffmann et al. (1981). Fresh tobacco is essentially free of nitrosamines but, as with other plant materials, nitrosamines are formed during curing, aging and fermentation procedures. Nitrosation occurs also during the smoking of tobacco, the concentration of nitrosamines in side-stream smoke, emitted from the smouldering end of the cigarette between puffs, being higher than that of the main-stream smoke which is drawn through the cigarette. As more tobacco is burnt between puffs than during smoking, the side-stream smoke may well be a hazard for non-smokers inhaling polluted air. As nitrosamines are destroyed by photolysis, significant exposure from inhaling outside air is unlikely. In certain indoor atmospheres, however, for example in bars frequented by smokers, the level of NDMA can reach 0.24 ng/litre. During 1 hour's inhalation in this environment the exposure to volatile nitrosamines could be 'substantial' (Preussmann et al. 1984b).

The nitrosamines in tobacco are formed by a variety of routes, including N-nitrosation of amines by nitrite originating in nitrate in the tobacco. Thus proteins and amines in the tobacco give rise to the esophageal carcinogens NDEA and N-PIP. A second source of nitrosatable substrates is the residue of agricultural chemicals, e.g. amines, amides and carbamates, present in the harvested tobacco. The main nitrosamine originating in an agricultural chemical is N'-nitrosodiethanolamine (NDELA), which is formed from the diethanolamine salt of maleic acid. But the major source of TSN is the alkaloids present in tobacco. The predominant alkaloid is nicotine, which forms approximately 90 % of the total content, but smaller amounts of nornicotine, anatabine and anabasine are also important (Fig. 5.3). Both nicotine and nornicotine give rise to N-nitrosonornicotine. The nitrosamine content of cigarettes can vary widely, depending mainly on the alkaloid and nitrate content of the tobacco. Thus N'-nitroso-nornicotine (NNN) can range from 11.9 to 0.22 ppm in different types of cigarette (Hoffmann et al. 1981).

It has not been established unequivocally whether or not smoking in non-drinkers is a cause of esophageal cancer, but it is certain that tobacco and alcohol consumption together have a synergistic effect on the incidence of esophageal cancer (Doll *et al.* 1981). The question of the role of tobacco in causing esophageal cancer is discussed together with the alcohol problem in Chapter 6.

Fig. 5.3. Tobacco-specific alkaloids and their nitrosation products.

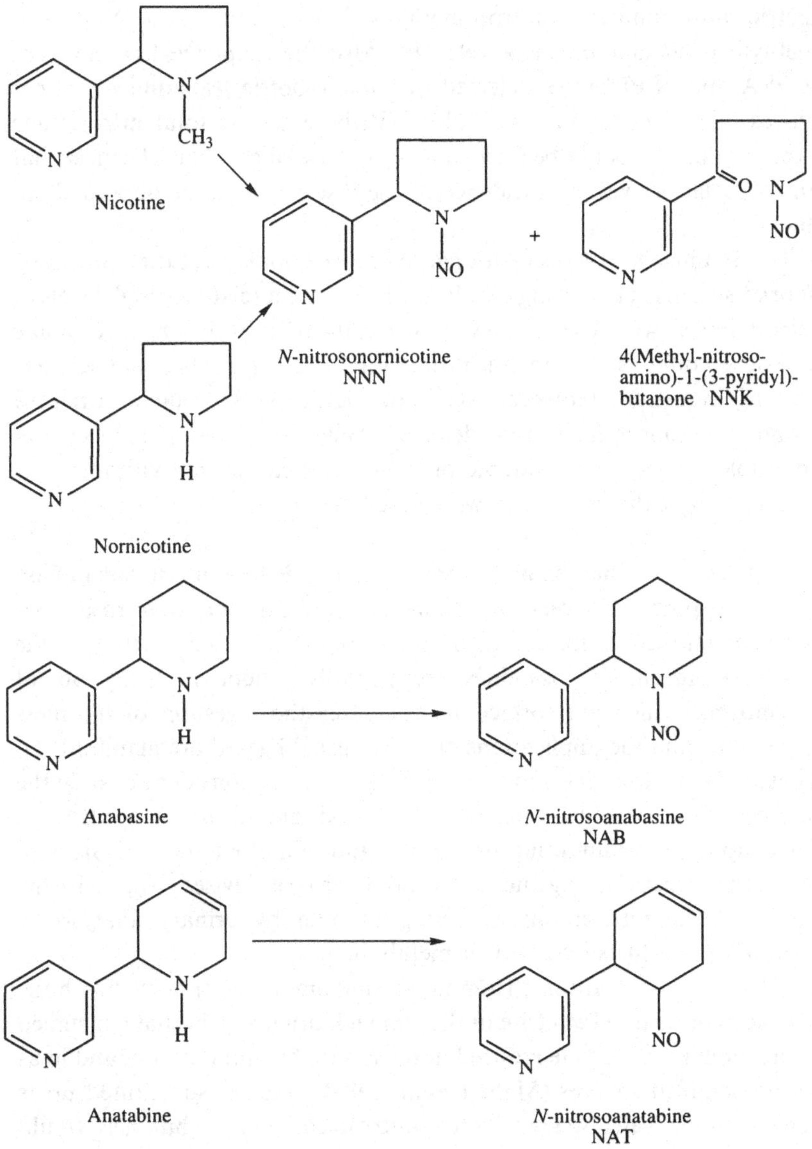

Nicotine

N-nitrosonornicotine
NNN

4(Methyl-nitroso-
amino)-1-(3-pyridyl)-
butanone NNK

Nornicotine

Anabasine

N-nitrosoanabasine
NAB

Anatabine

N-nitrosoanatabine
NAT

Occurrence in industrial products and occupational exposure

As nitrosamine formation is a possibility wherever amines and nitrite come together, various nitrosamines occur in a variety of industrial products. These include food packaging materials, rubber products, pesticides, cosmetics and shampoos (Preussmann *et al.* 1984*b*). With reference to esophageal cancer, the detection in cosmetics of the asymmetric nitrosamines *N*-nitrosomethyl-*n*-dodecylamine and *N*-nitrosomethylbenzylamine could be relevant. Also the esophageal carcinogens NDEA and N-PIP were detected in nursing-bottle teats and in rubber gloves. These nitrosamines would contribute to the total nitrosamine exposure, and so could be important as a cause of esophageal cancer, but any association with an incidence of the disease would be impossible to detect.

The significance of occupational exposure should be easier to assess. Workers exposed to cutting oils, known to contain relatively high levels of nitrosamines, would be at risk. Other industries in which nitrosamine exposure could occur are fish-processing, and the rubber and leather-tanning industries. However, very few instances of occupation-related esophageal cancer have been detected. Whether nitrosamines were responsible for the high incidence of esophageal cancer in a vulcanization factory in Stockholm is unknown (Norell 1983).

In vivo **formation of *N*-nitroso compounds from precursors in food**

A potentially very important source of exposure to nitrosamines results from their formation from precursors which react together in the human stomach. Nitrosamines are possibly unique in being potent carcinogens which are formed *in vivo* after the ingestion of harmless precursors, and the implications of this unusual hazard are manifold. To assess total nitrosamine exposure, it is necessary to consider not only the preformed nitrosamines consumed in food and drink, but also the consumption of amines, nitrate, nitrite, and inhibitors and activators of nitrosation reactions. Ingenious methods have been devised to measure the extent of the nitrosations occurring in man by urinary analysis of nitrosation products and of their metabolites.

Nitrosamines are formed from nitrite and amines when mixed with the stomach contents. The nitrite in the stomach originates in that consumed in the food, in the nitrate reduced in the mouth by oral bacteria, and in as yet unidentified sources (Mallett *et al.* 1985). Amides, substituted ureas and guanidines can also give rise to *N*-nitroso compounds, but these would react locally with the gastric mucosa and are a possible cause of stomach cancer. In contrast, the amines in the stomach can form nitrosamines which would be absorbed into the circulation, and could reach all organs of the body including the esophagus. The first evidence that this could occur was the induction of esophageal cancer when rats were fed a diet containing nitrite and N-methylbenzylamine (Sander *et al.* 1969). As the contents of the normal human stomach are acidic, the most basic amines, for example dimethylamine, methylbenzylamine, morpholine, piperazine and sarcosine, are the most readily nitrosated. The optimum pH for these nitrosations is pH 2.5–3.0. Many products of nitrosation are potent carcinogens for the esophagus. In achlorhydrics, however, the neutral stomach becomes colonized with bacteria, which not only catalyze various N-nitrosation reactions, but also reduce nitrate to nitrite (Leach *et al.* 1987). Although there is an increased risk of gastric cancer in achlorhydrics, there appears to be no evidence for an association with esophageal cancer.

The consumption of nitrosatable compounds and of nitrite, and the kinetics of nitrosation under conditions similar to those of the human stomach contents, have been reviewed (Mirvish 1972), and many experiments have been carried out in which food items have been nitrosated under simulated stomach conditions and the products analyzed for nitrosamines (Siddiqi *et al.* 1988). In addition to studying nitrosation reactions in animals and under simulated stomach conditions *in vitro*, the nitrosation of administered proline has been used to study endogenous nitrosation in man (Ohshima *et al.* 1981). The product of nitrosation, N-nitroso-proline, has not been shown to be carcinogenic, and is excreted almost quantitatively in the urine, where it can be measured. This technique allowed study of the capacity to carry out endogenous N-nitrosation of individuals consuming different diets and populations from high and low esophageal cancer regions. It is possible that thioproline would be a more useful substrate, as nitrosation occurs more rapidly than with proline (Tahira *et al.* 1984). Instead of being a cancer hazard, thioproline could have a protective effect by acting as a nitrite scavenger. Another potentially very useful method for estimating the capacity of an individual to carry out N-nitrosation in the gastrointestinal tract is the use of magnetic semi-permeable polyethleneimine microcapsules which can be swallowed and recovered from the feces (O'Neill *et al.* 1987). These capsules contained a polymer of the readily nitrosatable amine, piperazine, which traps nitrosating agents, and the extent of nitrosation could be determined in capsules recovered.

An important influence on *in vivo* N-nitrosation is the occurrence in normal foods of substances which can inhibit or increase the rate of nitrosation. The substances and mechanisms involved and the implications for human cancer have recently been reviewed (Bartsch *et al.* 1988). Using *in vitro* studies and *in vivo* tests with experimental animals, it was shown that the nitrosation of several amines can be modified. *In vivo* tests with man have been limited, for obvious reasons, to work with nitrosation of proline given in the absence and presence of additional nitrate, usually supplied in the form of beetroot juice. By decreasing or increasing the formation of nitrosamines, constituents of the diet could contribute to the protective effect of certain foods, or to their being secondary risk factors.

Ascorbic acid and α-tocopherol have been most widely studied, as these antioxidants inhibit nitrosation of amines *in vitro* (Mirvish 1986) and *in vivo* (Wagner *et al.* 1985), and could in part be responsible for the well-established protective effect of fresh fruit for many cancers including esophageal cancer. The compounds act mainly by reducing nitrite to nitrogen oxide (NO), a poor nitrosating agent, but certain phenols such as catechin can react with nitrite to form *C*-nitroso compounds which are themselves potent nitrosating agents, and thereby can increase the nitrosation of amines. The overall effect of the numerous polyphenols present in food therefore cannot be predicted. Chlorogenic acid, a polyphenol present in many vegetables, inhibits *N*-nitrosation (Pignatelli *et al.* 1982). Other inhibitory polyphenols are caffeic and ferulic acids, which occur in coffee beans and cereals as well as in fruit and vegetables (Kuenzig *et al.* 1984).

The effect of treatment with ascorbic acid on the levels of *N*-nitroso compounds in human urine was obviously of great interest. Initial observations showed that daily supplementation with ascorbic acid reduced the urinary *N*-nitrosamino acid levels in human subjects living on a Western diet (Ohshima *et al.* 1984). This confirmed the concept of the endogenous synthesis of nitrosamines, and also suggested a means for reducing the level of exposure. The results justified studies in Linxian, a region of China with a high esophageal cancer rate. Treatment with ascorbic acid lowered the high levels of urinary nitrosamino acids, and intervention studies were initiated. This work is discussed in detail by Bartsch *et al.* (1988).

One of the smaller number of chemicals which catalyze *N*-nitrosation is thiocyanate (Boyland 1972). This could be of relevance for esophageal cancer in man, as the high level of thiocyanate in the saliva of smokers could be responsible for their increased ability to nitrosate administered proline (Hoffmann *et al.* 1983). A plausible concept was that the increased risk of esophageal cancer associated with the consumption of alcoholic beverages was due to catalysis of *in vivo* nitrosation by one of the many constituents of the drinks. However, it was found that ethanol (Shendrikova *et al.* 1984), lyophilized beer (Pignatelli *et al.* 1983) and those constituents in beer which were investigated (Pignatelli *et al.* 1984) all inhibited rather than stimulated nitrosation. Chemicals occurring in spirits, however, which present a much higher risk of esophageal cancer than does beer, do not appear to have been studied in this way. Polyphenols extracted from the wooden casks in which the spirits are matured may inhibit or catalyse nitrosation. The tannins present in tea, which are of a different type from those extracted from wood, have been shown to inhibit nitrosation (Bogovski *et al.* 1972). This may be due to competition between tannins and secondary amines for nitrite.

In addition to nitrosation of food components in the stomach, there are several other sites in the human body at which the formation of nitroso compounds can take place. Oral bacteria not only convert nitrate to nitrite, but also catalyze *N*-nitrosation. On incubation of saliva with secondary amines, nitrosamine synthesis took place (Tannenbaum *et al.* 1978). With food which is chewed in the mouth for a considerable period, the amount of nitroso compounds formed may not be negligible, and after being swallowed, these nitrosamines would come into contact first with the esophagus. The colon is another possible site of nitrosamine formation by bacteria which has been considered, but the occurrence of nitrosation has not been demonstrated. On the other hand, nitrosation in the infected bladder is known to occur (Tricker *et al.* 1989), but no association has been noticed between bladder infection and esophageal cancer. Finally, activated macrophages can reduce nitrate to nitrite, and also catalyze *N*-nitrosation (Miwa *et al.* 1989). This property of macrophages could well be of importance in an esophagus damaged by trauma.

The hazard presented by betel quid chewing

A special case in which the *in vivo* formation of nitrosamines is very likely to be an important cause of esophageal cancer occurs in betal quid chewers. The habit of chewing betel quid has been widespread in the Orient since antiquity. An association with oral cancer, however, was not noticed until 1860 (Tennent 1980), and later an addiction to betel quid chewing was found to be related to a high incidence of cancer of the esophagus and stomach also.

The betel quid is composed of the nut of the betel palm, *Areca catechu*, which is wrapped in the leaf of the betel vine, *Piper betel*. This is smeared with lime, which has been prepared from whatever happens to be available locally (i.e. limestone, shells of snails or coral), and with catechu, a resinous extract isolated from the matrix of the tree. Pieces of the nut, which has been flaked, cracked or sliced, are placed on the leaf, and this is then folded and placed in the mouth and chewed. The nut contains alkaloids which are cholinergic and produce pleasant stimulatory effects, while the lime masks the bitter taste and astringency of the nut. Additional items may be added to the quid, the exact composition depending on the locality, socio-economic status and personal preference of the chewer. Tobacco is commonly added, especially in India, and spices, for example cloves, aniseed, nutmeg and turmeric, are also popular. The quid may be chewed for several hours and retained in the mouth overnight, and as a result the esophagus as well as the mouth is exposed for long periods to anything extracted from the quid or formed from the quid by the action of saliva. Where the habit is prevalent, betel chewing may begin at 10–14 years of age.

Carcinogenicity of betel quid

The biological effects in man and in experimental animals of exposure to the betel quid and to its constituents have been discussed in detail (IARC 1985). Epidemiological surveys associated first oral and then esophageal cancer with betel chewing (for review see Mori 1987). Evidence for an association with esophageal cancer came from case–control studies in Sri Lanka (Stephen *et al.* 1970), and from surveys of chewers and non-chewers in Bombay (Jussawalla *et al.* 1970, 1971) and in South Africa (Schonland *et al.* 1969). The cancer risk is present even when tobacco is not added to the quid, as has been shown for oral cancer in New Guinea (Atkinson *et al.* 1964), and for esophageal cancer in Bombay (Jussawalla *et al.* 1971). The latter study showed surprisingly that the risk for esophagus was greater when tobacco was not present in the quid. It was suggested that the explanation lies in the habit of spitting out the saliva when tobacco is present, so that less of the liquid extracted from the quid would reach the esophagus. When tobacco is not present, the saliva is more often swallowed and passes down the esophagus. Chewing and smoking, however, interacted synergistically to increase the risk of esophageal cancer (Jayant *et al.* 1977).

The results of experiments in which betel nut was fed in the diet to experimental animals have given less positive results. Many experiments were carried out in which extracts of the nut were administered by intraperitoneal or subcutaneous injection, by skin painting, or by gastric intubation, i.e. by routes less likely to affect the esophagus than the usual route of exposure from the mouth. The carcinogenicity of betel nut, betel leaf and lime, fed separately or in combination, was studied in rats (Mori *et al.* 1979). No malignant tumors were induced, but thickening of the epidermis was observed in the tongue, esophagus and forestomach. The effect was enhanced by the presence of lime. Unprocessed nuts, when fed in the diet to mice, displayed only weak carcinogenicity when given at high dose levels (Rao *et al.* 1989). In animal experiments, however, food passes rapidly down the esophagus, and exposure time is brief, while with human subjects betel chewing can continue for long periods. In addition, the effect of quid chewing in man in South-East Asia could well be potentiated by malnutrition and poor oral hygiene.

Suspect chemicals present in betel quid

Several components of the betel quid were shown to be carcinogenic for a number of organs, including the esophagus, when fed in the diet to experimental animals. The major constituents which are likely to be involved in carcinogenesis are the alkaloids, nitrosamines which may be formed in the oral cavity from the alkaloids, polyphenols, polymerized polyphenols (tannins) and, when tobacco is included in the quid, preformed nitrosamines. Alkaloids present in the highest concentrations are arecoline and its hydrolysis products, arecaidine, guvacoline and guvacine (Fig. 5.4).

Arecoline was found to be carcinogenic for the stomach and liver when fed in the diet to mice (Bhide *et al.* 1984) and for the esophagus when the alkaloid mixed with lime was placed in the cheek pouch of hamsters (Dunham *et al.* 1984). Another component of the quid, the leaf, has been shown repeatedly to have a protective effect (Shirname *et al.* 1983).

The molecular mechanisms involved in the association with carcinogenicity in man are not understood. Arecoline is metabolized to form

Fig. 5.4. Betel nut alkaloids.

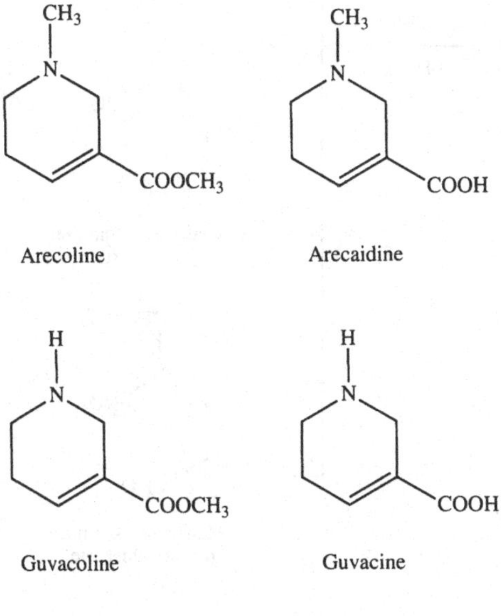

Arecoline

Arecaidine

Guvacoline

Guvacine

arecaidine, and *in vivo* and *in vitro* these compounds have been shown to react at the double bond to alkylate sulfhydryl groups (Boyland *et al.* 1969). There is evidence that betel nut chewing can damage chromosomes of the oral mucosa (Stich *et al.* 1982), and that the betel quid, the betel nut (but not the leaf) and betel nut alkaloids are mutagenic (Shirname *et al.* 1983). As yet, however, there is no evidence for a reaction with DNA (IACR 1985).

Possible nitrosamine involvement

Another way in which the betel quid could cause cancer is by nitrosation in the mouth of certain components of the quid to form nitrosamines. As arecoline and its hydrolysis products are tertiary amines, they are susceptible to nitrosation by the nitrite present in saliva. The quids are retained in the mouth for a considerable time, and any amines present

Fig. 5.5. Nitrosation of arecoline.

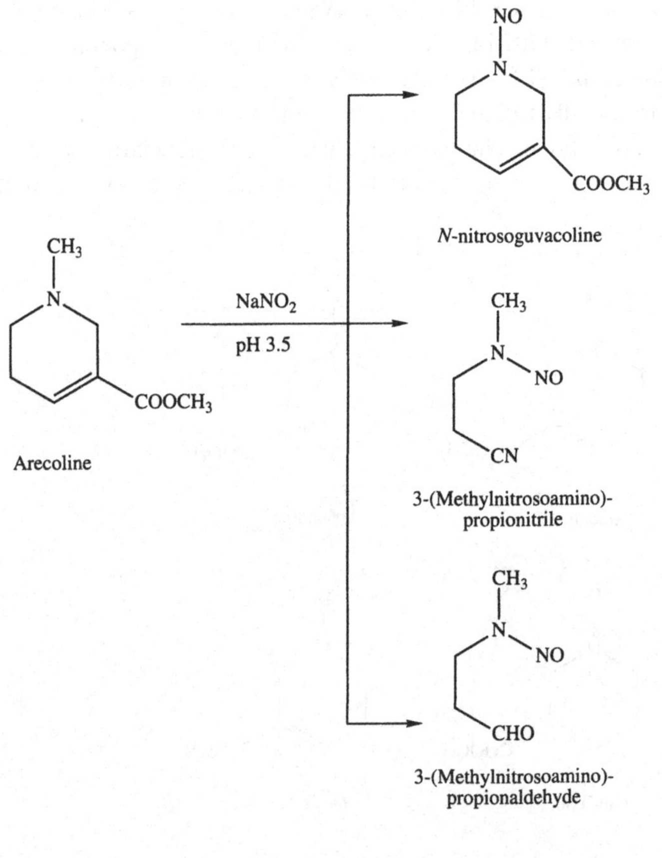
NO
N
COOCH3
N-nitrosoguvacoline
CH3
N
COOCH3
Arecoline
NaNO2
pH 3.5
CH3
N
NO
CN
3-(Methylnitrosoamino)-propionitrile
CH3
N
NO
CHO
3-(Methylnitrosoamino)-propionaldehyde

could become more extensively nitrosated than those which occur in food and therefore are rapidly swallowed.

The *in vitro* nitrosation of arecoline has been studied (Wenke *et al.* 1983) (Fig. 5.5). The nitrosation product, 3-(methylnitrosoamino)-propionitrile, was found to be a potent carcinogen for the esophagus when given subcutaneously to rats (Wenke *et al.* 1984). The nitrosamine was detected in the saliva of betel quid chewers, and 7-methylguanine and O^6-methylguanine were detected in the DNA, mainly of liver and nasal mucosa, of rats after its administration (Prokopczyk *et al.* 1987). Cyanoethylation was also shown to take place, mainly in the major target organ, the nasal mucosa, but also in the liver and esophagus (Prokopzyk *et al.* 1988). A metabolite of nitrosated alkaloids, *N*-nitrosopipecolic acid, was detected in the urine of treated rats (Ohshima *et al.* 1989). As most of the saliva is spat out by chewers, assay of urinary metabolites may give a better measure of the extent of exposure of the esophagus than does study of the saliva.

Other components of the betel quid which are candidates for involvement in carcinogenesis are the polyphenols and the tannins which occur in the betel nut, and in the catechu. A polyphenolic fraction was shown to induce tumors in the stomach and liver of mice when given by the intragastric route (Shirname *et al.* 1983), and to induced hepatomas after oral administration (Bhide *et al.* 1979). It is likely that the tannins are a greater hazard for the esophagus than are the simple polyphenols. The situation is complex, however, as there is evidence that tannins from the betel nut could have a protective action, as they can reduce the nitrosation of amines in man *in vivo* (Stich *et al.* 1983).

In summary, the epidemiological evidence strongly suggests that betel quid chewing is associated with cancer of the esophagus as well as of the mouth. The constituents most likely to be involved are the alkaloids and their nitrosation products. As it has been estimated that more than 250 million people in South-East Asia are addicted to chewing betel quid (Hirondo 1975) there is an urgent need to elucidate the mechanisms involved in the association with cancer, so that preventive measures can be taken. For example, there exists the possibility of promoting a safer quid, in which the protective components of the leaf have been added. Simple compounds which inhibit nitrosation of the alkaloids could also be included in the quid. Reduction of the extent of a long-standing addiction in populations that have few other pleasures would be a formidable task, but the use of less hazardous betel quids may well be possible.

Risk assessment

To determine whether nitrosamine exposure alone is sufficient to represent a feasible cause of human esophageal cancer, it is necessary to know the identity of the mixture of nitrosamines to which any population is exposed, the total level of exposure to nitrosamines preformed in the environment and to those formed *in vivo*, and to have dose–response curves for the human esophagus to each nitrosamine. In addition, there is very probably a large range of individual susceptibility, depending on the ability of the esophageal mucosa to metabolize the nitrosamines and to repair DNA damage, and on the rate of basal cell replication in the individual. All these factors are influenced by diet, the protective effect of fresh fruit and vegetables being counteracted by factors enhancing nitrosation of precursors, or by increasing either the metabolism of nitrosamines or the rate of replication of basal cells in the esophagus. Obviously anything like a quantitative assessment is impossible at present.

One of the few cases in which an attempt has been made to assess the daily intake of nitrosamines was carried out for males in former West Germany (Preussmann *et al.* 1984*b*). As shown in Table 5.5, the per capita intake of NDMA per day was about 1 μg, but if beer was omitted, this would be reduced to 0.3 μg. With reference to one of the few adequate dose–response curves obtained from animal experiments, biological effects of NDMA were measurable in rats at 0.01 mg/kg per day, or approximately 3 μg/rat per day (Peto *et al.* 1984). As the life span of man is very approximately 30 times that of a rat, the amounts of NDMA consumed are obviously well within levels which could be hazardous. However, in view of the multiplicity of factors involved and the lack of adequate information, especially for nitrosamines carcinogenic for the esophagus, in my view the situation regarding assessment of risk has been well expressed by Preussmann *et al.* (1984*b*): 'Sufficient data do not exist for a meaningful evaluation. Premature calculations are liable to be misinterpreted by those who are not familiar with the multitude of uncertainties and difficulties inherent in such calculations, especially when estimates of lifetime risks are based on such figures'.

In spite of this depressing state of affairs, the fact remains that nitrosamines are the only potent carcinogens for the esophagus which have yet been discovered, and they are widely distributed in the environment. Obviously there is a good case for taking action now, by limiting exposure as far as is practically possible. The reduction of the levels in beer by altering the brewing process is a good example of how this can be achieved. Reduction of the nitrite content of cured meat is more difficult, as slight reductions cause complaints about a loss of flavour, and further reductions

Table 5.5. *Daily per capita intake of NDMA for males in FRG*
(*Preussmann* et al. *1984b*)

Food	Intake (μg)	% total intake
Beer	0.7	64
Meat and meat products	0.1	10
Cheese	0.01	1
Others	0.2	25
	1.01	100

allow a risk of botulism. Changing the habits of people who over the centuries have sun-dried their fish or meat, or pickled their vegetables, and have no ready alternative methods of preservation, is difficult. Possibly giving these populations a supply of ascorbic acid with a view to reducing nitrosation would be a more feasible approach. In most situations, however, the levels of exposure to nitrosamines are low, and esophageal cancer is associated with the secondary risk factors, such as vitamin and mineral deficiencies, consumption of mycotoxins and, in Western countries, of alcohol. A more effective approach may be to provide adequate supplies of uncontaminated diets, to reduce alcohol consumption, and to increase consumption of the protective factors present in fresh fruit and vegetables. The protective effect of consumption of normal foods, for example garlic, merits further study. Although the need for more information on all aspects of the problem is obvious, there is much which can be done now on the part of industry and of individuals to reduce the risk of esophageal cancer.

References
Ahmad, M.U., Libbey, L.M., Barbour, J.F. and Scanlan, R.A. (1985) *Food Chem. Toxicol.* **23**, 841–847. Isolation and characterization of products from the nitrosation of the alkaloid gramine.

Anderson, D., Blowers, S.D. and Craddock, V.M. (1985) *Mutation Res.* **142**, 13–18. The effects of S9 mix from rat esophagus, salivary gland and liver on the mutagenicity of the rat esophageal carcinogen N-nitroso-N-methylaniline in the *Salmonella typhimurium* assay.

Archer, M.C. and Labuc, G.E. (1985) In: *Bioactivation of Foreign Compounds* (Anders, M.W. ed.). New York: Academic Press, 403–431, Nitrosamines.

Atkinson, L., Chester, I.C., Smyth, F.C. and Ten Seldam, R.E.L. (1964) *Cancer* **17**, 1289–1298. Oral cancer in New Guinea. A study in demography and etiology.

Autrup, H. and Stoner, G.D. (1982) *Cancer Res.* **42**, 1307–1311. Metabolism of N-nitrosamines by cultured rat and human esophagus.

Autrup, H., Harris, C.C., Wu, S., Bao, L., Pei, X., Lu, S., Sun, T. and Hsia, C. (1984) *Chem. Biol. Int.* **50**, 15–25. Activation of chemical carcinogens by cultured human fetal liver, esophagus and stomach.

Barch, D.H. and Fox, C.C. (1987) *Carcinogenesis* **8**, 1461–1464. Dietary zinc deficiency increases the N-methylbenzylnitrosamine-induced formation of O^6-methylguanine in the esophageal DNA of the rat.

Barch, D.H. and Fox, C.C. (1989) *Cancer Lett.* **44**, 39–44. Dietary ellagic acid reduces the esophageal microsomal metabolism of methylbenzylnitrosamine.

Bartsch, H., Oshima, H., Munoz, N., Crespi, M. and Lu, S.H. (1983) In: *Human Carcinogenesis* (Harris, C.C. and Autrup, H.M. eds.). New York: Academic Press, 833–856. Measurement of endogenous nitrosation in humans: potential applications of a new method and initial results.

Bartsch, H. and Montesano, R. (1984) *Carcinogenesis* **5**, 1381–1393. Relevance of nitrosamines to human cancer.

Bartsch, H., Ohshima, H. and Pignatelli, B. (1988) *Mutation Res.* **202**, 307–324. Inhibitors of endogenous nitrosation. Mechanisms and implications in human cancer prevention.

Bertram, B., Frei, E. and Wiessler, M. (1985) *Biochem. Pharmacol.* **34**, 387–388. Influence of disulfiram on glutathione, glutathione-S-transferase, and on nitrosamine dealkylase of liver, kidney and esophagus of the rat.

Bhide, S.V., Shivapurkar, N.M., Gottoskar, S.V. and Ranadive, K.J. (1979) *Br. J. Cancer* **40**, 922–926. Carcinogenicity of betel quid ingredients: feeding mice with aqueous extract and the polyphenol fraction of betel nut.

Bhide, S.V., Gothoskar, S.V. and Shivapurkar, N.M. (1984) *J. Cancer Res. Clin. Oncol.* **107**, 169–171. Arecoline tumorigenicity in Swiss strain mice on normal and vitamin B-deficient diet.

Bogovski, P., Castegnaro, M., Pignatelli, B. and Walker, E.A. (1972) In: *N-Nitroso Compounds: Analysis and Formation.* IARC Scientific Publ. No. 3,127–129. The inhibiting effect of tannins on the formation of nitrosamines.

Boyland, E., Roe, F.J.C., Gorrod, J.W. and Mitchley, B.C.V. (1964) *Br. J. Cancer* **23**, 265–270. The carcinogenicity of nitrosanabasine, a possible constituent of tobacco smoke.

Boyland, E. and Nery, R. (1969) *Biochem. J.* **113**, 123–130. Mercapturic acid formation during the formation of arecoline and arecaidine in the rat.

Boyland, E., Nice, E. and Williams, K. (1971) *Food Cosmet. Toxicol.* **9**, 639–643. The catalysis of nitrosation by thiocyanate from saliva.

Boyland, E. (1972) IARC Scientific Publ. No. 3, 124–126. The effect of some ions of physiological interest on nitrosamine synthesis.

Bradshaw, E. and Schonland, M. (1974) *Br. J. Cancer* **30**, 157–163. Smoking, drinking and esophageal cancer in African males of Johannesburg, South Africa.

Brady, J.F., Li, D., Ishizaki, H. and Yang, C.S. (1988) *Cancer Res.* **48**, 5937–5940. Effect of diallyl sulfide on rat liver microsomal nitrosamine metabolism and other monooxygenase activities.

Brent, T.P., Dolan, M.E., Fraenkel-Conrat, H., Hall, J., Karran, P., Lavall, F., Magison, G.P., Montesano, R., Pegg, A.E., Poller, P.M., Singer, B., Swenberg, J.A., Yarosh, D.B. (1988) *Proc. Natl. Acad. Sci.* **85**, 1759–1762. Repair of O-alkyl-pyrimidines in mammalian cells: a present consensus.

Camels, S., Ohshima, H., Vincent, P., Gounot, A.M. and Bartsch, H. (1985)

Carcinogenesis 6, 911–915. Screening of microorganisms for nitrosation catalysis at pH 7 and kinetic studies on nitrosamine formation from secondary amines by *E. coli* strains.

Castonguay, A., Stoner, G.D., Schut, H.A. and Hecht, S.S. (1983) *Proc. Natl. Acad. Sci.* **80**, 6694–6697. Metabolism of tobacco-specific N-nitrosamines by cultured human tissues.

Chung, F.L., Juchatz, A., Vitarius, J. and Hecht, S.S. (1984) *Cancer Res.* **44**, 2924–2928. Effects of dietary compounds on α-hydroxylation of *N*-nitroso-pyrrolidine and *N'*-nitrosonornicotine in rat target tissues.

Collins, C.H., Cook, P.J., Forman, J.K. and Palframan, J.F. (1971) *Gut* **12**, 1015–1018. A search for nitrosamines in East African spirit samples from area of varying oesophageal cancer frequency.

Craddock, V.M. (1971) *J. Natl. Cancer Inst.* **47**, 889–907. Liver carcinomas induced in rats by single administration of dimethylnitrosamine after partial hepatectomy.

Craddock, V.M. (1976) In: *Liver Cell Cancer* (Cameron, H.M., Linsell, C.A. and Warwick, G.P. eds.). Amsterdam: Elsevier, pp. 153–201. Cell proliferation and experimental liver cancer.

Craddock, V.M. and Henderson, A.R. (1982) *Carcinogenesis* **3**, 747–750. The activity of 3-methyladenine-DNA-glycosylase in animal tissues in relation to carcinogenesis.

Craddock, V.M. and Henderson, A.R. (1986) *J. Cancer Res. Clin. Oncol.* **111**, 229–236. Effect of N-nitrosamines carcinogenic for esophagus on O^6-alkyl-guanine-DNA-methyl transferase in rat esophagus and liver.

Craddock, V.M., Hill, R.J. and Henderson, A.R. (1987) *Cancer Lett.* **38**, 199–208. Stimulation of DNA replication in rat esophagus and stomach by the trichothecene mycotoxin diacetoxyscirpenol.

Daniel, E.M. and Stoner, G.D. (1991) *Cancer Lett.* **56**, 117–124. The effects of ellagic acid and 13-cis-retinoic acid on *N*-nitrosobenzylmethylamine-induced esophageal tumorigenesis in rats.

Dirsch, O.R., Koenigsmann, M., Ludeke, B.I., Scherer, E. and Kleihues, P. (1990) *Carcinogenesis* **11**, 1583–1586. Bioactivation of *N*-nitrosomethylbenzylamine and *N*-nitrosomethylamylamine in esophageal papillomas.

Doll, R. (1967) *Prevention of Cancer: Pointers from Epidemiology.* London: Nuffield Provincial Hospitals Trust.

Doll, R. and Peto, R. (1981) *J. Natl. Cancer Inst.* **66**, 1193–1308. The causes of cancer: quantitative estimates of avoidable risks of cancer in the United States.

Druckrey, H. and Preussmann, R. (1962) *Naturwissenschaften* **49**, 498–499. On the formation of carcinogenic nitrosamines in tobacco smoke.

Druckrey, H., Preussmann, R., Ivankovic, S. and Schmahl, D. (1967) *Z. Krebsforsch.* **69**, 103–201. Organotrope carcinogene wirkungen bei 65 Ver-schiedenen *N*-nitroso-Verbindungen an BD-ratten.

Dunham, L.J., Sheets, R.H. and Morton, J.F. (1974) *J. Natl. Cancer Inst.* **53**, 1259–1269. Proliferative lesions in cheek pouch and esophagus of hamsters treated with plants from Curaçao, Netherland Antilles.

Dyroff, M.C., Richardson, F.C., Popp, J.A., Bedell, M.A. and Swenberg, J.A. (1986) *Carcinogenesis* **7**, 241–246. Correlation of O^6-ethyldeoxythymidine accumulation, hepatic initiation and hepatocellular carcinoma induction in rats continuously administered diethylnitrosamine.

Enders, F., Havre, A., Helgebastad, A., Koppang, M., Madsen, R. and Ceh, L. (1964) *Naturwissenschaften* **51**, 637–638. Isolation and identification of a hepatotoxic factor in herring meal produced from sodium nitrite-preserved herring.

Fine, D., Rufeh, F. and Lieb, D. (1974) *Nature* **247**, 309–310. Group analysis of volatile and non-volatile *N*-nitroso compounds.

Fine, D.H., Lieb, D. and Rufeh, F. (1975) *J. Chromatogr.* **107**, 351–357. Principle of operation of the thermal energy analyzer for the trace analysis of volatile and non-volatile *N*-nitroso compounds.

Foiles, P.G., Trushin, N. and Castonguay, A. (1985) *Carcinogenesis* **6**, 989–993. Measurement of O^6-methyldeoxyguanosine in DNA methylated by the tobacco-specific carcinogen 4(methylnitrosoamino)-1-(3-pyridyl)-1-butanone using a biotin-avidin enzyme-linked immunosorbent assay.

Freund, H.A. (1937) *Ann. Intern. Med.* **10**, 1144–1155. Clinical manifestations and studies in parenchymatous hepatitis.

Garro, A.J., Seitz, H.K. and Lieber, C.S. (1981) *Cancer Res.* **41**, 120–124. Enhancement of dimethylnitrosamine metabolism and activation to a mutagen following chronic ethanol consumption.

Ghaisas, S., Sarananth, D. and Deo, M.G. (1989) *Carcinogenesis* **10**, 1847–1854. ICRC mouse with congenital mega-esophagus as a model to study esophageal tumorigenesis.

Goff, E.V. and Fine, D.H. (1979) *Food Cosmet. Toxicol.* **17**, 569–573. Analysis of volatile N-nitrosamines in alcoholic beverages.

Grice, H.C. (1988) *Food Chem. Toxicol.* **26**, 717–723. Safety evaluation of butylated hydroxyanisole from the perspective of effects on forestomach and esophageal squamous epithelium.

Haas, H., Mohr, V. and Kruger, F.W. (1973) *J. Natl. Cancer Inst.* **51**, 1295–1301. Comparative studies with different doses of *N*-nitrosomorpholine, *N*-nitroso-piperidine, *N*-nitrosomethylurea, and dimethylnitrosamine in Syrian Golden hamsters.

Hagan, E.C., Jenner, P.M., Jones, Wm. I., Fitzhugh, O.G., Long, E.L., Brouwer, J.G. and Webb, W.K. (1965) *Toxicol. Appl. Pharmacol.* **7**, 18–24. Toxic properties of compounds related to safrole.

Heath, D.F. and Dutton, A. (1958) *Biochem. J.* **70**, 619–626. Detection of metabolic products from dimethylnitrosamine in rats and mice.

Herrold, K. (1966) *J. Natl. Cancer Inst.* **37**, 389–394. Epidermoid carcinomas of esophagus and forestomach induced in Syrian hamsters by *N*-nitroso-*N*-methylurethane.

Hirono, I. (1975) In: Annual Report of Mutagenicity and Carcinogenicity Testing Group of US–Japan Cooperative Medical Sciences Program (Yamamoto, T. ed.). Tokyo, pp. 51–58. 1975 report of the actual surveys on cancer causation in south-eastern Asia.

Hirose, M., Maekawa, A., Kamiya, Y.S. and Odashima, S. (1979) *Gan No Rinsho* **70**, 653–662. Carcinogenic effect of *N*-ethyl and *N*-amyl-*N*-nitrosourethanes on female Donryu rats.

Hodgson, R.M., Wiessler, M. and Kleihues, P. (1980) *Carcinogenesis* **1**, 861–866.

Preferential methylation of target organ DNA by the esophageal carcinogen *N*-nitrosomethylbenzylamine.

Hoffmann, D., Raineri, R., Hecht, S.S., Maronpot, R.R. and Wynder, E.L. (1975) *J. Natl. Cancer Inst.* **55**, 977–981. Effects of *N'*-nitrosonornicotine and *N'*-nitrosoanabasine in rats.

Hoffmann, D., Adams, J.D., Brunnemann, K.D. and Hecht, S.S. In: *N-Nitroso Compounds* (1981) ACS Symposium No. 174 (Scanlan, P. and Tannenbaum, S. eds.). Washington DC.: ACS, pp. 247–273. Formation, occurrence and carcinogenicity of *N*-nitrosamines in tobacco products.

Hoffmann, D. and Brunneman, K.D. (1983) *Cancer Res.* **43**, 5570–5574. Endogenous formation of *N*-nitrosoproline in cigarette smokers.

Hoffmann, D., Rivenson, A., Amin, S. and Hecht, S.S. (1984) *J. Cancer Res. Clin. Oncol.* **108**, 481–486. Dose–response study of carcinogenicity of tobacco-specific nitrosamines in F-344 rats.

Horie, A., Kohchi, S. and Kuratsune, M. (1965) *Jpn. J. Cancer Res.* **56**, 429–441. Carcinogenesis in the esophagus. II. Experimental production of esophageal cancer by administration of ethanolic solution of carcinogens.

International Agency for Research on Cancer (1978) IARC Monographs on the Evaluation of the Carcinogenic Risk of Chemicals to Humans 1978, vol. 17. Some *N*-nitrosocompounds (IARC, Lyon, France).

International Agency for Research on Cancer (1985) IARC Monographs on the Evaluation of the Carcinogenic Risk of Chemicals to Humans, vol. 37. Tobacco habits other than smoking; betel-quid and Areca-nut chewing; and some related nitrosamines (IARC, Lyon, France).

Jayllant, K., Balakrishnan, V., Sanghvi, L.D. and Jussawalla, D.J. (1977) *Br. J. Cancer* **35**, 232–235. Quantification of the role of smoking and chewing tobacco in oral, pharyngeal, and esophageal cancers.

Ji, C., Li, M.H., Li, J.L. and Lu, S.J. (1986) *Carcinogenesis* **7**, 301–303. Synthesis of nitrosomethylisoamylamine from isoamylamine and sodium nitrite by fungi.

Joyce, C. (1986) *New Sci.* **1492**, 30–31. Cancer without smoke.

Jussawalla, D.J., Deschpande, V.A., Haenzel, W. and Natekar, M.V. (1970) *Br. J. Cancer* **24**, 56–66. Differences observed in the site incidence of cancer between the Parsi community and the total population of Greater Bombay: A critical appraisal.

Jussawalla, D.J. and Deschpande, V.A. (1971) *Cancer* **28**, 244–252. Evaluation of cancer risk in tobacco chewers and smokers: an epidemiological assessment.

Kleihues, P., Veit, C., Wiessler, M. and Hodgson, R. (1981) *Carcinogenesis* **2**, 897–899. DNA methylation by *N*-nitroso-*N*-methylbenzylamine in target and non-target tissues of NMRI mice.

Knight, T.M., Forman, D., Al-Dabbagh, S.A. and Doll, R. (1981) *Food Chem. Toxicol.* **25**, 277–285. Estimation of dietary intake of nitrates and nitrite in Great Britain.

Koenegsmann, M., Schmerold, I., Jeltsch, W., Lindeke, B., Kleihues, P. and Wiessler, M. (1988) *Cancer Res.* **48**, 5482–5486. Organ and cell specificity of DNA methylation by *N*-nitroso-*N*-methylamylamine in rats.

Koepke, S.R., Tondeur, Y., Farrelly, J.G., Stewart, M.L., Michejda, C.J. and Kroeger-Koepke, M.B. (1984) *Biochem. Pharmacol.* **33**, 1509–1513. Metabolism of ^{15}N-labelled *N*-nitrosodimethylamine and *N*-nitrosomethylaniline by isolated rat hepatocytes.

Kraft, P.L. and Tannenbaum, S.R. (1980*a*) *Cancer Res.* **40**, 1921–1927. Distribution of *N*-nitrosomethylbenzylamine evaluated by whole-body autoradiography and densitometry.

Kraft, P.L., Skipper, P.L. and Tannenbaum, S.R. (1980*b*) *Cancer Res.* **40**, 2740–2742. *In vivo* metabolism and whole-blood clearance of *N*-nitroso-*N*-methylbenzylamine in the rat.

Kuenzig, W., Chain, J., Norkis, E., Holowaschenko, H. and Newmark, H. (1984) *Carcinogenesis* **5**, 309–313. Caffeic and ferulic acid as blockers of nitrosamine formation.

Labuc, G.E. and Archer, M.C. (1982) *Cancer Res.* **42**, 3181–3186. Esophageal and hepatic microsomal metabolism of *N*-nitroso-*N*-methylbenzylamine and dimethylnitrosamine in the rat.

Leach, S.A., Thompson, M. and Hill, M. (1987) *Carcinogenesis* **8**, 1907–1912. Bacterially catalysed *N*-nitrosation reactions and their relative importance in the human stomach.

Li, M., Ji, C. and Cheng, S. (1986) *Nutr. Cancer* **8**, 63–69. Occurrence of nitroso compounds in fungi-contaminated foods: a review.

Lijinsky, W. (1980) In: *N-Nitroso Compounds: Analysis formation and occurrence.* IACR Scientific Publication No. 31 (Walker, E.A., Castegnaro, M., Griciute, L. and Borzsonyi, M. eds.). Lyon: IACR Press, pp. 745–751. Comparative carcinogenicity of *N*-nitroso compounds on different species.

Lijinsky, W., Singer, G.M., Saavedra, J.E. and Reuber, M.D. (1984) *Cancer Lett.* **22**, 281–288. Carcinogenesis in rats by asymmetric nitrosamines containing an allyl group.

Lijinsky, W. and Kovatch, R.M. (1988) *Cancer Res.* **48**, 6648–6652. Comparative carcinogenesis by nitrosomethylalkylamines in Syrian hamsters.

Lindahl, T. (1982) *Ann. Rev. Biochem.* **51**, 61–87. DNA repair enzymes.

Liu, J.G. and Li, M.H. (1989) *Carcinogenesis* **10**, 617–620. Roussin red methyl ester, a tumor promoter isolated from pickled vegetables.

Lu, S.H., Ohshima, H., Fu, H.M., Tian, Y., Li, F.M., Blettner, M., Wahrendorf, J. and Bartsch, H. (1986) *Cancer Res.* **46**, 1485–1491. Urinary excretion of *N*-nitrosoamino acids and nitrate by inhabitants of high and low risk areas for esophageal cancer in Northern China: endogenous formation of *N*-nitrosoproline and its inhibition by Vitamin C.

Mackawa, A., Onodera, H., Matsushima, Y., Nagaoka, T., Todate, A., Shilutani, M., Kodama, Y. and Hayashi, Y. (1989) *Jpn. J. Cancer Res.* **80**, 632–636. Dose–response carcinogenicity in rats on low-dose levels of *N*-ethyl-*N*-nitrosourethane.

MAFF (Ministry of Agriculture, Fisheries and Food) (1987) Food Surveillance Paper No. 20. Nitrate, nitrite and *N*-nitroso compounds in food. London: HMSO.

Magee, P.N. and Barnes, J.M. (1956) *Br. J. Cancer* X, 114–122. The production of malignant primary hepatic tumours in the rat by feeding dimethylnitrosamine.

Magee, P.N. and Barnes, J.M. (1959) *Acta Union Int. Contre Cancer* XV, 187–190. The experimental production of tumours in the rat by dimethylnitrosamine.

Magee, P.N. and Barnes, J.M. (1967) *Adv. Cancer Res.* **10**, 163–246. Carcinogenic nitroso compounds.

Mallett, A.K., Rowland, I.R., Walters, D.G., Gangolli, S.D., Cottrell, R.C. and Massay, R.C. (1985) *Carcinogenesis* **6**, 1585–1588. The role of oral nitrate in the nitrosation of [¹⁴C]proline by conventional microflora and germ-free rats.

Mandal, S., Shivapurkar, N., Superczynski, M. and Stoner, G.D. (1986) *Proc. Am. Assoc. Cancer Res.* Abstract No. 489. Inhibition of nitrosomethylbenzylamine-induced esophageal tumors in rats by ellagic acid.

Mandal, S., Shivapurkar, N.M., Galati, A.J. and Stoner, G.D. (1988) *Carcinogenesis* **9**, 1313–1316. Inhibition of nitrosomethylbenzylamine metabolism and DNA binding in cultured rat esophagus by ellagic acid.

Mandal, S. and Stoner, G.D. (1990) *Carcinogenesis* **11**, 55–61. Inhibition of *N*-nitrosobenzylmethylamine-induced esophageal tumorigenesis in rats by ellagic acid.

Marasas, W.F.O., Wehner, F.C., van Rensburg, S.J. and Schalkwyk, D.J. (1981) *Phytopathology* **71**, 792–796. Mycoflora of corn produced in human esophageal cancer areas in Transkei, Southern Africa.

Masuda, Y., Mori, K., Hiroshata, T. and Kuratsune, M. (1966) *Jpn. J. Cancer Res.* **57**, 549–557. Carcinogenesis in the esophagus. III. Polycyclic aromatic hydrocarbons and phenols in whiskey.

Masui, T., Shirai, T., Takahashi, S., Mutai, M. and Furushima, S. (1988) *Carcinogenesis* **9**, 1918–1985. Summation of effect of uracil on two-stage and multiple models of urinary bladder carcinogenesis in F344 rats initiated by *N*-butyl-*N*-(4-hydroxybutyl)nitrosamine.

McGlashan, N.D., Walters, C.L. and McLean, A.E.M. (1968) *Lancet* **ii**, 1017. Nitrosamines in African alcoholic spirits and esophageal cancer.

Mehta, R., Labuc, G.E., Urbanshi, S.J. and Archer, M.C. (1984*a*) *Cancer Res.* **44**, 4017–4022. Organ specificity in the microsomal activation and toxicity of N-nitroso-N-methylbenzylamine in various species.

Mehta, R., Labuc, G.E. and Archer, M.C. (1984*b*) *J. Natl. Cancer Inst.* **72**, 1443–1447. Induction and suppression of *N*-nitroso-*N*-methylbenzylamine activation by microsomes from rat liver and esophagus.

Mirvish, S.S. (1972) In: *Topics in Chemical Carcinogenesis* (Nakahara, W., Takayama, S., Sugimura, T. and Odashima, S. eds.). Baltimore: University Park Press, pp. 279–295. Studies on *N*-nitrosation reactions: kinetics of nitrosation, correlation with mouse feeding experiments, and natural occurrence of nitrosatable compounds (ureides and guanidines).

Mirvish, S.S., Wang, M., Smith, J.W., Deshpande, A.D., Makary, M.H. and Issenberg, P. (1985) *Cancer Res.* **45**, 577–583. β- to ω-hydroxylation of the esophageal carcinogen methyl-*n*-amylnitrosamine by the rat esophagus and related tissues.

Mirvish, S.S. (1986) *Cancer* **58**, 1842–1850. Effects of vitamins C and E on *N*-nitroso compound formation, carcinogenesis and cancer.

Mirvish, S.S., Ji, C. and Rosinsky, S. (1988) *Cancer Res.* **48**, 5663–5668. Hydroxymetabolites of methyl-*n*-amylnitrosamine produced by esophagus, stomach, liver and other tissues of the neonatal to adult rat and hamster.

Miwa, M., Tsuda, M., Kurashima, Y., Hara, H., Tanaka, Y. and Shinohara, K.

(1989) *Biochem. Biophys. Research Comm.* **159**, 373–378. Macrophage-mediated *N*-nitrosation of thioproline and proline.

Mohr, U., Reznik-Schuller, H., Reznik, G. and Hilfrich, J. (1975) *J. Natl. Cancer Inst.* **55**, 681–683. Transplacental effects of nitrosodiethanolamine in Syrian golden hamsters as related to different days of administration during pregnancy.

Mori, H., Matsubara, N., Ushimaru, Y. and Hirono, I. (1979) *Experientia* **35**, 384–385. Carcinogenicity examination of betel nuts and piper betel leaves.

Mori, H. (1987) In: *Naturally Occurring Carcinogens of Plant Origin* (Hirono, I. ed.). Elsevier, Amsterdam: pp. 167–180. Betel nut.

Morris, J.E., Price, J.M., Lalich, J.J. and Stein, R.J. (1969) *Cancer Res.* **29**, 2145–2156. The carcinogenic activity of some 5-nitrofuran derivatives in the rat.

Morse, M.A., Hecht, S.S. and Chung, F.L. (1989) Proceedings of Tenth International Meeting on *N*-nitroso compounds, mycotoxins and tobacco. Lyon: IACR, p. 94. Chemoprevention of tobacco-specific nitrosamine 4-(methyl-nitrosoamino)-1-(3-pyridyl)-1-butanone tumorigenesis with aromatic isothiocyanates.

Murphy, S.E., Heiblum, R. and Trushin, N. (1990) *Cancer Res.* **50**, 4685–4691. Comparative metabolism of *N'*-nitroso-nornicotine and 4-(methylnitroso-amino)-1-(3-pyridyl)-1-butanone by cultured F344 rat oral tissue and esophagus.

Nakamura, T., Matsuyama, M. and Kishimoto, H. (1974) *J. Natl. Cancer Inst.* **52**, 519–522. Tumors of the esophagus and duodenum induced in mice by oral administration of *N*-ethyl-*N*-nitro-*N*-nitroso-guanidine.

Neurath, G.B., Dunger, M., Pein, F.G., Ambrosius, D. and Schreiber, O. (1977) *Food Chem. Toxicol.* **15**, 275–282. Primary and secondary amines in the human environment.

Norell, S., Ahlbom, A., Lipping, H. and Osterblom, L. (1983) *Lancet* **i**, 462–463. Oesophageal cancer and vulcanization work.

Ohshima, H. and Bartsch, H. (1981) *Cancer Res.* **41**, 3658–3662. Quantitative estimation of endogenous nitrosation in humans by monitoring *N*-nitrosoproline excreted in urine.

Ohshima, H., O'Neill, I.K., Friesen, M., Bereziat, J.C. and Bartsch, H. (1984) *J. Cancer Res. Clin. Oncol.* **108**, 121–128. Occurrence in human urine of new sulphur-containing *N*-nitroso amino acids, *N*-nitrosothioazolidine 4-carboxylic acid and its 2-methyl derivative, and their formation.

Ohshima, H., Friesen, M. and Bartsch, H. (1989) *Cancer Lett.* **44**, 211–216. Identification in rats of *N*-nitroso-nipecotic acid as a major urinary metabolite of the areca-nut alkaloid-derived nitrosamines, N-nitroso-guvacoline and N-nitroso-guvacine.

O'Neill, I.K., Castegnaro, M., Brouet, I. and Povey, A.C. (1987) *Carcinogenesis* **8**, 1469–1474. Magnetic semipermeable poly ethyleneimine microcapsules for monitoring of *N*-nitrosation in the gastrointestinal tract.

Peto, R., Gray, R., Brantom, P. and Grasso, P. (1984) In: *N-Nitroso Compounds: Occurrence, Biological Effects and Relevance to Human Cancer.* IACR Scientific Publications No. 57 (O'Neill, I.K., von Borstel, R.C., Miller, C.T., Long, J. and Bartsch, H. eds.). Lyon: IACR, pp. 627–665. Nitrosamine carcinogenesis in 5120 rodents: chronic administration of sixteen different concentrations of NDEA, NDMA, NPYR and NPIP in the water of 4440 inbred rats, with parallel studies on NDEA alone of the effect of age of starting (3, 6 or 20 weeks) and of species (rats, mice or hamsters).

Pignatelli, B., Bereyiat, J.C., Descotes, G. and Bartsch, H. (1982) *Carcinogenesis* 3, 1045–1049. Catalysis of nitrosation *in vivo* and *in vitro* in rats by catechin and resorcinol and inhibition by chlorogenic acid.

Pignatelli, B., Scriban, R., Descotes, G. and Bartsch, H. (1983) *Carcinogenesis* 4, 491–494. Inhibition of endogenous nitrosation of proline in rats by lyophilized beer constituents.

Pignatelli, B., Scriban, R., Decotes, G. and Bartsch, H. (1984) *J. Am. Soc. Brew. Chem.* 42, 18–23. Modifying effects of polyphenols and other constituents of beer on the formation of N-nitroso compounds.

Poirier, S., Ohshima, H., de The, G., Hurbert, A., Bourgde, M.C. and Bartsch, H. (1987) *Int. J. Cancer* 39, 293–296. Volatile nitrosamine levels in common foods from Tunisia, South China, and Greenland, high-risk areas for nasopharyngeal carcinoma.

Preussmann, R. and Stewart, B.W. (1984a) In: *Chemical Carcinogens*, vol. 2, ACS Monograph 182 (Searle, C.E. ed.). San Diego: ACS Press, pp. 643–828. N-nitroso carcinogens.

Preussmann, R. and Eisenbrand, G. (1984b) In: *Chemical Carcinogens*, vol. 2, ACS Monograph 182 (Searle, C.E. ed.). San Diego: ACS Press, pp. 829–868. N-nitroso carcinogens in the environment.

Prokopczyk, B., Rivenson, A., Bertinato, P., Brunnemann, K.D. and Hoffmann, D. (1987) *Cancer Res.* 47, 467–471. 3-(methylnitrosoamino)-propionitrile: occurrence in saliva of betel quid chewers, carcinogenicity, and DNA methylation in F344 rats.

Prokopczyk, B., Bertinato, P. and Hoffmann, D. (1988) *Cancer Res.* 48, 6780–6784. Cyanoethylation of DNA *in vivo* by 3-(methylnitrosoamino)-propionitrile, an *Areca*-derived carcinogen.

Rajewsky, M.F. (1972) *Z. Krebsforsch* 78, 12–30. Proliferative parameters of mammalian cell systems and their role in tumor growth and carcinogenesis.

Rao, A.R. and Das, P. (1989) *Int. J. Cancer* 43, 728–732. Evaluation of the carcinogenicity of different preparations of areca nut in mice.

Rogers, A.E. (1982) In: *Trace Substances and Health. A Handbook*, part II (Newberne, P.M. ed.). New York: Marcel Dekker, pp. 47–80. Nitrosamines.

Saffhill, R., Margison, G.P. and O'Connor, P.J. (1985) *Biochim. Biophys. Acta* 823, 111–145. Mechanisms of carcinogenesis induced by alkylating agents.

Sakar, S., Nagabhushan, M., Soman, C.S., Tricker, A.R. and Bhide, S.V. (1989) *Carcinogenesis* 10, 733–736. Mutagenicity and carcinogenicity of smoked meat from Nagaland, a region of India prone to a high incidence of nasopharyngeal cancer.

Sander, J. and Burkle, G. (1969) *J. Cancer Res. Clin. Oncol.* 73, 54–66. Induction of malignant tumors in rats by simultaneous feeding of nitrite and secondary amines.

Scherer, E., Van Den Berg, T., Vermeulen, E., Winterwerp, H.H.K. and Den Engelse, L. (1989) *Cancer Lett.* 46, 21–29. Immunocytochemical analysis of O^6-alkylguanine shows tissue specific formation in and removal from esophageal and liver DNA in rats treated with methylbenzylnitrosamine, dimethylnitrosamine diethylnitrosamine, and ethylnitrosourea.

Schoental, R. and Magee, P.N. (1962) *Br. J. Cancer* **XVI**, 92–101. Induction of squamous carcinoma of lung and stomach and esophagus by diazomethane and *N*-methyl-*N*-nitrosourethane respectively.

Sen, N.P., Baddoo, P.A., Weber, D. and Helgason, T. (1990) *J. Agric. Food Chem.* **38**, 1007–1011, Detection of a new nitrosamine, *N*-nitroso-*N*-methylaniline, and other nitrosamines in Icelandic smoked mutton.

Sen, N.P. (1991) In: *Relevance to Human Cancer of N-Nitroso Compounds, Tobacco Smoke and Mycotoxins.* IACR Scientific Publication No. 105 (O'Neill, I.K., Chen, J. and Bartsch, H. eds.). Lyon: IACR, pp. 232–234. Recent studies in Canada on the occurrence and formation of *N*-nitroso compounds in foods and food contact materials.

Shank, R.C. (1981) In: *Mycotoxins and N-Nitroso Compounds, Environmental Risks,* vol. 1 (Shank, R.C. ed.). Boca Raton: CRC Press, pp. 155–183. Occurrence of *N*-nitroso compounds in the environment.

Shendrikova, I.A., Ermilov, V.B. and Dikum, P.P. (1984) *Cancer Lett.* **25**, 49–54. The influence of ethanol on synthesis of *N*-nitrosodimethylamine *in vivo* and *in vitro*.

Shirname, L.P., Menon, M.M., Nair, J. and Bhide, S.V. (1983) *Nutr. Cancer* **5**, 87–91. Correlation of mutagenicity and tumorigenicity of betel quid and its ingredients.

Siddiqi, M., Tricker, A.R. and Preussmann, R. (1988*a*) *Cancer Lett.* **39**, 37–43. The occurrence of preformed *N*-nitroso compounds in food samples from a risk area of esophageal cancer in Kashmir, India.

Siddiqi, M., Tricker, A.R. and Preussmann, R. (1988*b*) *Cancer Lett.* **39**, 259–265. Formation of *N*-nitroso compounds under simulated gastric conditions from Kashmir foodstuffs.

Siddiqi, M. and Preussmann, R. (1989) *J. Cancer Res. Clin. Oncol.* **115**, 111–117. Esophageal cancer in Kashmir – an assessment.

Singer, G.M. and Lijinsky, W. (1976) *J. Agric. Food Chem.* **24**, 550–553. Naturally occurring nitrosatable compounds. I. Secondary amines in foodstuffs.

Singer, G.M., Chuan, J., Roman, J., Min-Hsin, L. and Lijinsky, W. (1986) *Carcinogenesis* **7**, 733–736. Nitrosamines and nitrosamine precursors in foods from Linxian, China, a high incidence area for esophageal cancer.

Song, P.J. and Hu, J.F. (1988) *Food Chem. Toxicol.* **26**, 205–208. *N*-nitrosamines in Chinese food.

Spiegelhalder, B., Eisenbrand, G. and Preussmann, R. (1982) In: *N-Nitroso Compounds: Occurrence and Biological Effects.* (Bartsch, H., O'Neil, I.K., Castegnaro, N. and Okada, M. eds.). IACR Scientific Publication No. 41. Lyon: IACR Press, pp. 443–449. Urinary excretion of *N*-nitrosamines in rats and humans.

Stephen, S.J. and Uragoda, C.G. (1970) *Br. J. Cancer* **24**, 11–15. Some observations on esophageal carcinoma in Ceylon, including its relationship to betel chewing.

Stich, H. and Stich, W. (1982) *Cancer Letters* **15**, 193–202. Chromosome-damaging activity of saliva of betel nut and tobacco chewers.

Stich, H.F., Ohshima, H., Pignatelli, B., Michelson, J. and Bartsch, H. (1983) *J. Natl. Cancer Inst.* **70**, 1047–1050. Inhibitory effect of betel nut extracts on endogeneous nitrosation in humans.

Stoner, G.D., Morrissey, D.T., Heur, Y.H., Daniel, E.M., Galati, A.J. and Wagner, S.A. (1991) *Cancer Res.* **51**, 2063–2068. Inhibitory effects of phenethyl isothiocyanate on N-nitrosobenzylmethylamine carcinogenesis in rat esophagus.

Tahira, T., Tsuda, M., Wakabayashik, K., Nagao, M. and Sugimura, T. (1984) *Jpn. J. Cancer Res.* **75**, 889–894. Kinetics of nitrosation of thioproline, the precursor of a major nitroso compound in human urine, and its role as a nitrite scavenger.

Takahasi, M., Shirai, T., Fukushima, S., Hosoda, K., Yoshida, K. and Ito, N. (1978) *Cancer Lett.* **4**, 265–270. Carcinogenicity of 8-nitroquinoline in Sprague–Dawley rats.

Tang, W.C., Lin, P.Z., Frank, N. and Wiessler, M. (1984) *J. Cancer Res. Clin. Oncol.* **108**, 221–226. Metabolism of, and DNA methylation by, N-nitrosomethylbenzylamine in chicken.

Tannenbaum, S.R., Archer, M.C., Wishnok, J.S. and Bishop, W.W. (1978) *J. Natl. Cancer Inst.* **60**, 251–253. Nitrosamine formation in human saliva.

Tennent, J.E. (1860) *Ceylon. An Account of the Island, Physical, Historical and Topographical*, vol. 1. London: Longman, Green, Longman and Roberts.

Terracini, B. and Magee, P.N. (1964) *Nature* **202**, 502–503. Renal tumors in rats following injection of dimethylnitrosamine at birth.

Tricker, A.R., Perkins, M.J., Massey, R.C., Bishop, C., Key, P.E. and McWeeny, D.J. (1984) *Food Addit. Contam.* **1**, 245–252. The incidence of some non-volatile N-nitroso compounds in cured meats.

Tricker, A.R., Wacker, C.D. and Preussmann, R. (1987a) *Cancer Lett.* **35**, 199–206. Nitrosation products from the plant Ephedra altissima and their potential endogenous formation.

Tricker, A.R., Wacker, C.D. and Preussmann, R. (1987b) *Toxicol. Lett.* **8**, 45–50. 2-(N-nitroso-N-methylamine)propiophenone, a direct-acting bacterial mutagen found in nitrosated Ephedra altissima tea.

Tricker, A.R., Mostafa, M.H., Spiegelhalder, B. and Preussmann, R. (1989) *Carcinogenesis* **10**, 547–552. Urinary excretion of nitrate, nitrite and N-nitroso compounds in schistosomiasis and bilharzia bladder cancer patients.

Umbenhauer, D., Wild, C.P., Montesano, R., Saffhill, R., Boyle, J.M., Huh, N., Kirstein, U., Thomale, J., Rajewsky, M.F. and Lu, S.H. (1985) *Int. J. Cancer* **36**, 661–665. O^6-methyldeoxyguanosine in esophageal DNA among individuals at high risk of esophageal cancer.

von Hofe, E., Schmerold, J., Lijinsky, W. and Kleihues, P. (1987) *Carcinogenesis* **8**, 1337–1341. DNA methylation in rat tissues by a series of homologous aliphatic nitrosamines ranging from N-nitrosodimethylamine to N-nitrosomethyldodecylamine.

Waddell, W.J. and Marlowe, C. (1980) *Cancer Res.* **40**, 3518–3523. Localization of [^{14}C]nitrosonornicotine in tissues of the mouse.

Wagner, D.A., Shuker, D.E.G., Bilmazes, C., Obiedyinski, M., Baker, I., Young, U.R. and Tannenbaum, S.R. (1985) *Cancer Res.* **45**, 6519–6522. Effects of vitamins C and E on endogenous synthesis of N-nitrosoamino acids in humans: precursor – product studies with [^{15}N]nitrate.

Walker, E.A., Castegnaro, M. and Griciute, L. (1979a) *Cancer Lett.* **6**, 175–178. N-nitrosamines in the diet of experimental animals.

Walker, E.A., Castegnaro, M., Garren, L., Touissaint, G. and Kowalski, B.

116   *The nitrosamines*

(1979*b*) *J. Natl. Cancer Inst.* **63**, 947–951. Intake of volatile nitrosamines from consumption of alcohols.
Wargovich, M.J., Woods, C., Eng, U.W.S., Stephens, L.C. and Gray, K. (1988) *Cancer Res.* **48**, 6872–6875. Chemoprevention of nitrosomethylbenzylamine-induced esophageal cancer in rats by the naturally occurring thioether, diallylsulfide.
Wattenberg, L.W. (1979) In: *Environmental Carcinogenesis* (Emmelot, P. and Kriek, E. eds). Amsterdam: Elsevier-North-Holland Biomedical Press, pp. 241–263. Inhibitors of chemical carcinogens.
Wattenberg, L.W. (1980) In: *Naturally-Occurring Carcinogens-Mutagens and Modulators of Carcinogenesis* (Miller, E.C., Miller, J.A., Hiromo, I., Sugimura, T. and Takayama, S. eds.). Baltimore: University Park Press, pp. 315–329. Naturally-occurring inhibitors of chemical carcinogens.
Wenke, G. and Hoffmann, D. (1983) *Carcinogenesis* **4**, 167–172. A study of betal quid carcinogenesis. 1. On the *in vitro* nitrosation of arecoline.
Wenke, G., Rivenson, A. and Hoffman, D. (1984) *Carcinogenesis* **5**, 1137–1140. A study of betel quid carcinogenesis. 3. 3-(methyl-nitrosoamino)propionitrile, a powerful carcinogen in F344 rats.
Wiessler, M., Romruen, K. and Pool, B.L. (1983) *Carcinogenesis* **4**, 867–871. Biological activity of benzylating *N*-nitroso compounds: models of activated *N*-nitrosomethylbenzylamine.
Woo, Y-T., Lai, D.Y., Arcos, J.C. and Argus, M.F. (1988) *Chemical Induction of Cancer*, vol. IIIC. *Natural, Metal, Fibre, and Macromolecular Carcinogens*. New York: Academic Press, pp. 357–435. Betel nut carcinogens.
Wurtzen, G. and Olsen, P. (1986) *Food Chem. Toxicol.* **24**, 1229–1233. Butylated hydroxyanisole study in pigs.
Yu, M.C., Mo, C.C., Chong, W.X., Yeh, F.C. and Henderson, B.E. (1988) *Cancer Res.* **48**, 1954–1959. Preserved foods and nasopharyngeal carcinoma: a case-control study in Guaigxi China.
Zucker, P.F., Giles, A., Chaulk, E.J. and Archer, M.C. (1991) *Carcinogenesis* **12**, 405–408. Selective cytotoxicity of *N*-nitrosamines to cultured rat esophageal epithelial cells.

6

Alcoholic beverages and tobacco

Introduction

The consumption of beer and wine was popular in biblical times and was documented in ancient Egypt, and surprisingly strong drink as distinct from wine is described in The Old Testament Book of Proverbs around 500 BC. Distilled rice and barley liquors were enjoyed in India at approximately the same time (Prakash 1961), but the knowledge remained isolated for more than 1000 years. Distillation was described by the Greeks (Barbor 1986), but although Aristotle in his Meteorology Book 2 (quoted in McGee 1984) detailed the distillation of wine and sea-water with the formation of potable water, the brandy and salt were regarded as useless impurities and were discarded. Plato knew the difference between wine and strong drink, but widespread consumption of distilled liquors did not occur until much later, and then at first as a medicine. Episodes of very heavy drinking have occurred in certain populations, as during the gin epidemic in London, when 1 in 4 of the adult population is said to have consumed a bottle of gin a day (Robinson 1988). In spite of this, the ill effects of chronic heavy consumption, as described by careful observers from Plato to Hogarth, have not included cancers. Apparently there was no conspicuously high incidence of esophageal cancer similar to that which has been recognized by the community to occur in certain areas in China since antiquity. The first evidence that alcoholic beverages might cause esophageal cancer was possibly the report of an association of the disease with consumption of absinth (Lamy 1910). Other more commonly consumed beverages were implicated in 1921, when a two-fold excess mortality from cancer of the upper alimentary tract was recorded in barmen and waiters in England and Wales (Stocks et al. 1933). It is now well established that consumption of alcoholic beverages is the major cause of esophageal cancer in the Western world, being responsible for 75 % of the incidence in the USA (Rothman 1980). The evidence for associating alcoholic beverages with cancer was concluded to be 'compelling' for mouth, larynx, pharynx, esophagus and liver, 'moderately' strong for lung, breast, stomach and colorectum, and 'suggestive' for pancreas (Ziegler 1986).

The fact that the incidence of esophageal cancer in the USA and in Europe is higher in men than in women (Table 4.2) is probably due largely to the higher alcohol consumption by men. Thus in France men drink four times as much alcohol as do women (Picheral 1986), while in England and Wales the consumption by men is three times that of women (Wilson 1980). As a result, alcohol is the predominating cause of cancer for men, while for women other factors, notably dietary deficiencies, are usually more important (Chapter 10). This results in a different geographical distribution of high-incidence areas within each country for men and women. The effect is especially obvious in the UK, where the distribution of high-incidence areas for men is scattered, while for women the high cancer rate down the west coast and especially in remote regions of Scotland has been postulated to be due to a low consumption of fresh fruit and vegetables in these areas (Kemp *et al.* 1985). Therefore in most of the following discussion on the effect of alcohol, reference is made especially to consumption and cancer incidence in men.

Although alcohol consumption is now generally believed to be the major cause of esophageal cancer in men in Europe and in the USA, there are several factors which have complicated the effects of consumption of alcoholic beverages and have obscured an obvious association. One such factor is the dependence of the degree of risk on the nature of the alcoholic drink. Spirits were found to present a much greater hazard than that resulting from consumption of the same amount of ethanol in the form of wine or beer (Tuyns *et al.* 1979). This could be due to the higher ethanol concentration in spirits (40 %) compared with wine (13 %) or beer (4 %), or else it could imply that some of the many non-ethanolic constituents of the drinks are important. There is evidence that certain higher alcohols, for example 3-methylbutanol, which occur in especially high concentrations in the more hazardous drinks, may be involved (Craddock 1989).

Another factor which has obscured the importance of alcohol consumption is the dramatic synergistic effect of tobacco smoking on alcohol-related esophageal cancer. For each level of alcohol consumed, the risk of esophageal cancer was found to increase with the number of cigarettes smoked (Tuyns *et al.* 1977). The effect of tobacco was synergistic rather than additive, but alcohol consumption was the more important hazard in the population in France under survey (Tuyns *et al.* 1977). As a result of a survey limited by the very low numbers of non-drinkers available for study in the Calvados region of France, it was suggested that tobacco smoking in the absence of alcohol was not a risk factor (Tuyns 1983*a*). More recent work in Italy, however, has given evidence for an independent action of tobacco (La Vecchia *et al.* 1989; Franceschi *et al.* 1990). By contrast, in a group of black men with a very different life style, studied in Washington, DC, the very high consumption of alcohol apparently obscured any additional effect of smoking (Pottern *et al.* 1981). In most situations, however, the synergistic effect of tobacco smoking is likely to be important, as simultaneous exposure to alcohol and tobacco is a common occurrence. People tend to smoke while drinking beer or spirits, although possibly wine is consumed more often with meals.

The most convincing evidence that alcohol consumption is the major cause of esophageal cancer for men in the West has come from case–control studies in high-incidence areas. These surveys have been carried out mainly in the USA (Martinez 1969; Ziegler *et al.* 1981; Yu *et al.* 1988*b*; Brown *et al.* 1988) and in France (Tuyns *et al.* 1977). However, although these studies gave compelling evidence implicating alcohol consumption, the explanation of the association with esophageal cancer remains obscure. There is no experimental evidence for the carcinogenicity of alcohol or of alcoholic beverages, and although the biological and biochemical effects of alcohol treatment are very extensive (Lieber 1982*c*) there is no obvious reason why they should cause cancer in certain organs. The alcohol consumed comes into contact first and in highest concentration with the mucosa of the mouth and esophagus, but contact is transient and of very short duration, especially in the esophagus. Swallowed liquid remains in contact with the gastric mucosa for a much longer period, and yet the evidence for an association with stomach cancer is very much less certain than that for cancer of the esophagus. In spite of the fact that alcohol in the stomach is usually diluted by gastric juice and by food, and the mucosa is protected also be a mucous barrier, consumption of alcohol has been shown to cause lesions in the gastric mucosa in man and in experimental animals at concentrations which do not affect the esophagus (Glass 1979). The direct damaging effect of alcohol on epithelia seems not to be related to its carcinogenic potential. Following its absorption into the circulation, alcohol is distributed throughout the body in the body water, and all organs might be expected to be exposed in proportion to their water content.

Apart from its effect on the nervous system, the biological effects of ethanol might be expected to be due not to the ethanol *per se*, but to depend on the metabolism of the compound. Ethanol is metabolized mainly in the liver in man, not only by the cytosolic alcohol dehydrogenase, but also by the microsomal P450 group of enzymes, which metabolize many endogenous chemicals and xenobiotics. Therefore, as might be expected, ethanol has a profound effect on the metabolism of many hormones, metabolic intermediates, toxic chemicals and carcinogens, and it is as a result of these interactions that ethanol may enhance the effect of environmental carcinogens. Thus levels of nitrosamines consumed in food or formed *in vivo* may be too low to cause esophageal cancer unless their carcinogenicity is potentiated, possibly in some way by alcohol consumption.

Another important indirect way in which alcohol consumption could cause esophageal cancer is as a result of its adverse effect on nutritional status. For a variety of reasons alcohol consumption can lead to a deficiency of certain micronutrients and, as discussed elsewhere (Chapter 10), the effect of certain dietary deficiencies is to increase the vulnerability of the esophagus to carcinogens.

Several attractive mechanisms have been proposed to account for the association between alcohol consumption and esophageal cancer, and it is possible that they may each be operative, the relative importance of each varying with the population under consideration. Thus the adverse effects of alcohol on nutrition would be more important in the black population of Washington, DC, already existing on a relatively poor diet as a result of low economic status (Pottern et al. 1981) than in the affluent inhabitants of Normandy (Tuyns et al. 1987). The as yet unresolved problem of how consumption of alcoholic beverages causes esophageal cancer is discussed in this chapter.

Epidemiological evidence
Europe
Time trends in the pattern of esophageal cancer mortality in various European countries show mortality to increase with increasing consumption of alcohol, except where the starting levels were very low (Moller *et al.* 1990). Thus countries with high and increasing levels of consumption (Denmark, Hungary, Federal Republic of Germany and Czechoslovakia) showed an increase in mortality after about 1910. In contrast, countries with low starting levels of consumption (Sweden, Norway, Finland, The Netherlands, Poland and UK) and those with high but stable levels of consumption (France, Italy and Portugal) did not show an increase in mortality over the period studied.

France

Esophageal cancer has been called 'the French disease' (Picheral 1986), as France has the highest incidence of the disease of any Western country (see Fig. 4.2). France also has the highest per capita consumption of alcohol of any country (Table 6.1). Study of geographical variations in cancer rate throughout the country have shown the incidence to be much higher in Brittany and Normandy than elsewhere (see Fig. 4.5), and that this distribution correlates with the incidence of mortality due to alcoholism (Tuyns 1970). The cancer incidence map of France shows that the high-incidence areas occur in the regions where the weather is more suitable for the cultivation of apples than of grapes, and as a result cider and apple brandy are consumed more than wine and grape brandies. The exceptional high cancer incidence in these regions justified case–control studies, which were carried out in the Ille-et-Vilaine (Tuyns *et al.* 1977). It was found that the logarithm of the relative risks of developing esophageal cancer increased linearly with daily consumption of alcohol and tobacco independently, and the combined effect suggested a multiplicative action.

The importance of the nature of the alcoholic beverage consumed was studied using an ingenious technique (Tuyns *et al.* 1979). As very few people consume only one type of drink, a comparison was made for people consuming the same total amount of ethanol but who never consumed one particular drink. The risk of cancer associated with a mixture of the other drinks could then be assessed (Table 6.2). It was found that apple brandy presented a much greater risk than did cider, which in turn was more hazardous than wine or beer. The world record for the sex ratio of esophageal cancer, men/women 20/1, could be explained by the fact that men in this region drink four times more alcohol than do women (Picheral 1986). After careful consideration of diet in further case–control studies, alcohol consumption remained the predominant hazard for esophageal cancer (Tuyns *et al.* 1987). The apparent association with salt consumption disappeared when corrections were made for alcohol consumption (Tuyns 1983).

Britain

Although the incidence of esophageal cancer in men in England and Wales (5.02/100000) and in Scotland (7.10/100000) is higher than in the USA (4.3/100000) (Table 6.1), very little has been done to investigate the causes in the UK. The esophageal cancer map for Scotland for men shows three main high-incidence areas (see Fig. 4.8; Kemp *et al.* 1985), none of which corresponds to the Spey Valley where the majority of the whisky distilleries are situated. A Family Expenditure Survey showed that in Scotland more

Table 6.1. *Alcohol consumption in litres ethanol per year per person over 15 years (Passmore et al. 1986) in relation to male esophageal cancer mortality rates per 100 000 (Tuyns 1982)*

Country	Alcohol consumption	Esophageal cancer mortality rate
France	22.6	13.53
Italy	15.0	4.45
Austria	14.4	3.96
Germany	13.5	3.44
Portugal	13.4	4.51
Switzerland	13.0	7.79
USA	10.1	4.3
UK	7.2	
Scotland		7.10
England and Wales		5.02

Table 6.2. *Relative risks of esophageal cancer in relation to the type of alcoholic beverage consumed, in the Calvados region of France (after Tuyns et al. 1979)*

		Relative risks[a]		
Daily alcohol consumption:		1–40 g	41–80 g	≥ 81 g
Beer	Consumers	0.98	1.82	10.50
	Non-consumers	0.72	2.97	12.69
Cider	Consumers	0.90	3.07	16.44
	Non-consumers	0.71	1.87	5.53
Wine	Consumers	0.70	2.33	10.35
	Non-consumers	1.00	2.89	18.72
Aperitifs	Consumers	0.71	2.31	10.43
	Non-consumers	0.83	2.55	13.69
Digestives	Consumers	1.53	2.92	13.79
	Non-consumers	0.52	1.76	3.68

[a] Relative to the risk of 1.0 for abstainers.

is spent per family on alcoholic drink than in the UK as a whole, and that the rate of admission to psychiatric institutions due to alcoholism or alcoholic psychoses is more than five times that in England (Kemp *et al.* 1985). This implies that the higher cancer rate in Scotland could be a result of a higher consumption of spirits.

In England and Wales, the high-incidence areas for women are clearly located down the west coast from Cumberland through Wales to the western counties, while pockets of high-incidence rates for men are widely distributed, including a high rate in the western counties (see Fig. 4.10; Gardner *et al.* 1983). Traditionally Devon and Somerset were the home of cider making, and consumption was excessive in the days when cider was accepted as part of the farm labourer's weekly wage. However, in contrast to the situation in Normandy, it is dubious whether consumption of cider or apple brandy contributes to the risk of esophageal cancer in the UK at present. The facts that the esophageal cancer rate is higher for men, and that men, married, single, or divorced, drink three times more alcohol than do women (Wilson 1980), are consistent with alcohol being a cancer risk. However, study of the regional distribution of alcohol consumption (Wilson 1980) was not sufficiently detailed for comparison with the esophageal cancer map (see Figs 4.9 and 4.10; Gardner *et al.* 1983). There is obviously an urgent need for a survey similar to that carried out in the USA (Schoenberg *et al.* 1971) in which the esophageal cancer rate and consumption of cigarettes and of alcohol in different forms could be compared county by county. This would be of especial interest in Scotland, where the incidence varies from 10.5 to 3.5/100000 in different regions of the country (Kemp *et al.* 1985).

Italy
In contrast to the situation elsewhere, a study in the north-east region of Italy, an area where there is a high incidence of esophageal cancer, suggests that wine is the most hazardous type of drink (Barra *et al.* 1990). It is possible that, in each district, the most popular type of drink is the most hazardous, even when the cancer risks are compared on the basis of the amount of ethanol consumed in each type of drink.

United States
Studies in the USA of the geographic distribution of esophageal cancer and alcohol consumption and case–control studies have shown again that the consumption of alcoholic beverages is the predominant cause and, as in France, a higher risk is more often associated with spirits than with other beverages. An extensive survey was carried out in which the esophageal cancer mortality rate and the per capita sales of distilled spirits and of cigarettes were determined for each state (Schoenberg *et al.* 1971). It was found that the cancer rate was highest in the north-east of the USA, and that this correlated with alcohol intake. Thus Connecticut was found to have the highest cancer rate (4.46/10000) for any state, and also, with the exception of Alaska, the highest alcohol consumption. The survey

did not, however, include consumption of beer and wine. As with other studies, it did not imply that alcohol consumption was the sole cause of esophageal cancer. Other factors are obviously involved, but alcohol was by far the predominant cause.

More detailed case–control studies have been carried out in several high-incidence regions in the USA. Thus in New York it was found that in the absence of heavy alcohol consumption, the risk among smokers of developing esophageal cancer was relatively small, but that for heavy drinkers the risk was 25 times higher than in non-drinkers (Wynder *et al.* 1961). The risk associated with whisky consumption was greater than that for wine or beer. In Puerto Rico, consumption of rum was suggested to be the predominant cause (Martinez 1969). The concentration of ethanol in rum, which is produced from by-products of sugar-cane mills in many Caribbean countries, is said to reach 90% (Barbor 1988). In Washington, DC, where the cancer rate for black men (28.6/100000) was twice the national average for non-white males and 7 times that for white males, the predominant cause was again alcohol consumption (Pottern *et al.* 1981). Although the relative risk increased with consumption of ethanol in any form, the increase was highest among drinkers of whisky or bourbon. The amount consumed was so large that the effect overwhelmed any additional risk associated with cigarette smoking. A case–control study in Los Angeles also showed that the risk associated with consumption of spirits was more than twice that for the same amount of ethanol in the form of beer (Yu *et al.* 1988).

In South Carolina, the cancer rate for men living in the coastal region was higher than that for the state as a whole (Brown *et al.* 1988). Consumption of beer and/or wine was associated with only a slightly increased cancer risk, while the major determinants were tobacco and consumption of spirits, especially moonshine. Eighty-five per cent of the black male cases were reported to be regular users of moonshine.

The above studies provide compelling evidence that hard liquor presents a greater hazard for esophageal cancer than does the consumption of the same amount of ethanol as beer or wine. It is of interest that the highest esophageal cancer rates in the USA occur in New England (Schoenberg *et al.* 1971), and that this region, as with the high-incidence region in France, has a long association with a high consumption of cider. Before the nineteenth century cider was the main drink of the region, apparently being given to each member of the family at breakfast, dinner and supper and to people working in the fields (Barbor 1988). Apple brandy, or applejack, is still prepared by leaving the cider outside through the cold New England winter, when the water freezes, and the concentrated liquor can be decanted. Hence, the colder the winter, the stronger the liquor. Applejack would therefore have a very different composition from the apple brandy drunk in Normandy, where it is prepared by distillation of the cider. It would be of interest to assess the risk of esophageal cancer associated with consumption of applejack in New England.

South Africa

In South Africa an attempt has been made to determine whether the alarming increase in incidence of esophageal cancer in men in certain regions in recent decades is related to alcohol and tobacco use. In contrast to the situation in France and the USA, alcohol has not been shown to be the predominant cause. Studies in South Africa are especially difficult on account of the variety of home-brewed alcoholic beverages which are consumed, each tribe often having its own traditional method of preparation (Warwick *et al.* 1973). For example, the Pedi tribe use fruit in addition to cereals, and beer prepared from the prickly pear fruit is especially popular, in spite of the inflammation in the esophagus caused by the spines from the cacti lodging in the esophagus. Commercially prepared beverages are also consumed, and increasingly Western drinks are imported. Also the effect of a poor diet plays a greater role than in France or the USA, and factors such as *Fusaria* contamination of the maize used for brewing purposes could be important. The extent of contamination each year depends on the weather at the time of harvest. It is therefore not surprising that no clear overall picture of the etiology of esophageal cancer in South Africa has emerged.

In contrast to the situation elsewhere, in South Africa there is evidence that consumption of certain types of beer constitutes a major hazard (Cook 1971; McGlashan *et al.* 1982; Segal *et al.* 1988). Beer prepared from maize appears to be a risk factor, while beer prepared from sorghum is not (Broitman 1984). It is of interest that in Kenya, where the government encouraged the cultivation of maize, the incidence of esophageal cancer is high, while in Uganda, where maize cultivation has been officially discouraged, esophageal cancer rates are low (Haas 1978). This must be one of the rare instances where a cancer rate changes abruptly at a political boundary. The increase in cancer incidence in South African black males which has occurred over the last few decades could be due to the decrease in the amount of sorghum and increase in the proportion of maize used in brewing. The explanation of the deleterious effect of this change could be the decrease in riboflavin content of the beer, which could reduce the vitamin status of people whose customary intake is minimal (Segal *et al.* 1988), or it could lie in the fact that some types of Kaffir beer, in contrast to European beer, can contain high levels of certain congeners, the higher alcohols (O'Donovan 1966). These long-chain alcohols may be implicated in causing esophageal cancer (see later). The fusel alcohols are formed by yeast during fermentation. When maize is used, a fermenting agent, sometimes yeast, is added, but no additional fermenting agent is necessary when sorghum is used. It would be of interest to know the fusel alcohol contents of maize- and sorghum-brewed beers.

With reference to the interplay between alcohol and tobacco use in Africa, it has been suggested that, as the epidemiology of lung cancer differed from that of esophageal cancer, tobacco was not a major hazard for cancer of the esophagus (Cook 1971). In contrast, a study of six major tribes in Johannesburg in which 80 % of the smokers used pipes concluded that pipe smoking but not cigarette smoking was a cancer risk (Bradshaw *et al.* 1974). There appeared to be no association between cancer and alcohol consumption, but in this study only the type and not the amount of alcohol was considered. Later studies have also implicated smoking as a risk factor (McGlashan *et al.* 1982). It could be that the predominating effect of alcohol over smoking on esophageal cancer which applies in Europe and in the USA does not apply in South Africa. In the West tobacco is consumed mainly in the form of cigarettes, while in South Africa pipe smoking predominates, at least in certain regions. The condensates in the stem of the pipe are sucked out and swallowed, and the residues in the bulb are removed and chewed. These habits, which result in a flow of smoked tobacco condensates down the esophagus, could well increase the effect of smoking on the esophagus, but possibly not the effect on the lung.

It can therefore only be concluded that alcohol, tobacco, poor diet, and other factors including mycotoxin consumption, are operative in producing the high cancer rate in certain areas of South Africa, the relative importance of each factor changing over the years and varying with the locality.

Alcohol-related occupations

The incidence of esophageal cancer associated with alcohol-related occupations merits further study, if only to allow warnings based on the facts to be given to those at risk. A striking association was suggested in a study (Hurst 1939) which showed the relative rates of esophageal cancer in cellarmen, barmen, waiters, the general population and Anglican clergymen to be 46:43:41:10:2.

Brewery workers, especially those given a free allowance of beer, should provide another suitable population for study, but the results of investigations in different breweries have given results which are superficially conflicting. Thus workers in a Danish brewery were found to have an increased risk of contracting esophageal cancer of 2.09, but no increased risk for colorectal cancer (Jensen 1979), while men in a Dublin brewery showed no increase in risk for cancer of esophagus but did have a significantly increased risk of rectal cancer (Dean *et al.* 1979). However, the Danish workers were allowed six bottles, equivalent to 78 g ethanol, of light pilsner beer per day, while the Dublin workers were given only 2 pints of stout, amounting to 58 g ethanol. The difference in risk could be due to the different amounts of ethanol consumed, to differences in the nature of the drink, or to the fact that the evening consumption of alcohol by the two groups of men studied are unlikely to have been similar. A study of brewery workers in Sweden showed an increased risk for cancer of the esophagus, rectum, lung and pancreas (Carstensen *et al.* 1990). The excess in lung and pancreatic cancers was thought to be the result of differences in smoking habits of the brewery workers from those of the general male population.

Between-country comparisons

In contrast to the situation in Europe, the USA and South Africa, esophageal cancer in high-incidence areas in most Eastern countries does not in general appear to be related to alcohol consumption. Studies in Japan, the most Westernized of the Far Eastern countries, confirmed work in Europe and the USA, in showing that esophageal cancer risk increased with consumption of alcohol, the risk being lowest for beer, and increasing for saki and whisky, being highest for shochu, a strong liqueur (Hirayama 1979). In China, however, although consumption of pai kan, a very potent spirit containing 60–80 % ethanol, has been incriminated, it is unlikely that the very high cancer rates in certain regions are caused by alcohol consumption (quoted in Warwick *et al.* 1973).

Although the evidence is compelling that in the West alcohol is the major cause of esophageal cancer, the cancer rate for European countries does not correspond to the per capita alcohol consumption (Table 6.1). This is very probably due mainly to the fact that the type of beverage determines the extent of the risk, and each country has its own order of preference for consumption of different types of drink. Although France has by far the highest consumption and the highest esophageal cancer rate in men, the rate in Switzerland may be higher than might have been expected from the amount of ethanol drunk on account of the high proportion consumed in the form of spirits. Italy on the other hand may have a rate lower than expected, as in Italy wine is the most popular drink. The relative cancer rates in Austria and Germany may be low as a result of the fact that beer accounts for a high proportion of the ethanol consumed in these countries.

A 'safe' level of consumption?

In spite of many confounding factors, the conclusion cannot be avoided that consumption of even moderate amounts of any alcoholic beverage constitutes a risk of contracting esophageal cancer. A very important question is whether very small levels of consumption, which may be acceptable for many people, do constitute an appreciable hazard. Studies in France showed that 4–6 units per day, i.e. two pints of beer, four glasses of wine, or four measures of spirit, constituted a substantial risk (Tuyns *et al.* 1979). Further work from the USA, Japan and Europe has very approximately given similar data.

In a California population a cohort study was carried out in which the mortality from oral plus esophageal cancer was related to the number of 'drinks' per day consumed, either as beer, wine, spirits or cocktails (Klatsky *et al.* 1981). The data showed that as the number of drinks increased from 0, to less than 2, to 3–5, and finally to more than 6, the percentage mortality was respectively 2, 0, 5 and 8, i.e. non-drinkers had a slightly higher mortality from upper aerodigestive cancer than those who consumed less than 2 drinks per day, while 3–5 drinks roughly doubled the mortality of those who consumed very little, and more than 6 drinks (about 72 g alcohol) quadrupled the mortality. Study of a Japanese population showed a dose-related association of deaths from upper aerodigestive tract cancers, with an incidence of 16/100000 for drinkers of fewer than 2 go/day, and 95/100000 for those who drink more than two go/day (Kono *et al.* 1986). (A 'go' is a Japanese measure of alcohol of approximately 21 g.)

The previously mentioned study in Europe (Moller *et al.* 1990) also showed that esophageal cancer mortality is only slightly affected by moderate doses of alcohol, but rises steeply with consumption of large quantities, with an apparent threshold of 8 litres of alcohol per capita per year. For comparison, this works out to 17 g alcohol per day.

Overall, the data confirm the current advice given in the UK, that the maximum consumption should be 14 units per week for women and 21 units for men, a unit being $\frac{1}{2}$ pint beer, 1 measure of spirits, or 1 glass of wine. Mercifully, in contrast to the situation relating to tobacco use, there is no justification for complete prohibition, except for those who, once they have started to drink, are unable to stop.

Evidence for the carcinogenicity and genotoxicity of ethanol

In view of the absence of evidence to the contrary, it is generally agreed that ethanol *per se* is not carcinogenic. In most experiments, however, ethanol has been administered to animals at relatively low concentrations in drinking water. This method approximately mimics consumption of alcohol in beer, but as spirits present a very much higher risk for esophageal cancer than does beer, the technique is not the most appropriate for studies on esophagus. More relevant would be intubation, using a short tube, of ethanol at 40%, two or three times daily for life – a demanding experiment which does not appear to have been recorded. However, ethanol at this concentration has been given in 'forced drinking' experiments (Kuratsune *et al.* 1971), in which the water bottles of mice were replaced intermittently by alcohol solutions throughout the life of the animals. There was no evidence that alcohol given in this way was carcinogenic. Certain alcoholic beverages, i.e. Japanese and Scotch whisky, sherry and sake, were tested in the same manner, and again there was no evidence for carcinogenicity. Also, when brandy was given orally to rats throughout their life, there were no treatment-related cancers (Habs *et al.* 1982). Thus although certain drinks may on occasions contain carcinogens (see next section), ethanol and the industrially manufactured beverages which have been tested have not been found to be carcinogenic.

Mutagenicity and genotoxicity of chemicals may provide a rough guide to their carcinogenic potential. Excellent reviews of the genetic effects of ethanol have been published recently (Obe *et al.* 1979, 1987). While there is no evidence to suggest that ethanol *per se* is genotoxic, its major metabolite, acetaldehyde, is mutagenic. Also methanol, a natural component of many alcoholic beverages, can be mutagenic on account of its metabolic conversion to formaldehyde. Other genetic damage, such as the induction of sister chromatid exchange in lymphocytes *in vitro*, also depends on the metabolism of ethanol. An effect on esophagus would therefore depend on the alcohols being metabolized in the esophagus, an important point which was not studied until recently (see later), or on aldehydes formed by metabolism in the liver reaching the esophagus via the circulation. At present it can be concluded that, although alcoholics show a higher frequency of chromosomal aberrations and sister chromatid exchange in peripheral lymphocytes than normal, there is no evidence to suggest that alcoholic beverages *per se* are carcinogenic.

Non-ethanolic constituents of alcoholic beverages

The vast majority of alcoholic beverages contain a large number of a variety of different types of chemicals in addition to ethanol. Most of these constituents are either harmless, or are present in such low concentrations that they are unlikely to constitute a hazard. However, a small number of compounds which occur in a range of drinks could well be relevant in causing esophageal cancer. As the levels of non-ethanolic constituents vary widely from one type of drink to another, their involvement could explain why the degree of cancer risk depends on the type of beverage consumed.

Components other than ethanol are often referred to as 'congeners'. Strictly speaking, this term defines chemicals in the same genus as ethanol, i.e. homologous straight-chain primary alcohols such as *n*-butanol and *n*-propanol. In practice the term is often used to include all volatile components other than ethanol, for example other alcohols, carbonyls, esters and phenols. The term 'congeners' has also been used to cover any non-ethanolic components, such as sugars and tannins. In view of the ambiguity, the term is best avoided.

Apart from the restricted composition of a small number of spirits, the array of chemicals which occur in alcoholic beverages is very diverse. Some of these components originate in the starting materials used for fermentation, either from natural components of the cereals, grapes, apples, cacti, or whatever fermentable material is employed, or from contaminants, such as insecticides or mycotoxins. These chemicals may be altered and others added during preliminary treatments before fermentation, as in the malting of barley, a process in which nitrosamines can be formed, and in the mashing of cereals and maceration of fruits. The yeasts then not only convert fermentable materials into alcohols, but also carry out various synthetic and degradative reactions, when the possibly hazardous higher alcohols are produced. Extraneous materials may be added, either deliberately, as with the addition of hops, clearing agents or colour to beer, or inadvertently, as in the contamination of beer in asbestos fibres during filtration.

During storage of alcoholic beverages in wooden casks, various chemicals are extracted from the wood into the alcoholic solutions. Tannins, long suspected of being associated with esophageal cancer, can reach relatively high concentrations. The development of subtle aromas and bouquets illustrates the fact that the components continuously alter or react together during maturation. In the final stages of the manufacturing process various extraneous chemicals may be added, common examples being the addition of preservatives, antioxidants, antifoaming agents and stabilizers in the wine industry. The variety of techniques used in the preparation of alcoholic beverages varies from the accepted procedures used in industrial manufacture to the localized practices used in home brewing and distillation, when discarded car exhausts may be employed for distillation and disused oil drums for storage of the drinks. Polycyclic hydrocarbon contamination from such procedures may explain the high

Table 6.3. *Volatile components of Calvados* (*Postel* et al. *1981*)

Component	Content (mg/100 ml Calvados)
Acids	6–24
Aldehydes	2–26
Esters	43–158
Methanol	35–73
Higher alcohols	152–308
Ethanol	32000

levels of esophageal cancer in certain localized regions of the world. In spite of the complexity of the situation, it is possible to assess those chemicals which might constitute a major hazard to the majority of consumers.

A number of tabulations of the compounds identified in alcoholic beverages have been published (Kahn 1969; Leake *et al.* 1971; Nykanen *et al.* 1983). The major components occurring in varying concentrations in different drinks are alcohols, acids, esters, carbonyls, phenolics including tannins, lactones, sugars, sulfur compounds, and hydrocarbons. Chemicals with a more restricted distribution are the low levels of certain vitamins which originate in the materials used for fermentation and may occur in non-distilled drinks, the large variety of spices added to liqueurs, and compounds from peat smoke in Scotch whisky, to mention a few. Only the non-ethanolic constituents which may be operative in causing esophageal cancer are discussed here.

Alcohols
The volatile components of the beverage carrying the highest risk for esophageal cancer, i.e. the apple brandy Calvados, are shown in Table 6.3. The compounds present in the highest concentrations after ethanol are the higher alcohols, esters and methanol. The esters are generally regarded to be innocuous, but the higher alcohols and methanol may well play a role in causing esophageal cancer.

Methanol
Methanol is formed by hydrolysis of pectins by the enzyme pectinase present in the macerated fruits used for fermentation. The alcohol therefore occurs only in very small quantities in beer and whisky, but is found in larger amounts in wines and those distilled beverages prepared from fermented fruits. The concentrations found in different samples of the

same type of drink are very variable, but roughly wines can contain up to 238 mg/l and brandies up to 750 mg/l (Nykanen *et al.* 1983). The content of methanol in the drinks therefore correlates with the risks they present for esophageal cancer, although the concentration in the most hazardous beverage, apple brandy, is not especially high (Postel *et al.* 1981). There is apparently no evidence to suggest that chronic ingestion of methanol can cause cancer. Its major metabolite, formaldehyde, is carcinogenic for nasal mucosa when inhaled by rats in the gaseous form, but the evidence is inadequate to assess its carcinogenicity in man (IACR 1982). It is possible that methanol is oxidized to formaldehyde in esophagus and that, in contrast to the situation in liver, the aldehyde is not rapidly oxidized further to form formic acid and carbon dioxide. It may therefore react with cellular macromolecules in the esophagus. When given by intubation to rats formaldehyde increases the rate of DNA synthesis in the gastric mucosa (Furihata *et al.* 1988). If formed *in situ* in the esophagus, formaldehyde could increase the rate of cell proliferation, a situation well known to increase the vulnerability of various organs to carcinogens.

Fusel alcohols
The volatile components present in alcoholic beverages in the highest concentration after ethanol are certain higher alcohols (Table 6.3; Postel *et al.* 1981). The term 'fusel oil' is sometimes applied to this group of alcohols. In the trade, however, the term refers to a cut of the distillate collected within a certain range of boiling points, and therefore includes volatile acids, esters, carbonyls, etc., while elsewhere it has been taken to mean contaminating oils from external sources. In view of the ambiguity, it is preferable to use the term 'fusel alcohols'.

The higher alcohols are well recognized as important contributors to the flavour of certain spirits, but their presence in beer is generally undesirable. They are formed by yeast during fermentation. In part they arise as a result of deamination and decarboxylation of amino acids, as in the formation of 3-methylbutanol from leucine, 2-methylbutanol from isoleucine, and β-phenethylalcohol from phenylalanine (Webb *et al.* 1963). Higher alcohols are also formed in biosynthetic reactions via various metabolic routes. The amounts formed depend on the nature of the fermented material, the strain of yeast used, and factors such as the duration and temperature of fermentation (Beech 1972; Williams 1974). The amount in the final product is determined also by the distillation and ageing procedures. During maturation of wines and spirits, the alcohols react with acids to form esters, and therefore the concentrations of the higher alcohols decrease.

Table 6.4. *Approximate fusel alcohol contents of alcoholic beverages*
(*references in text*)

Beverage	Content (mg/100 ml beverage)
Beer	
Top fermentation	4–23
Lager	4–5
Kaffir	3–20
European	10
Wine	
Californian red and white	25
South African red	29
South African white	23
Cider	
English	15–60
Spirits	
Gin	0
Vodka	0.4
Rum	4–100
Scotch whisky	42–114 (often over 200)
Bourbon	120
Cognac	96
Grape brandy	90
Apple brandy (Calvados)	152–308

Evidence suggests that these alcohols could well be a cause of esophageal cancer. Thus the levels of higher alcohols which occur in different types of drink vary very widely with the nature of the drink (Table 6.4), and show a striking correlation with the risk presented by the drink for causing esophageal cancer (see previous section). The concentrations found in beer vary within relatively low limits (Hough *et al.* 1961), the levels in Kaffir beer falling in the higher part of the range (O'Donovan 1966). This is a result of a more prolonged period of fermentation. The relatively high level is of interest as South Africa is one of the few regions where beer is especially associated with esophageal cancer (see previous section). Wines from different regions of the world contain slightly higher levels (Guymon 1952; O'Donovan 1966), while non-distilled apple-based alcoholic drinks contain up to 60 mg/100 ml drink (Beech 1972). The content in spirits ranges from essentially zero in gin and vodka to more than 200 mg/100 ml whisky and more than 300 mg/100 ml apple brandy (Postel 1983).

The range of higher alcohols which occur in apple brandy is shown in Table 6.5 (Postel *et al.* 1983). 3-Methylbutanol and 2-methylbutanol are

Table 6.5. *Fusel alcohol content of Calvados* (*Postel* et al. *1983*)

Alcohol	Content (mg/100 ml ethanol)
Propanol-1	24–165
Allylalcohol	2.2–13
Butanol-1	13–28
Butanol-2	10–242
2-Me-propanol-1	39–70
2-Me-butanol-1	38–58
3-Me-butanol-1	170–261
Pentanol-1	0.2–0.5
Hexanol-1	7.7–21
Octanol-1	0.1–0.3
Decanol-1	0.05–0.15
Benzylalcohol	0–0.25
2-Phen-ethanol	3.4–11

among the most abundant aliphatic higher alcohols, while β-phenethyl-alcohol is the aromatic alcohol which occurs at the highest levels. A similar spectrum of alcohols occur in brandies, whiskies and wines (Postel *et al.* 1985), in cider, sake and rum (Rose 1977), and in beer (Engan 1981). The hazard is therefore more likely to be due to the higher alcohols as a group, rather than to any particular member of the group.

To test the idea that higher alcohols are important causes of esophageal cancer, it would be of interest to know whether consumption of gin, which contains essentially zero levels of these alcohols, is associated with the disease. In most epidemiological studies, however, consumption of spirits has been assessed without special reference to the type of spirit consumed. During the notorious gin epidemic which occurred in Britain around 1750, it has been estimated that a quarter of the population of London consumed a pint of gin each day (Robinson 1988). It would be of interest to look for any evidence of a high incidence of esophageal cancer in London which might have ensued. This may not be as unfeasible as it may at first appear, as evidence has suggested that an epidemic of esophageal cancer occurred in The Netherlands during a period in which tea drinking was excessive, and ended when inexpensive coffee became available and replaced tea as the more popular drink (Morton 1972).

It has been claimed that the 'fusel oil' fraction prepared from fermented potatoes, when given to rats by intubation three times weekly for life, produced papillomas and tumors in the forestomach (Gibel *et al.* 1968). However, as explained by the authors, the distillate which was used contained components in addition to higher alcohols. Treatment of animals with specific higher alcohols, propan-1-ol, 2-methylpropanol and 3-methylbutanol, was said to cause a low incidence of leukemia, liver cell cancer, and one forestomach tumor, but no esophageal cancers were induced (Gibel *et al.* 1975). Thus there is no evidence to suggest that the higher alcohols are carcinogenic *per se.*

In addition to the fact that the higher concentrations of higher alcohols occur in the more hazardous drinks, a second line of evidence which implicates higher alcohols in esophageal cancer is the fact that, on intubation into rats, they have been shown to increase the rate of basal cell replication in the esophagus (Craddock and Edwards, unpublished). Higher alcohols have also been shown to alter the metabolism by esophageal microsomes of a nitrosamine, methylbenzylnitrosamine, which is carcinogenic for the esophagus (Craddock *et al.* 1989), and to be metabolized by the esophagus (Craddock 1991). The possible importance of these facts is discussed in later sections of this chapter.

Tannins

The question of whether tannin consumption is an important cause of esophageal cancer has been discussed most widely in relation to tea drinking. The problem is relevant to consumption of alcoholic beverages, as tannins occur in relatively high concentrations in certain drinks. Thus red wines often contain high levels of tannins which originate in the skins of the grapes. Although tannins are not volatile they occur also in certain distilled spirits, as they are extracted by the alcoholic solutions from the wooden casks in which the spirits are matured. The tannins found in wood, in fruits used in the preparation of wines, and in leaves used for brewing tea are chemically very different, and may well have different biological effects. The possibility that they are a cause of esophageal cancer is discussed in Chapter 7.

Mycotoxins

While the question of tannins applies mainly to wines and spirits, mycotoxins, apart from the liver carcinogen aflatoxin, are more likely to be a hazardous constituent in beer. Work carried out mainly in South Africa has for a long time associated consumption of certain mycotoxins with esophageal cancer. The mold concerned, various species of *Fusaria*, grows on maize, and when contaminated maize is used in the preparation of beer the mycotoxins produced, notably trichothecenes and Fusaria C, occur in the beer. While the better grades of the harvest are used for direct human consumption, contaminated crops tend to be used for brewing beer. In Britain, where maize honey is imported from Africa for sweetening beer, a close check is made of its possible contamination by mycotoxins. The complex question of whether mycotoxins are implicated in esophageal cancer is discussed in Chapter 9.

Nitrosamines

Certain nitrosamines are by far the most potent chemicals known which are carcinogenic for the esophagus, and the discovery of relatively high concentrations of nitrosamines in beer was therefore a considerable cause for concern. Beer constituted the major source of dietary nitrosamine consumption for men in Germany (Preussmann *et al.* 1984*b*). The nitrosamines were formed during the malting of barley, and changes in the malting procedures have now reduced very considerably the levels of nitrosamines which occur in beer. However, as the high levels were found especially in beer, the beverage which presents the lowest risk for esophageal cancer, and usually low levels were found in the more hazardous drinks (Preussmann *et al.* 1984*b*), it seems unlikely that nitrosamines in alcoholic beverages were a cause of esophageal cancer. This certainly does not imply that nitrosamines are not important. However, those nitrosamines which occur in the beverages might be prevented from being effective by the ethanol which is consumed at the same time. Good evidence that this is the case has now been presented by Mufti *et al.* (1989), who showed that treatment of animals simultaneously with alcohol and nitrosamine protected against esophageal cancer, presumably as a result of inhibition of metabolism of the nitrosamine. Alcohol given after nitrosamine exposure enhanced carcinogenesis. In addition, the main nitrosamine found in beer is dimethylnitrosamine, which has not been shown to be carcinogenic for the esophagus in animal experiments. It can therefore be tentatively concluded that the nitrosamines occurring in alcoholic beverages are not especially implicated in esophageal cancer, but that alcohol enhances the carcinogenicity of nitrosamines consumed in food, formed *in vivo*, or absorbed from other environmental sources. The complex question of the effect of ethanol on nitrosamine carcinogenicity and metabolism is discussed later in this chapter, and of the levels of nitrosamine exposure from various sources, including alcoholic beverages, in Chapter 5.

Miscellaneous

Several additional carcinogenic chemicals have been detected in alcoholic beverages, foremost among these being asbestos and urethane.

The well-established fact that inhalation of certain types of asbestos causes mesothelioma led to the suggestion that oral consumption of fluids containing asbestos might cause cancer in the gastrointestinal tract. Asbestos has been detected in beer (Biles *et al.* 1968), in gin (Wehman *et al.* 1974), and in other beverages (Cunningham *et al.* 1971). Both the potentially hazardous amphibole asbestos and the apparently harmless chrysotile form of asbestos have been detected. Asbestos can originate in the filters used for clarifying the beverages, or in asbestos-cement water pipes. However, widespread surveys of drinking water have not produced any evidence of carcinogenicity. The use of asbestos for filtering beverages has now been prohibited in most European countries.

Urethane (ethyl carbamate) can induce lung adenomas and lymphomas in rodents, but apparently the chemically has not been shown to be carcinogenic for the esophagus, possibly because it has not been administered by the appropriate route. It occurs at low levels in most fermented foods, including bread, and in many alcoholic beverages (Lau *et al.* 1987). However, the concentration in certain beverages may be relatively high. Thus in wine urethane may occur at more than 150 μg/l (Waddell *et al.* 1987), and in certain brandies it can reach 10 mg/l (IACR 1988). These high levels are due to the use of urea as a fermentation 'booster', and to the addition of diethyldicarbonate to wine to inhibit spoilage by yeasts and other fungi (Ough 1987). The carcinogenicity of urethane has been studied after administration of aqueous solutions, in contrast to exposure as a result of its presence in alcoholic beverages. Treatment of mice with urethane in 12% ethanolic solutions altered the localization of urethane in certain mouse tissues (Waddell *et al.* 1987). Ethanol may inhibit the metabolism of urethane, and thereby inhibit its carcinogenicity. The risk presented by urethane in alcoholic beverages is therefore impossible to assess. However, the use of urea and of diethyldicarbonate has now been banned in the USA and certain other countries (Ough 1987).

The question of the phenolics which occur in red wine is discussed in Chapter 7.

Metabolism of ethanol and higher alcohols
In liver

Ethanol *per se*, without metabolism, probably has a significant action only in the brain, where it is thought to interfere with neurotransmission. The alcohol may interact with a subunit of the γ-aminobutyric acid receptor, and thereby boost the response of the receptor to the transmitter. The deleterious effects on other organs are more likely to depend on their ability to metabolize alcohols. In man the major part of the ethanol ingested is metabolized in the liver, but in the rat the intestine and lung each have approximately 10% of the activity of liver, while in the chicken it is over 20%, and in the frog the stomach and intestine each have approximately 60% the activity of liver (von Wartberg 1971). The metabolism in rat esophagus has recently been studied (see later). These species variations should be borne in mind during work on the effects of alcohol in different experimental animals, and the situation in hamsters and minipigs should be investigated.

In rat liver, approximately 80% of the ethanol ingested is oxidized in the cytoplasm by the alcohol dehydrogenase/nicotinamide adenine dinucleotide (ADH/NAD$^+$) system, and 20% by the microsomal ethanol oxidizing system (MEOS/NADPH). A small proportion, possibly 2%, is metabolized in the peroxisomes by catalase and hydrogen peroxide (Lieber 1982a). In each case, acetaldehyde is the product of oxidation, as shown in the following equation:

$$1. \quad CH_3CH_2OH + NAD^+ \xrightarrow{ADH} CH_3CHO + NADH + H^+$$
$$2. \quad CH_3CH_2OH + NADPH + H + O_2 \xrightarrow{MEOS}$$
$$CH_3CHO + NADP^+ + 2H_2O$$
$$3. \quad CH_3CH_2OH + H_2O_2 \xrightarrow{catalase} CH_3CHO + 2H_2O$$

As a result of the fact that the Michaelis constant of ADH (K_m 0.5–1.0 mmol/l) is lower than that of the MEOS (K_m 8–10 mmol/l) (Lieber 1982a), the proportion of a dose of ethanol metabolized by the MEOS increases with an increase in the circulating concentration of ethanol. For this reason a higher proportion of the ethanol ingested would be metabolized by the MEOS after consumption of spirits, containing 40% ethanol, than after consumption of wine or beer, when the resulting blood concentrations are lower. This could in part explain the greater risk of esophageal cancer associated with spirits than with other alcoholic drinks.

The acetaldehyde formed from ethanol in the liver is rapidly metabolized further to form acetic acid (Lieber 1982b). The question of how much if any aldehyde escapes into the circulation during intoxication or in alcoholics is still a matter of debate, owing to difficulties experienced in measuring small amounts of aldehyde in blood (Eriksson 1987). Alcohol-fed animals show an increased capacity to metabolize ethanol, while the mitochondria have a decreased capacity to oxidize acetaldehyde (Lieber 1982b), so that the likelihood of the aldehyde escaping into the circulation and reaching other organs is increased. Exposure of non-hepatic organs to this reactive metabolite could well have deleterious consequences, as other organs generally have a much lower capacity than liver for the metabolism of aldehydes (Deitrich 1966). Thus it has been suggested that acetaldehyde is responsible for the flushing of the skin which sometimes occurs after alcohol consumption, especially in Orientals (Lieber 1982*b*). The renal cortex of the human and of the baboon, however, have been reported to have a high capacity for aldehyde metabolism (Michoudet *et al.* 1987). The level in rat esophagus is described in the section on non-hepatic metabolism.

The MEOS is of special interest in the current context, as it forms part of the P450 microsomal system which is responsible for the metabolism of many xenobiotics, including certain carcinogens (Lieber 1983; Lieber *et al.* 1987). A unique isozyme was isolated from liver microsomes of ethanol-treated rabbits which had a high activity for the oxidation of ethanol and aniline (Koop *et al.* 1982). The ethanol-oxidizing P450 isozyme has been referred to as rat P450j, P450ac and P450et and rabbit P450LM3a, but it has been concluded that each refers to the identical isozyme, and the official terminology is now P450IIEI (Nebert *et al.* 1987).

The fact that chronic ingestion of ethanol by animals or man results in an increase in the ability of liver to metabolize the drug is due entirely to an induction of the MEOS (Lieber 1982*a*). There is no increase in the activity of ADH. In man, the increased capacity for metabolism is said to persist for 4–9 weeks after cessation of alcohol consumption (Seitz 1985). An important consequence of the induction of the MEOS is that a higher proportion of a dose of ethanol consumed would be metabolized by the MEOS as compared with ADH, i.e. by the P450 system responsible for the metabolism of many carcinogenic nitrosamines. The same amount of drink could therefore be more hazardous for chronic than for occasional consumers.

The chemicals other than ethanol which occur in exceptionally high levels in the more hazardous drinks are certain higher alcohols, especially the primary amyl alcohols, 2-methylbutanol and 3-methylbutanol. These alcohols are 12 times more toxic than is ethanol, and a high dose rapidly disappears from the blood when given to rats (Haggard *et al.* 1954) or to rabbits (Kamil *et al.* 1953). The limited number of *in vitro* studies of the metabolism of long chain alcohols which have been carried out were due to interest in enzyme kinetics rather than in carcinogenesis, and have not specifically included those alcohols most likely to be consumed in alcoholic drinks by man.

Liver ADH has a broad substrate specificity. The affinity of the enzyme for higher alcohols increases with increasing chain length, i.e. with increasing lipophilicity, but the maximum velocity of oxidation of the alcohol does not increase in parallel with the affinity (von Wartburg 1971).

The oxidation reactions of ethanol and of higher alcohols have similar values for V_{max}, but the K_m values decrease with increasing chain length. Ethanol, 1-butanol, 1-hexanol and 3-methylbutanol had V_{max} values within the range 12–9.6, but the range of values for K_m decreased from 0.4 for ethanol to 0.06 for 1-hexanol (Pietruszko *et al.* 1979; McCoy *et al.* 1981). However, the alcohols with a high affinity can be potent competitive inhibitors of the oxidation of ethanol (von Wartburg 1961) and presumably of other substrates. This has important implications for the effect of fusel alcohols on nitrosamine metabolism (see later).

In contrast to ADH, the MEOS of liver metabolized ethanol at a faster rate than propanol or butanol (Teschke *et al.* 1975), but butanol (10 mmol/l) inhibited the metabolism of ethanol (50 mmol/l) by 46.9 % (Teschke *et al.* 1976). It is very probable that, as with ADH, higher alcohols have a greater affinity for the MEOS than does ethanol, but are not necessarily metabolized faster.

In extra-hepatic organs

The ADH group of enzymes has been studied more often than the MEOS in extra-hepatic organs. In relation to oral cancer, there was found to be an active metabolism of ethanol and of certain higher alcohols in post-microsomal fractions isolated from the hamster cheek pouch epithelium, but the MEOS was not studied (McCoy *et al.* 1981). Very relevant to the problem of esophageal cancer was the discovery of a minor form of ADH in liver which, in contrast to the main ADH enzymes of liver with a K_m of around 7.5 mmol/l was active in 2 mol/l ethanol (Pares *et al.* 1981). A similar enzyme exists in human placenta (Pares *et al.* 1984), and in this organ it was the only ADH to be detected. Forms of ADH active in very high concentrations of ethanol were discovered in the cornea of the baboon (Holmes *et al.* 1986*b*), in the testis of the hamster (Keung 1988; Holmes *et al.* 1986*a*), and in stomach of the rat (Cederbaum *et al.* 1975), mouse (Algar *et al.* 1983) and baboon (Holmes *et al.* 1986*a*). An ADH, classified as ADH 1, was found in most organs directly exposed to external factors, including the esophagus (Boleda *et al.* 1989).

An ADH which metabolized ethanol at a concentration of 2 mol/l with a specific activity 40 times that of the liver enzyme at its optimum substrate concentration was discovered in the cytosol of rat esophageal mucosa (Craddock *et al.* 1990; Craddock 1991). The major fusel alcohols, 3-methylbutanol, β-phenethylalcohol and *n*-butanol, were also very actively metabolized by the cytosol fraction of rat esophageal mucosa.

An important aspect of the metabolism of alcohols is the rate of further metabolism of the toxic reactive aldehydes to which they give rise. While acetaldehyde was metabolized in esophagus at approximately the same rate as in liver, 3-methylbutaldehyde was oxidized more slowly (Craddock 1991). Therefore, although more of this metabolite would be formed from 3-methylbutanol in esophagus than in liver, it would not be eliminated more rapidly, and could have a more deleterious action on esophagus than on liver. The high K_m esophageal ADH was described also by Pares (1991).

The role of the high K_m ADH in organs such as placenta, testis and cornea is not immediately obvious, as these organs would never be exposed to concentrations of ethanol sufficiently high to be effective. Its normal function may be in the metabolism of some other substrate. The esophagus, however, could well be exposed to ethanol at concentrations approaching 2 mol/l, especially after consumption of spirits containing ethanol at 40 %, i.e. 7 mol/l. A plausible conclusion is therefore that the esophagus and stomach protect the internal organs from exposure to ethanol by metabolism while the alcohol is being absorbed through the wall of the alimentary canal. The ethanol which escapes this barrier and reaches the liver is metabolized by the liver enzymes with the much lower K_m of 7.5 mmol/l. The combined action of oral, esophageal, gastric and liver ADH enzymes therefore very greatly reduces the amount of ethanol which reaches the organ on which it has the most immediate devastating effect, i.e. the brain.

With reference to the MAOS in extra-hepatic organs, ethanol was shown to be metabolized by microsomes from rat lung (Seitz *et al.* 1981), but in contrast cytochrome P4503a was identified by immunological techniques in microsomes from rabbit nasal mucosa and from kidney, but not in those derived from intestine, lung, ovary, spleen, brain, heart, testis or uterus (Ding *et al.* 1986). Preliminary experiments have shown that esophageal microsomes oxidize ethanol and 3-methylbutanol, but less effectively than those derived from liver.

Effect of ethanol on carcinogenicity of nitrosamines

In view of the fact that ethanol *per se* and the alcoholic beverages which have been tested do not appear to be directly carcinogenic (see previous section), a plausible concept is that they act by enhancing in some way the carcinogenic potential of other chemicals. The effect of ethanol on the response to carcinogens has been studied in a number of organs for which the human disease has been associated with alcohol consumption. As nitrosamines are potent carcinogens for almost every organ in the body, and as human exposure to nitrosamines is widespread, the effect of alcohol on nitrosamine carcinogenicity has received the most attention. Disappointingly, the enhancement which might have been anticipated on the basis of induction of microsomal P450 systems, inhibition of repair of DNA damage, and deleterious effects on micronutrient status, in general has not been demonstrated. The effect of alcohol treatment on carcinogenesis in the pancreas initiated by *N*-nitroso-2-oxopropyl-(2-oxobutyl)amine (BOP) has revealed the complexity of the situation (Pour *et al.* 1983). In liver, simultaneous chronic administration of alcohol with *N*-nitroso-*N*-diethylamine (NDEA) resulted in a reduced rather than an enhanced cancer incidence (Habs *et al.* 1981). The acute inhibitory effect of ethanol on nitrosamine metabolism (see later) may be the determining factor even in experiments involving chronic treatment.

These effects of alcohol on liver and other target organs are relevant to carcinogenesis in the esophagus, as alcohol may not only increase or reduce the usual carcinogenic potential of the nitrosamine, but it has been shown also to cause a change in the target organ. Thus the carcinogenicity in mice of chronic treatment with low doses of *N*-nitroso-dimethylamine (NDMA) by intragastric intubation in ethanolic solutions differed from that of low doses given in water (Griciute *et al.* 1981). Ethanol decreased the morbidity resulting from liver tumors, but caused previously unseen olfactory epitheliomas to develop, some of which infiltrated the frontal lobe of the brain.

The effect of alcohol on carcinogenicity depends on the species and organ under study, on the nitrosamine used for initiation of cancer, on the absolute and relative doses of alcohol and carcinogen, and importantly on the regime used for the timing of treatment with alcohol and carcinogen. There are a large variety of schedules which can be implemented, some designed to mimic the situation as it occurs in man as nearly as is technically possible, others designed to elucidate the mechanisms involved in the modifying effect of alcohol on carcinogenesis. Among the schedules which could be employed to study the effect of ethanol on nitrosamine-induced cancer in the esophagus are the following:

1. A limited number of treatments with carcinogen and, simultaneously, with ethanol. Enhancement of carcinogenesis would imply a co-carcinogenic action of ethanol, possibly resulting from an increase in the metabolism of the nitrosamine by esophagus, a decrease in the rate at which the relevant DNA damage is repaired, or from an increase in the rate of replication of the target cells.
2. A limited number of treatments with nitrosamine, and treatment with ethanol before and/or during and/or after treatment with carcinogen. This type of schedule would detect a co-carcinogenic or a promotional effect of ethanol.

3. Chronic treatment concurrently with low doses of nitrosamine and with ethanol. Repeated small oral doses of carcinogen given at approximately the same time as small oral doses of a high concentration of ethanol as it occurs in spirits would be the situation most akin to the type of human exposure which correlates with esophageal cancer.

Although experimental evidence has shown that ethanol treatment can modify nitrosamine-induced cancer in certain organs, including liver (Habs *et al.* 1981), nasal cavity and trachea (McCoy *et al.* 1981), and pancreas (Pour *et al.* 1983), until recently there was little firm data to show that it could enhance esophageal carcinogenesis. Some experimental data suggested that ethanol given by intubation increased the incidence of NDEA-induced esophageal cancer (Gibel 1967). However, ethanol given in the drinking water did not enhance the esophageal carcinogenicity of *N*-nitroso-methylphenylamine (NMPhA) (Schmahl 1976). This could be due to the very likely possibility that different enzyme systems are involved in the metabolism of the two nitrosamines, or that the high concentration of ethanol given by intubation was more effective than the lower concentration given in drinking water. Later experiments, however, did not support the limited evidence that ethanol given by intubation enhanced the esophageal carcinogenicity of NDEA (Habs *et al.* 1981).

The possibility of indirect effects of alcohol consumption must be considered. Thus in work with hamsters it was found that, as the caloric intake from alcohol increased, the amount of chow consumed decreased so that the total calorie intake remained constant (McCoy *et al.* 1986). This could result in micronutrient deficiencies, which in turn would alter nitrosamine metabolism, and also cause adaptive metabolic changes to occur in the animals. Evidence for the importance of this effect of alcohol on micronutrient intake came from experiments in which it was found that esophageal cancer induced by *N*-nitroso-methylbenzylamine (NMBzA) was enhanced by feeding a zinc-deficient diet for 4 weeks before nitrosamine treatment, and that this enhancement was increased by giving ethanol at 4 % in the drinking water during the same period (Gabrial *et al.* 1982). As alcohol ingestion is known to increase the excretion of zinc in urine and feces (Newberne *et al.* 1983), the effect on NMBzA carcinogenicity could have been secondary to enhancement of zinc deficiency.

The effect of alcohol consumption on nutrition can be avoided in testing for a more direct action of alcohol on carcinogenesis by use of isocaloric liquid diets containing ethanol (DeCarli *et al.* 1967). However, these diets are not ideal for studying the effect of alcohol consumption on esophageal cancer, as high risk associates with consumption of spirits containing approximately 40 % ethanol in a relatively simple aqueous solution. With spirit drinkers, the concentration of ethanol coming into contact with the esophageal epithelium and the blood levels of ethanol reached after consumption would be much higher than those attained in experimental animals consuming a liquid feed containing ethanol. Use of isocaloric diets, however, has given much interesting information. Using this technique, it has recently been shown (Mufti *et al.* 1989) that treatment with ethanol before and during a course of injections with NMBzA decreased the incidence of esophageal tumors, while treatment after the cessation of the NMBzA injections increased the tumor incidence. It is probable that simultaneous exposure to ethanol inhibited the metabolism and carcinogenicity of NMBzA, while treatment at the later stage promoted carcinogenesis by increasing the rate of basal cell replication.

The effect of ethanol on squamous forestomach of rodents has sometimes been taken as evidence for an effect on esophagus. Thus *N*-nitroso-dipropylamine (NDPA) has been shown to be carcinogenic for the esophagus in rats but not in Syrian hamsters, while mice have not been tested (Preussmann *et al.* 1984*a*). When NDPA was given to mice by repeated intragastric intubation, solution of the NDPA in 40 % ethanol increased the incidence of forestomach tumors above those induced by aqueous solutions of NDPA (Griciute *et al.* 1982). Any effect on esophagus as distinct from forestomach was not clearly defined, but nevertheless it was suggested that ethanol increased the potential of the nitrosamine to induce esophageal cancer. However, it is well established that the effects of ethanol, NDMA, NDEA and NMBzA on forestomach are very different from those on esophagus. In spite of the histological similarity between the two organs, there is no basis for assuming a biochemical similarity, or a similarity in response to toxic compounds.

In view of the synergistic effect of tobacco smoking on alcohol-related esophageal cancer (Tuyns *et al.* 1977), the effect of alcohol on the carcinogenicity of tobacco-specific nitrosamines is of special interest. Nitrosonornicotine (NNN) is the major tobacco-specific nitrosamine, occurring in main-stream and side-stream tobacco smoke. The main target organ for NNN in the rat is the nasal cavity, but tumors are induced also in esophagus (Hoffman *et al.* 1975, 1984). The incidence at each site depends on the route of administration. Ethanol administered in a liquid diet had not effect on tumor incidence at either site when NNN was given by subcutaneous injection, but when the nitrosamine was given orally ethanol increased the incidence of tumors in the nasal cavity but decreased those in the esophagus (Castonguay *et al.* 1984). The evidence was that ethanol induced the metabolism of NNN in the nasal mucosa, but not in esophageal mucosa. The increased rate of removal of NNN from the circulation by the nasal mucosa could therefore reduce the exposure of the esophagus to the circulating carcinogen. When NNN was given to rats dissolved in 40% ethanol, again the incidence of esophageal cancer was not increased (Griciute *et al.* 1986). The effect of alcohol on carcinogenicity of 4(methyl-nitroso-amino)-1-(3 pyridyl)-butanone (NNK), another major component known to be carcinogenic for lung, liver and nasal cavity in F344 rats (Hoffmann *et al.* 1984), has apparently not yet been studied. The effect of alcohol on *N*-nitrosoanabasine (NAB), a nitrosamine occurring in tobacco smoke and carcinogenic for the esophagus (Boyland *et al.* 1964), would be of special interest.

Effect of ethanol and higher alcohols on nitrosamine metabolism
In vitro

As ethanol and many of the carcinogenic nitrosamines are metabolized by the microsomal P450 system, it was anticipated that a study of the effect of ethanol on nitrosamine might explain the association between consumption of alcoholic beverages and cancer in various organs. However, in spite of the fact that each organ apparently has its own spectrum of P450 isozymes, until recently experiments have been limited almost exclusively to microsomes of liver.

Addition of ethanol, *n*-propanol or *n*-butanol to a suspension of liver microsomes reduced the metabolism of NDMA (Peng *et al.* 1982). Inhibition was competitive. This suggests that a low concentration of ethanol would be sufficient to inhibit metabolism of the very low concentrations of NDMA to which human liver is likely to be exposed.

With reference to esophagus, NDMA is carcinogenic for liver and is metabolized by liver microsomes, but this nitrosamine is not carcinogenic for or metabolized by esophagus. NMBzA is carcinogenic only for esophagus, and is metabolized by esophagus at a greater rate than by liver *in vivo* (Hodgson *et al.* 1980). Therefore it seems very likely that different P450 isozymes are involved. As the isozyme responsible for metabolism of ethanol is identical to that which metabolizes NDMA (Park *et al.* 1986), it is very improbable that it is identical to the esophageal NMBzA-metabolizing species of P450.

A study was made of the effect of ethanol on the metabolism of NMBzA using both esophageal and liver microsomes (Craddock 1989; Craddock *et al.* 1991). A very much higher concentration of ethanol was necessary to inhibit metabolism in esophagus than in liver. As the degree of risk of esophageal cancer associates especially with drinks containing the highest concentrations of certain higher alcohols, the effect of commonly occurring branched chain alcohols was studied (Craddock 1989). It was found that 2- and 3-methylbutanol and β-phenethylalcohol were more than 1000 times more inhibitory for esophageal microsomes than was ethanol. This supports the concept that the fusel alcohols may well be the more important components of alcoholic beverages.

Studies have been made of the metabolism of nitrosamines in microsomes isolated after treatment of rats with ethanol. Acute effects cannot be studied in this way, as the alcohol is washed out of the microsomes during the preparative procedures. An apparent rapid induction of NDMA metabolism in liver was shown to occur after 2–3 days' treatment with ethanol, the level of induction being higher after 3 days than after 6 days (Peng *et al.* 1982). It had been suggested that this increase in activity could have been due to the effect of stress and adrenal stimulation rather than to a genuine induction of P450 by the action of ethanol on liver microsomes, but it has now been shown that a rapid increase in P450IIEI can be detected by immunological assay (Li *et al.* 1987).

In vivo

Induction of P450 in liver microsomes by chronic consumption of ethanol has been studied both by feeding rats a liquid diet containing ethanol and by administration of ethanol in the drinking water. These treatments were shown to induce metabolism of NDMA in liver microsomes (Schwarz *et al.* 1980; Garro *et al.* 1981). As chronic consumption of ethanol is known to induce the MEOS, and as ethanol and NDMA are metabolized by the identical P450 isozyme, this result was not unexpected. However, ethanol treatment induced also the liver microsomal metabolism of nitrosopyrrolidine (McCoy *et al.* 1979), and of tobacco-related nitrosamines (McCoy *et al.* 1982) in hamsters.

Although the alcohol-inducible form of cytochrome P450, P4503a, has been detected in extra-hepatic tissues, there is very little data on the question of whether the cytochrome is induced in these tissues by chronic treatment with ethanol, and of whether there is a corresponding increase in their ability to metabolize nitrosamines. Thus P4503a was detected in microsomes prepared from rabbit kidney and nasal mucosa, but not in those isolated from the other organs studied (Ding *et al.* 1986). This distribution was supported by the evidence that ethanol given in the drinking water at 10% for 15 days increased the activity of aniline hydroxylase in kidney but not in lung microsomes (Ueng *et al.* 1987). However, ethanol treatment induced the metabolism of NDMA in lung as well as in liver in rats (Carlson 1990). Apparently the only information on the esophagus is the evidence that chronic alcohol consumption for 4 weeks increased the ability of microsomes from liver, lung and esophagus, but not from stomach, to metabolize nitrosopyrrolidine to form a mutagenic product (Farinati *et al.* 1985). This result is unexpected as nitrosopyrrolidine has not been shown to be carcinogenic for esophagus in rats, a fact usually taken to imply that the nitrosamine is not metabolized by this organ.

In the intact animal, there are a variety of ways in which ethanol consumption could alter nitrosamine metabolism in esophagus other than by a direct action on esophageal microsomes. The effect of ethanol on the absorption, distribution and metabolism of nitrosamines in other organs is relevant, and several techniques have been used to study these questions. Among these giving data relevant to the esophagus are the following:

1. Determination of the effect of ethanol on the rate of disappearance of unmetabolized nitrosamine from the blood or the appearance of the nitrosamine in urine. In experiments with human volunteers, it was found that after an oral dose of NDMA, 13–23 μg, a small proportion of the dose (1.8–2.4%) was detectable in urine only if the NDMA had been given in a solution of 6% ethanol (Spiegelhalder *et al.* 1982). As NDMA is metabolized mainly by the liver, inhibition of metabolism by ethanol would result not only in detectable excretion in the urine, but also in an increase in exposure of non-hepatic organs to the NDMA. Although this nitrosamine is not carcinogenic for esophagus, this type of effect of ethanol could well apply to the metabolism of other nitrosamines. However, there appear to be no reports on the effect of ethanol on the rate of clearance from blood of a nitrosamine carcinogenic for the esophagus, although the disappearance of NMBzA from the circulation was slowed down by treatment of the animals with disulfiram (Schweinsberg *et al.* 1984, 1986). This drug interferes with the metabolism of ethanol and acetaldehyde and is used in the treatment of alcoholics.

2. Determination of the rate of expiration of $^{14}CO_2$ after treatment with ethanol and a ^{14}C-labelled nitrosamine. Again, while $^{14}CO_2$ exhalation after NMBzA treatment was inhibited by disulfiram (Schweinsberg *et al.* 1984, 1986), there is no evidence that ethanol has a similar effect.

3. The localization of ^{14}C label after injection of labelled nitrosamines can be studied by autoradiography of sagittal sections of the whole body of the animal. After treatment of rats with [^{14}C]NMBzA, labelling was especially high in esophageal epithelium (Kraft *et al.* 1980). Unfortunately the effect of ethanol on the distribution of label has not yet been studied.

In experiments with [^{14}C]NNN in mice, although initially the degree of labelling was highest in liver, kidney and parotid gland, after 24 hours the label was visible only in nasal, bronchial and esophageal epithelia and in salivary glands (Waddell *et al.* 1980). It was suggested that radioactivity is eliminated by renal and hepatic secretion, while bound metabolites were retained at the sites of carcinogenic action. However, in mice, NNN is carcinogenic for lung and salivary gland rather than for esophagus (Preussmann *et al.* 1984*a*). Treatment with ethanol 20 minutes before injection of NNN reduced the localization in salivary duct, bronchial epithelia and liver, but not in nasal and esophageal epithelia (Waddell *et al.* 1983). Interestingly *n*-butanol and *t*-butanol had a greater effect than ethanol. It was suggested that treatment with alcohols might reduce carcinogenicity of NNN in certain organs and increase the incidence at other sites. This idea was validated in the experiments, described in the previous section, on the effect of alcohol treatment on NNN carcinogenesis (Castonguay *et al.* 1984; Griciute *et al.* 1986). In view of the organ specificity of the alcohols and of their differences in potency, it is probable that the mechanism of action is through metabolic processes rather than through solvent effects. At one time it was thought that *t*-butanol was exceptional in not being metabolized, and that any biochemical effects must result from its solvent action. However, there is now evidence to show that even in this case the alcohol is metabolized, but by a system different from that oxidizing primary and secondary alcohols (Baker *et al.* 1982).

Effect of alcohols on DNA alkylation by nitrosamines

Probably the most relevant data on the effect of ethanol on nitrosamine metabolism comes from experiments involving the isolation of DNA from esophagus and other organs of animals treated with nitrosamines in the presence and absence of treatment with ethanol. Analysis of DNA for the identity, extent and duration of the DNA adducts formed should throw light on possible consequences for carcinogenesis. As discussed in Chapter 5, alkylation of DNA in the guanine residues is considered to be the relevant reaction for initiation of cancer, with O^6-methylguanine likely to be the adduct which mis-pairs at replication and 'fixes' a change in base sequence which can result in malignancy. 7-Methylguanine is also produced. Although this base may not be directly implicated in carcinogenesis, it is formed in proportion to the O^6-methylguanine and in ten times larger quantities, and so is a more easily determined measure of the extent of DNA alkylation.

Pioneering experiments showed that treatment of rats with alcohol simultaneously with NDMA increased the extent of formation of 7-methylguanine in DNA of liver and increased that in kidney (Swann 1982). The effect on methylation of DNA by NDMA appeared to be due to inhibition of first-pass clearance of NDMA from the circulation during its passage through the liver, resulting in an increased exposure of the kidney. It might be expected from this result that the long-term effect of treatment with alcohol and NDMA would be to increase the incidence of kidney tumors. Also, as NDMA is one of the most commonly occurring nitrosamines in the environment, an epidemiological association between consumption of alcohol and renal cancer might be anticipated. However, there seems to be no evidence for either of these effects on carcinogenesis. Administration of ethanol with [^{3}H]NDEA resulted in a decrease in the level of ethylation of liver DNA and an increase in that of esophagus (Swann *et al.* 1984, 1987). With NDEA, there was no evidence for a first-class clearance by liver even at very low doses, and it was suggested that the effect of ethanol on ethylation in esophagus was the result of a specific stimulatory effect on metabolism in esophagus. However, the amount of ethanol given to the animals, 1 ml of a 5% solution given to a 200 g rat, was said to be equivalent to 1 pint of beer for a 70 kg man, but it is the consumption of spirits (40% ethanol) rather than beer (5% ethanol) which is associated with esophageal cancer in man. The higher ethanol concentration would result in higher levels being reached in the blood, with the possibility that nitrosamine metabolism in esophagus would be inhibited also. In fact an oral dose of 40% ethanol given to animals simultaneously with NMBzA caused a decrease in the formation of 7-methylguanine in both esophageal and liver DNA (Craddock and Cary, unpublished).

The effect of chronic treatment with alcohol was studied by giving rats drinking water containing 30% ethanol for 3–4 weeks, followed by an injection of [^{14}C]NMBzA (Kouros *et al.* 1983). The alcohol treatment decreased the 7-methylguanine and O^6-methylguanine levels in liver, and increased those in lung and esophagus. It is rather surprising that chronic treatment with alcohol should decrease the extent of alkylation in liver, where induction of liver P450 might have been anticipated. The result may be due to the presence of ethanol in the circulation at the time of injection of [^{14}C]NMBzA. Until the alcohol consumed in the drinking water had been metabolized, the direct effect of inhibition of nitrosamine metabolism could predominate over the induced increase in P450. Further experiments along these lines, using ethanol, higher alcohols, and those alcoholic beverages which carry the highest risk for esophageal cancer, may well lead to an explanation at least in part of the association between alcohol consumption and esophageal cancer.

In addition to increasing the extent of formation of O^6-alkylguanine in esophageal DNA, there is evidence that, in liver, chronic treatment with ethanol can decrease the rate of DNA repair (Mufti *et al.* 1988). Replication of the alkylated DNA is considered to be an essential event in the initiation of cancer. By increasing the level of O^6-alkylguanine and decreasing the rate of its removal, ethanol would prolong the presence of the alkylated base in DNA, and thereby increase the possibility of replication occurring while the adduct was still present. The higher alcohols also increase the rate of replication of the basal cells in the esophagus (see following section).

Effect of ethanol and higher alcohols on basal cell replication

As with several other risk factors for esophageal cancer, such as riboflavin and zinc deficiencies and mycotoxin exposure, it is possible that alcohol consumption enhances the carcinogenicity of the primary carcinogen by producing an increase in the rate of replication of basal cells of the esophageal epithelium. To determine whether or not this occurs in people consuming hazardous amounts of alcohol, an epidemiological study should be made similar to that carried out in the areas in China with a high incidence of esophageal cancer (Yang *et al.* 1987). In this survey, biopsy material was incubated with [³H]thymidine, and labelling indices were studied. Unfortunately no such survey has been carried out in the regions where the high incidence rate is associated with alcohol consumption, as in the Calvados region of France or in the black population of Washington, DC. Evidence for an alcohol-induced increase in basal cell proliferation comes from animal experiments, but this work is difficult to relate to the human situation.

There are several ways in which consumption of alcohol could stimulate cell replication in esophagus. Under normal conditions, the passage of liquids through the esophagus is rapid, and the duration of contact with the surface epithelium is very brief. However, it has been shown using human volunteers that ethanol given orally or by intravenous injection decreases the frequency of peristalsis (Hogan *et al.* 1972). This would delay clearance of the esophagus, and prolong the time of contact of the contents with the lumen surface. Also, by the use of pH measurements in human volunteers it was shown that a 'relatively modest quantity of alcohol' (180 ml of 100 proof vodka) increased the frequency of gastric reflux (Kaufman *et al.* 1978). The acidic gastric contents are known to damage the esophagus which, unlike the stomach, is not protected by a film of mucus, and the epithelium attempts to heal the recurring wounds by restorative hyperplasia (see Chapter 3). In correlation with the association with esophageal cancer, strong liquor is said to produce more severe heartburn than does beer (Wienbeck *et al.* 1981). The high incidence of cancers in the lower region of the esophagus in men might well be explained in this way.

Animal experiments involving prolonged perfusion of the esophagus with alcoholic solutions are difficult to relate to the effect of alcohol consumption in man. For example, when an isolated rabbit esophagus was perfused for $3\frac{1}{2}$ hours, a solution containing 20% ethanol was 'relatively harmless' while 40% ethanol caused oedema and erythema (Salo 1983). However, $3\frac{1}{2}$ hours of continuous exposure would not occur in man. As the animals were killed at the end of the perfusion period, any effect on replication could not be assessed. Using a 20 minute perfusion period, rat esophagus was perfused with either 2 ml apple brandy or 2 ml ethanol of the equivalent concentration through a catheter sewn into position *in situ* (Haentjens *et al.* 1987). Animals were then killed at intervals, 1 hour after receiving an injection of [³H]thymidine. In both groups of animals the labelling index began to increase after 6–12 hours and the mitotic index after 12–18 hours. As there was no histological evidence for superficial desquamation, the proliferative response did not appear to be a reaction secondary to cellular shedding.

Chronic treatment of intact animals has also shown that ethanolic solutions can increase the rate of cell replication in the esophagus. Thus consumption for 8 weeks of a liquid diet containing 36% calories in the form of ethanol doubled the labelling index in the esophagus (Mak *et al.* 1987). The thickness of the epithelium was increased, but no changes in morphology were detected. This supports the suggestion by Haentjens *et al.* (1987) that the proliferative response is not the result of cell loss or of damage and restorative hyperplasia.

In man the esophagus is exposed to alcohol in the brief periodic episodes during which consumption of alcoholic beverages occurs, those drinks with the highest alcohol concentrations, i.e. spirits, being the most hazardous. The effect could well differ from that of a low concentration of ethanol present in a liquid diet. In an attempt to mimic more closely the situation as it occurs in man, alcoholic solutions were administered to rats using an intubation tube sufficiently long to prevent the solution from passing into the lungs, but as short as possible to allow maximum flow through the esophagus (Craddock 1991). One day after treatment the animals were given a 1-hour pulse of bromodeoxyuridine (BUdR) and were killed, and cell replication was studied by the BUdR–antibody technique. The most hazardous alcoholic beverages contain relatively high concentrations of certain higher alcohols, a regularly occurring example being 2-methylbutanol (Postel *et al.* 1981). It was found that intubation of 64% ethanol had no detectable effect on basal cell replication (Fig. 6.1*a*), but when 2-methylbutanol was dissolved in the ethanol the mixture produced a dramatic increase in replication (Fig. 6.1*b*). This effect could

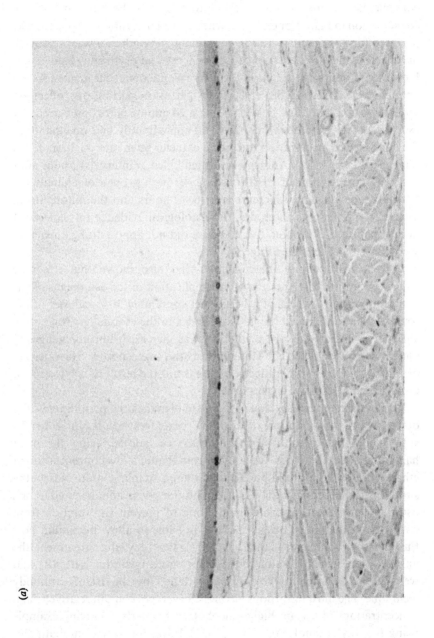

(b)

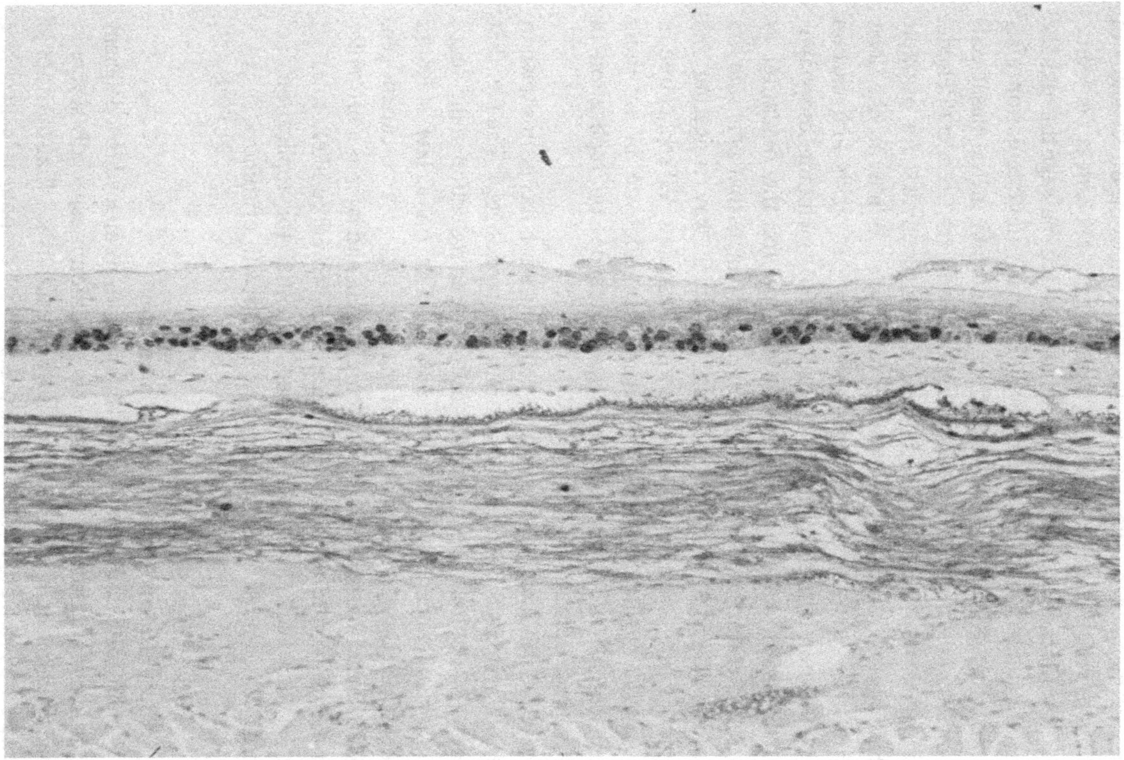

Fig. 6.1. DNA replication in esophagus visualized by the BUdR–antibody technique, 1 day after short-tube intubations of the following solutions: (a) 0.8 ml ethanol 64 %; (b) 0.8 ml of a solution containing ethanol 32 %, 2-methylbutanol 32 %, total alcohol concentration 64 %. × 300.

well explain the dependence of the degree of risk on the type of beverage consumed.

It is probable that the increase in cell proliferation produced by the various treatments mentioned above is not the result of the direct action of the alcohols *per se* on the esophagus, but that metabolism is necessary. Alcohols could reach the basal cells either as a result of passage through the superficial cellular layers of the epithelium, or via the circulation after absorption from the gastrointestinal tract. Oxidation in the basal cells would presumably form aldehydes, ethanol giving rise to acetaldehyde, and higher alcohols forming the corresponding aldehydes, for example 2-methylbutanol forming 2-methylbutyraldehyde. While in the liver aldehydes are generally rapidly oxidized further to acids and carbon dioxide, the non-hepatic organs (Deitrich 1966), including esophagus (Craddock 1991), have a much lower capacity for the oxidation of aldehydes. Therefore aldehydes formed in the esophagus may persist *in situ* and react with cellular macromolecules, in some way triggering cell replication. Formaldehyde has been shown to stimulate cell replication in rat stomach (Furihata *et al.* 1988) and benzaldehyde in rat lung (Schweinsberg *et al.* 1986). The effect of aldehydes on replication in esophagus merits study.

However it is induced, an increase in cell replication has been shown in a variety of systems to increase vulnerability to carcinogens. The fact that a reduction in alcohol consumption leads to a rapid reduction in incidence of esophageal cancer suggests that alcohol acts on a late stage in carcinogenesis (Day *et al.* 1982), i.e. it may act first as a co-carcinogen, altering the metabolism of the primary carcinogen, and later as a promoter by increasing the rate of cell proliferation. This would be likely to affect especially those cells with an increased potential for replication, i.e. malignant cells, and so to increase the rate of growth of tumors.

Effect of alcohol consumption on nutrition

There is no doubt that alcohol consumption can lead to a deficient micronutrient status in man, and that this condition is especially severe in alcoholics (Lieber *et al.* 1982*d*). It is also well established that nutritional deficiencies are often but not always associated with esophageal cancer (see Chapter 10). It therefore appears likely that a proportion of the cancer risk associated with alcohol consumption could be mediated through an adverse effect on micronutrient status. The proportion of the risk which originates in this way would depend on the population under consideration.

The fact that alcohol consumption can have an adverse effect on micronutrient status has been shown by a variety of methods of investigation, i.e. cohort studies, case–control studies and animal experiments. The evidence and the complex interrelationships involved have been discussed in several reviews (Lieber *et al.* 1982*d*; Seitz *et al.* 1987) and only those aspects which have a direct bearing on esophageal cancer will be discussed here.

There are several routes by which alcohol consumption can impair micronutrient status. Thus alcohol intake can reduce the absorption and increase the excretion of certain micronutrients. Secondly, in those sections of the population with a low socioeconomic status, the more spent on alcohol, the less can be spent on food. In addition, alcohol consumption can affect life-style of individuals in a way which affects nutrition. For example, in a study of the patterns of consumption of alcoholic beverages in England and Wales it was found that 63 % of the men's 'drinking occasions' took place in bars (Wilson 1980). Consumption of crisps and nuts, i.e. foods with a high fat and low micronutrient content, would be likely to replace traditional meals containing vegetables and fruit. Further, in order to avoid obesity, deliberate attempts may be made to compensate for the calories consumed in alcohol by reducing food intake (Sato *et al.* 1986).

Cohort and case–control studies have shown that the micronutrient deficiencies most likely to be associated with esophageal cancer are of zinc, magnesium, riboflavin, nicotinamide and vitamin C (Chapter 10). Of these, an adverse effect of alcohol consumption on zinc status has been most thoroughly documented. Thus in an experiment in which rats were fed a zinc-deficient diet containing ethanol, the urinary and fecal losses of zinc were higher than in the pair-fed controls and the tissue levels were lower in all tissues studied with the exception of bone (Russell 1980; Ahmed *et al.* 1982), but it is unfortunate that the esophagus was not among the organs studied. Human volunteers showed an increased excretion of zinc within 3 hours of consuming 6 oz vodka (Gudbjarnason *et al.* 1969), but again not data is available on zinc levels in the esophagus of people with a high alcohol consumption. The alcohol may affect zinc status by causing renal dysfunction with an increased loss of zinc from the renal tubules, by causing a release of zinc from the tissues and so making it available for excretion, or by altering the chemical state of zinc in the blood (Russell 1980).

Apart from the effect on zinc status, alcohol-related deficiencies mainly concern thiamin, pyridoxin, folate, vitamin B_{12}, and vitamin A (Lieber *et al.* 1982*d*; Seitz *et al.* 1987). There is little evidence to suggest that deficiencies of these vitamins are especially associated with esophageal cancer.

Two careful studies of populations with a high incidence of alcohol-associated esophageal cancer have investigated the interrelationships between alcohol consumption and nutrient deficiencies. A case–control study of black men in Washington, DC, showed that alcohol consumption was the major factor responsible (Pottern *et al.* 1981), but that the least well-nourished third of the population had twice the risk of developing esophageal cancer as the most well-nourished third. The foods considered in determining nourishment were the 'affluent foods', i.e. fresh or frozen meat or fish, vegetables, fruit, dairy produce and eggs (Ziegler *et al.* 1981). The high risk associated with poor diet remained after controlling for alcohol consumption, the two factors having additive effects. It was not determined how far the low micronutrient status was a result of the high alcohol consumption.

A contrasting population was studied in Calvados, France (Tuyns *et al.* 1987). This is a very rare example of a region in which an affluent population consuming a good diet has an exceptionally high incidence of esophageal cancer. In the black population studied in Washington, mentioned above, the esophageal cancer rate was 28.6/100000, twice the national average for black men in the USA (Pottern *et al.* 1981), while the incidence in Calvados was 45/100000 (Picheral 1986). As in Washington, alcohol consumption was the major risk factor, but again certain foods, especially fresh meat and citrus fruit, were found to be protective, after adjustment for alcohol and tobacco use (Tuyns *et al.* 1987).

As with studies of esophageal cancer in China and South Africa where alcohol consumption is not the major cause, the data at present show that certain foods are protective, but the nature of the micronutrients responsible is uncertain. As pointed out by Tuyns *et al.* (1987), the protective effect of vitamin C appears to be greater when consumed in citrus fruit than in potatoes and, although the effect of cooking potatoes is difficult to evaluate, the protective action of these foods could be due to some other factor the concentration of which parallels that of vitamin C. In any case, it is clear that a diet which is normally adequate cannot overcome the risk associated with high alcohol consumption. As stated by Tuyns *et al.* (1987), every known risk factor carries its own weight and must be taken into account. A poor diet can add to the risk associated with alcohol consumption, but a good diet cannot negate the risk.

Possible mechanisms involved in causing esophageal cancer

Alcohols can reach the basal cells of the esophagus either by passing through the narrow layers of superficial cells during the rapid transit of alcoholic drinks down the lumen, or after absorption from the stomach and small intestine into the circulation. Organs most at risk of cancer as a result of alcohol consumption, i.e. mouth, pharynx, larynx and esophagus, come into direct contact with alcoholic beverages, while those for which alcohol presents a lower risk, i.e. liver, pancreas and breast, come into contact with alcohol only after it has been absorbed into the circulation. This suggests that direct contact is the more hazardous route of exposure, and that the concentration of alcohol is critical.

Dependence on concentration may in part explain why spirits present a higher risk than does wine or beer. After consumption of spirits containing 40% ethanol (7 mol/l) the alcohol could reach the basal cells at only slightly lower concentrations. After drinking tequila, where the concentration can reach 80% ethanol, the cells could be exposed to 1400 mmol/l. In contrast, after absorption from the stomach and intestine into the circulation, the concentrations reached are much lower. The legal limit for alcohol in the bloodstream when driving in the UK is 17 mmol/l and 50 mmol/l is not usually exceeded during social drinking.

As neither ethanol nor fusel alcohols have been shown to be carcinogenic *per se*, enhancement of the carcinogenicity of a primary carcinogen is a reasonable concept, and a way in which this could be brought about is by increasing the rate of basal cell replication. It has been demonstrated in many systems, for example in liver (Craddock 1971), in stomach (Weisburger *et al.* 1989; Iishi *et al.* 1989), and in bladder (Masui *et al.* 1988) that an increase in the rate of cell replication enhances the carcinogenicity of *N*-nitroso compounds. Also it has been shown that ethanol (Mak *et al.* 1987) and fusel alcohols (Craddock 1991) increase the rate of replication of basal cells of the esophagus.

For reasons described in previous sections, certain nitrosamines are the most likely candidates for the role of primary esophageal carcinogens. Ethanol given simultaneously with a nitrosamine carcinogenic for esophagus reduced its carcinogenicity (Mufti *et al.* 1989), probably as a result of inhibition of metabolism of the carcinogen. Ethanol given after nitrosamine treatment increased carcinogenicity, in keeping with the concept that an increase in cell replication is the important factor. This increase could affect especially the initiated pre-malignant cells, and so increase the rate of appearance of tumors.

It is possible that chronic consumption of ethanol induces the microsomal metabolism of nitrosamines, but the effect would be apparent only when nitrosamine exposure occurred after the ethanol had been metabolized and had disappeared from the circulation. The dramatic effects of alcohol treatment on the metabolism of nitrosamines may therefore not be the relevant factor in the inhancement of their carcinogenicity.

An important problem is the synergistic action of tobacco smoking and alcohol consumption. One possibility is that the high content of nitrosamines in tobacco smoke increases the exposure of the esophagus to nitrosamines, so that there are an increased number of initiated cells present in the esophagus, and the action of alcohol is to increase the rate of replication of these cells. In addition, tobacco smoke acts as an irritant to the esophageal mucosa, and alcohol, acting on cells which are already damaged, could have an enhanced effect.

In conclusion, it is very likely that a variety of processes, including the induction of metabolism of carcinogens, micronutrient deficiency, or a damaging effect of tannins, may play a role in causing alcohol-associated esophageal cancer. However, the major factor may be that initiated cells, formed during exposure to nitrosamines, are later stimulated to replicate by exposure to ethanol and to fusel alcohols. The exceptionally high risk of esophageal cancer presented by certain drinks could be due to their especially high content of fusel alcohols.

References

Ahmed, S.B. and Russell, R.M. (1982) *J. Lab. Clin. Med.* **100**, 211–217. The effect of ethanol feeding on zinc balance and tissue levels in rats maintained on zinc deficient diets.

Alexandrov, V.A., Novikov, A.I., Zabezhinsky, M.A., Stlyarov, V.I. and Petrov, A.S. (1989) *Cancer Lett.* **47**, 179–185. The stimulating effect of acetic acid, alcohol and thermal burn injury on esophagus and forestomach carcinogenesis induced by *N*-nitrososarcosin ethyl ester in rats.

Algar, E.M., Seeley, T.L. and Holmes, R.S. (1983) *Eur. J. Biochem.* **137**, 139–147. Purification and molecular properties of mouse ADH isozymes.

Baker, R.C., Sorensen, S.M. and Deitrich, R.A. (1982) *Alcohol Clin. Exp. Res.* **6**, 247–251. The *in vivo* metabolism of tertiary butanol by adult rats.

Barbor, T. (1988) *Alcohol: Customs and Rituals*. London: Burke.

Barra, S., Francheschi, S., Negri, E., Talamini, R. and La Vecchia, C. (1990) *Int. J. Cancer* **46**, 1017–1020. Type of alcoholic beverage and cancer of the oral cavity, pharynx and oesophagus in an Italian area with high wine consumption.

Beech, F.W. (1972) *J. Inst. Brewing* **78**, 477–491. Cider making and cider research: a review.

Bartram, B., Frei, E. and Wiessler, M. (1985) *Biochem. Pharmacol.* **34**, 387–388. Influence of disulfiram on glutathione, glutathione-*S*-transferase, and on nitrosamine dealkylase of liver, kidney and esophagus of the rat.

Biles, B and Emerson, T.R. (1968) *Nature* **219**, 93–94. Determination of fibres in beer.

Boleda, M.D., Julia, P., Moreno, A. and Pares, X. (1989) *Arch. Biochem. Biophys.* **274**, 74–81. Role of extrahepatic alcohol dehydrogenase in rat ethanol metabolism.

Boyland, E., Roe, F.J.C., Gorrod, J.W. and Metchley, B.C.V. (1964) *Br. J. Cancer* **23**, 265–270. The carcinogenicity of nitrosoanabasine, a possible constituent of tobacco smoke.

Bradshaw, E. and Schonland, M. (1974) *Br. J. Cancer* **30**, 157–163. Smoking, drinking and esophageal cancer in African males of Johannesburg, South Africa.

Broitman, S.A. (1984) In: *Vitamins, Nutrition and Cancer* (Prasad, A.S. ed.). Basel: Karger, pp. 195–211. Relationship of ethanolic beverages and ethanol to cancers of the digestive tract.

Brown, L.M., Blot, W.J., Schuman, S.H., Smith, V.M., Ershow, A.G., Marks, R.D. and Fraumeni, J.F. (1988) *J. Natl. Cancer Inst.* **80**, 1620–1625. Environmental factors and high risk of esophageal cancer among men in coastal South Carolina.

Carlson, G.P. (1990) *Cancer Lett.* **54**, 153–156. Induction of N-nitrosodimethylamine metabolism in rat liver and lung by ethanol.

Carstensen, J.M., Bygren, L.O. and Hatschek, T. (1990) *Int. J. Cancer* **45**, 393–396. Cancer incidence among Swedish brewery workers.

Castonguay, A., Rivenson, A., Trushin, N., Reinhardt, J., Spathopoulos, S., Weiss, C.J., Reiss, B. and Hecht, S.S. (1984) *Cancer Res.* **44**, 2285–2290. Effects of chronic ethanol consumption on the metabolism and carcinogenicity of N′-nitrosonornicotine in F344 rats.

Cederbaum, A.I., Pietrusko, R., Hempel, J., Becker, F.F. and Rubin, E. (1975) *Arch. Biochem. Biophys.* **171**, 348–360. Characterization of non-hepatic ADH from rat hepatocellular carcinoma and stomach.

Collins, C.H., Cook, P.J., Forman, J.K. and Palframan, J.F. (1971) *Gut* **12**, 1015–1018. A search for nitrosamines in East African spirit samples from area of varying oesophageal cancer frequency.

Cook, P. (1971) *Br. J. Cancer* **25**, 853–880. Cancer of the esophagus in Africa: A summary and evaluation of the evidence for the frequency of occurrence, and a preliminary association with the consumption of alcoholic drinks made from maize.

Craddock, V.M. (1971) *J. Natl. Cancer Inst.* **47**, 889–907. Liver carcinomas induced in rats by single administration of dimethylnitrosamine after partial hepatectomy.

Craddock, V.M. (1989) *Br. J. Cancer* **59**, 823. Potent inhibition of esophageal metabolism of methylbenzylnitrosamine, an esophageal carcinogen, by higher alcohols present in alcoholic beverages.

Craddock, V.M. and Abbs, M. (1990) *Br. J. Cancer* **62**, 529. Metabolism of alcohol and of fusel alcohols by rat esophagus.

Craddock, V.M. (1991) In: *Alcoholism: A Molecular Perspective.* (T.N. Palmer ed.). New York: Plenum Press, pp. 283–287. Metabolism of ethanol and of higher alcohols present in alcoholic drinks and their corresponding aldehydes in subcellular components of rat esophageal mucosa, and relevance for esophageal cancer in man.

Craddock, V.M. and Henderson, A.R. (1991) In: *Relevance to Human Cancer of N-Nitroso Compounds, Tobacco Smoke and Mycotoxins* (O'Neill, T.K., Chen, J.

and Bartsch, H. eds.). Lyon: IARC Press, pp. 564–567. Potent inhibition of oesophageal metabolism of *N*-nitrosomethylbenzylamine, an oesophageal carcinogen, by higher alcohols present in alcoholic beverages.

Cunningham, H.M. and Pontefract, R. (1971) *Nature* 232, 332–333. Asbestos fibres in beverages and drinking water.

Day, N.E., Munoz, N. and Ghadirian, P. (1982) In: *Epidemiology of Cancer of the Digestive Tract* (Correa, P. and Haenszel, W. eds.). Dordrecht: Martinus Nijhoff, pp. 21–57. Epidemiology of esophageal cancer: a review.

Dean, G., MacLennan, R., McLoughlin, H. and Shelley, E. (1979) *Br J. Cancer* 40, 581–589. Causes of death in blue collar workers at a Dublin brewery 1954–1973.

DeCarli, L.M. and Lieber, C.S. (1967) *J. Nutr.* 91, 331–336. Fatty liver in the rat after prolonged intake of ethanol with a nutritionally adequate new liquid diet.

Deitrich, R.A. (1966) *Biochem. Pharmacol.* 15, 1911–1922. Tissue and subcellular distribution of mammalian aldehyde oxidizing capacity.

DeMeester, T.R. (1984) In: *Disorders of the Esophagus* (Watson, A. and Cestin, L.R. eds.). London: Pitman, pp. 73–93. Pathophysiology of gastroesophageal reflux.

Ding, X., Koop, D.R., Crump, B.L. and Coon, M.J. (1986) *Mol. Pharmacol.* 30, 370–378. Immunochemical identification of cytochrome P-450 isozyme 3a in rabbit nasal and kidney microsomes and evidence for differential induction by alcohol.

Engan, S. (1981) In: *Brewing Science*, vol 2. (Pollock, J.R.A. ed.). New York: Academic Press, pp. 93–165. Beer composition: volatile substances.

Eriksson, C.J.P. (1987) *Mutation Res.* 186, 235–240. Human acetaldehyde levels: aspects of current interest.

Farinati, F., Zhou, Z., Bellah, J., Lieber, C.S. and Garro, A.J. (1985) *Drug Metab. Dispos.* 13, 210–214. Effect of chronic ethanol consumption on activation of nitrosopyrrolidine to a mutagen by upper alimentary tract, lung and hepatic tissue.

Francheschi, S., Talamini, R., Barra, S., Baron, A.E., Negri, E., Bidoli, E., Serraino, D. and La Vecchia, C. (1990) *Cancer Res.* 50, 6502–6507. Smoking and drinking in relation to cancers of the oral cavity, pharynx, larynx and esophagus in northern Italy.

Furihata, C., Yamakoshi, A. and Matsushima, T. (1988) *Jpn. J. Cancer Res.* 79, 917–920. Induction of ornithine decarboxylase and DNA synthesis in rat stomach mucosa by formaldehyde.

Gabrial, G.N., Schrager, T.F. and Newberne, P.M. (1982) *J. Natl. Cancer Inst.* 68, 785–789. Zinc deficiency, alcohol and a retinoid: association with esophageal cancer in rats.

Gardner, M.J., Winter, P.D., Taylor, C.P. and Acheson, E.D. (1983) *Atlas of Cancer Mortality in England and Wales, 1968–1978.* Chichester: Wiley.

Garro, A.J., Seitz, H.K. and Lieber, C.S. (1981) *Cancer Res.* 41, 120–124. Enhancement of dimethylnitrosamine metabolism and activation to a mutagen following chronic ethanol consumption.

Gibel, von W. (1967) *Arch. Geschwulstforsch.* 30, 181–189. Experimentalle Untersuchungen zur Synkarzinogenes beim Osophaguskarzinom.

Gibel, von W., Wildner, G.P. and Lohs Kh. (1968) *Arch. Geschwulstforsch.* 32, 115–125. Carcinogenic and hepatotoxic action of fusel oils.

Gibel, von W. (1975) *Arch Geschwulstforsch* **45**, 19–24. Carcinogenicity of propanol, 2-methylpropanol and 3-methylbutanol.

Glass, G.B.J., Slomiany, B.L. and Slomiany, A. (1979) In: *Biochemistry and Pharmacology of Ethanol* (Majchracz, E. and Noble, E.P. eds.). New York: Plenum Press, pp. 551–586. Biochemical and pathological derangements of the gastrointestinal tract following acute and chronic ingestion of ethanol.

Goldberg, L. (1949) *Q. J. Stud. Alcohol* **10**, 279–288. Alcohol research in Sweden 1939–1948.

Griciute, L., Castegnaro, M. and Bereziat, J.C. (1981) *Cancer Lett.* **13**, 345–352. Influence of ethyl alcohol on carcinogenesis with dimethylnitrosamine.

Griciute, L., Castegnaro, M. and Bereziat, J.C. (1982) In: *N-Nitroso Compounds: Occurrence and Biological Effects*, IARC Scientific Publication No. 41 (Bartsch, H., O'Neill, I.K., Castegnaro, N., Okada, M. eds.). Lyon: IARC Press, pp. 643–648. Influence of ethyl alcohol on the carcinogenic activity of N-nitrosodipropylamine.

Griciute, L., Castegnaro, M., Bereziat, J.C. and Cabral, J.R.P. (1986) *Cancer Lett.* **31**, 267–275. Influence of ethyl alcohol on the carcinogenic activity of N-nitrosonornicotine.

Gudbjarnason, S. and Prasad, A.S. (1969) In: *Biochemical and Clinical Aspects of Alcohol Metabolism* (Sardesai, V.M. ed.). Springfield: C.C. Thomas, pp. 266–272. Cardiac metabolism in experimental alcoholism.

Guymon, J.F. and Heitz, J.E. (1952) *Food Technol.* **6**, 359–362. The fusel oil content of California wines.

Haas, J.F. and Schothenfeld, D. (1978) In: *Gastrointestinal Tract Cancer* (Lipkin, M. and Good, R.A. eds.). New York: Plenum Press, pp. 145–172. Epidemiology of esophageal cancer.

Habs, M. and Schmahl, D. (1981) *Hepatogastroenterology* **28**, 242–244. Inhibition of the hepatocarcinogenic activity of diethylnitrosamine by ethanol in rats.

Habs, M. and Schmahl, D. (1982) In: *Cancer of the Esophagus*, vol. 2 (Pfeffer, C.J. ed.). Boca Raton: CRC Press, pp. 229–239. Modifying factors of chemical carcinogenesis in the rat esophagus.

Haentjens, P., De Backer, A. and Willems, G. (1987) *Digestion* **37**, 184–192. Effect of an apple brandy from Normandy and of ethanol on epithelial cell proliferation in the esophagus of rats.

Haggard, H.W., Miller, D.P. and Greenberg, L.A. (1945) *J. Industr. Hyg.* **27**, 1–14. The amyl alcohols and their ketones: their metabolic fates and comparative toxicities.

Hamilton, S.R., Sohn, O.S. and Fiala, E.S. (1987) *Cancer Res.* **47**, 4305–4311. Effects of timing and quantity of chronic dietary ethanol consumption on azoxymethane-induced colonic carcinogenesis and azoxymethane metabolism in Fischer 344 rats.

Hellman, B. and Tjalve, H. (1986) *Acta Pharmacol. Toxicol.* **59**, 279–284. Effects of N-nitrosopyrrolidine and N-nitrosoproline on the incorporation of ^{3}H-thymidine into the DNA of various organs of the mouse: tissue specificity and effects of ethanol consumption.

Hirayama, T. (1979) *Nutr. Cancer* **1**, 67–81. Diet and cancer.

Hodgson, R.M., Wiessler, M. ad Kleihues, P. (1980) *Carcinogenesis* **1**, 861–866. Preferential methylation of target organ DNA by the esophageal carcinogen *N*-nitrosomethylbenzylamine.

Hoffmann, D., Raineri, R., Hecht, S.S., Maronpot, R.R. and Wynder, E.L. (1975) *J. Natl. Cancer Inst.* **55**, 977–981. Effects of *N'*-nitrosonornicotine and *N'*-nitrosoanabasine in rats.

Hoffmann, D., Rivenson, A., Amin, S. and Hecht, S.S. (1984) *J. Cancer Res. Clin. Oncol.* **108**, 81–86. Dose–response study of carcinogenicity of tobacco-specific nirosamines in F-344 rats.

Hogan, W.J., de Andrade, S.R.V. and Winship, D.H. (1972) *J. Appl. Physiol.* **32**, 755–760. Ethanol-induced acute esophageal motor dysfunction.

Holmes, R.S., Courtney, Y.R. and Van de Berg, J.L. (1983*a*) *Alcohol Clin. Exp. Res.* **10**, 623–630. Alcohol dehydrogenase isozymes in baboons: tissue distribution, catalytic properties, and variant phenotypes in liver, kidney, stomach and testis.

Holmes, R.S. and Van de Berg, J.L. (1986*b*). *Exp. Eye Res.* **43**, 383–396. Ocular NAD-dependent alcohol dehydrogenase in the baboon.

Horie, A., Kohchi, S. and Kuratsune, M. (1965) *Jpn. J. Cancer Res.* **56**, 429–441. Carcinogenesis in the esophagus. II. Experimental production of esophageal cancer by administration of ethanolic solution of carcinogens.

Hough, J.S. and Stevens, R. (1961) *J. Inst. Brew.* **67**, 488–494. Beer flavour. IV. Factors affecting the production of fusel oil.

Hudson, J.R. and Stevens, R. (1960) *J. Inst. Brew.* **66**, 471–474. Beer flavour. II. Fusel oil content of some British beers.

Hurst, A. (1939) *Lancet* **i**, 621–626. Cancer of the alimentary tract. II. Carcinoma of the esophagus.

IARC Monographs on the evaluation of the carcinogenic risk of chemicals to humans 1982, vol. 29. Some Industrial Chemicals and Dyestuffs. Lyon: IACR, pp. 345–389. Formaldehyde.

IARC Monographs on the evaluation of the carcinogenic risk of chemicals to humans 1988, vol. 44. Lyon: IACR. Alcohol Drinking.

Iishi, H., Tatsuta, M., Baba, M. and Taniguchi, H. (1989) *Br. J. Cancer* **59**, 719–721. Promotion by ethanol of gastric carcinogenesis induced by *N*-methyl-*N'*-nitro-*N*-nitrosoguanidine in Wistar rats.

Jensen, O.M. (1979) *Int. J. Cancer* **23**, 454–463. Cancer morbidity and causes of death among Danish brewery workers.

Kahn, J.H. (1969) *J. Assoc. Anal. Chem.* **59**, 1166–1178. Compounds identified in whisky, wine, and beer: a tabulation.

Kamil, I.A., Smith, J.N. and Williams, R.T. (1953) *Biochem. J.*, **53**, 129–136. Studies in detoxication 46. Metabolism of aliphatic alcohols.

Kaufman, S.E. and Kaye, M.D. (1978) *Gut* **19**, 336–338. Induction of gastro-oesophageal reflux by alcohol.

Kemp, I., Boyle, P., Smans, M. and Muir, C. (1985) *Atlas of Cancer in Scotland 1975–1980. Incidence and epidemiological perspective.* IARC Scientific Publication No. 72. Lyon: IARC.

Keung, W.M. (1988) *Biochem. Biophys. Res. Com.* **156**, 38–45. A genuine specific alcohol dehydrogenase from hamster testis: isolation, characterization and developmental changes.

Klatsky, A.L., Friedman, G.D. and Siegelaub, A.B. (1981) *Ann. Intern. Med.* **95**, 139–145. Alcohol and mortality.

Kono, S., Ikeda, M., Tokudome, S., Nishizumi, M. and Kuratsune, M. (1986) *Int. J. Epidemoli.* **15**, 527–532. Alcohol and mortality: a cohort study of male Japanese physicians.

Koop, D.R., Morgan, E.T., Tarr, G.E. and Coon, M.J. (1982) *J. Biol. Chem.* **257**, 8472–8480. Purification and characterization of a unique isozyme of cytochrome P450 from liver microsomes of ethanol-treated rabbits.

Kouros, M., Monch, W., Reiffer, F.J. and Dehnen, W. (1983) *Carcinogenesis* **4**, 1081–1084. The influence of various factors on the methylation of DNA by the esophageal carcinogen *N*-nitrosomethylbenzylamine. I. The importance of alcohol.

Kraft, P.L. and Tannenbaum, S.R. (1980(1)) *Cancer Res.* **40**, 1921–1927. Distribution of *N*-nitrosomethylbenzylamine evaluated by whole-body autoradiography and densitometry.

Kraft, P.L., Skipper, P.L. and Tannenbaum, S.R. (1980(2)) *Cancer Res.* **40**, 2740–2742. *In vivo* metabolism and whole-blood clearance of *N*-nitroso-*N*-methylbenzylamine in the rat.

Kuratsune, M., Kohchi, S., Horie, A. and Nishizumi, M. (1971) *Jpn. J. Cancer Res.* **62**, 395–405. Test of alcoholic beverages and ethanol solutions for carcinogenicity and tumor-promoting activity.

Lamy, L. (1910) *Arch. Mal. Appar. Dig. Mal Nutr.* **4**, 451–475. Etude de statistique clinique de 131 cas de cancer de l'esophage et du cardia.

Lau, B.P.Y., Weber, D. and Page, B.D. (1987) *J. Chromatog.* **402**, 233–241. Gas chromatographic–mass spectometric determinations of ethyl carbamate in alcoholic beverages.

La Vecchia, C. and Negri, E. (1989) *Int. J. Cancer* **43**, 784–785. The role of alcohol in esophageal cancer in non-smokers, and of tobacco in non-drinkers.

Leake, C.D. and Silverman, M. (1971) In: *The Biology of Alcoholism*, vol. 1. *Biochemistry* (Kissin, B. and Begleiter, H., eds.). New York: Plenum Press, pp. 575–612. The chemistry of alcoholic beverages.

Leclerc, A., Brugere, J., Luce, D., Point, D. and Guenel, P. (1987) *Eur. J. Cancer Clin. Oncol.* **23**, 529–534. Type of alcoholic beverage and cancer of the upper respiratory and digestive tract.

Levi, F., DeCarli, A. and La Vecchia, C. (1988) *Rev. Epidemiol. Sante Publique* **36**, 15–25. Trends in cancer mortality in Switzerland, 1951–1984.

Li, D., Brady, J.F., Lee, M.J. and Yang, C.S. (1989) *Toxicol. Lett.* **45**, 141–147. Effect of 1,3-butanediol in rat liver microsomal NDMA demethylation and other monooxygenase activities.

Lieber, C.S. (1982*a*) In: *Medical Disorders of Alcoholism*, vol. XXII. Philadelphia: Saunders, pp. 1–42. Metabolism of ethanol.

Lieber, C.S. (1982*b*) In: *Medical Disorders of Alcoholism*, vol. XXII. Philadelphia: Saunders, pp. 43–64. Acetaldehyde and acetate.

Lieber, C.S. (1982*c*) *Medical Disorders of Alcoholism*, vol. XXII. Philadelphia: Saunders.

Lieber, C.S. and Shaw, S. (1982*d*) In: *Medical Disorders of Alcoholism*, vol. XXII. Philadelphia: Saunders, pp. 551–568. General nutritional status in the alcoholic, including disorders of minerals and vitamins.

164   *Alcohol and tobacco*

Lieber, C.S. (1983) *Pharmacol Biochem. Behav.* **18**, Suppl 1, 181–187. Microsomal ethanol oxidizing system MEOS: interaction with ethanol, drugs and carcinogens.

Lieber, C.S., Baraona, E., Leo, M.A. and Garro, A. (1987) *Mutation Res.* **186**, 201–233. Metabolism and metabolic effects of ethanol, including interaction with drugs, carcinogens and nutrition.

Mak, K.M., Leo, M.A. and Leiber, C.S. (1987) *Gastroenterology* **93**, 362–370. Effect of ethanol and vitamin A deficiency on epithelial cell proliferation and structure in the rat esophagus.

Martinez, I. (1969) *J. Natl. Cancer Inst.* **42**, 1069–1094. Factors associated with cancer of the esophagus, mouth and pharynx in Puerto Rico.

Masuda, Y., Mori, K., Hiroshata, T. and Kuratsune, M. (1966) *Jpn. J. Cancer Res.* **57**, 549–557. Carcinogenesis in the esophagus. III. Polycyclic aromatic hydrocarbons and phenols in whiskey.

Masui, T., Shirai, T., Takahashi, S., Mutai, M. and Furushima, S. (1988) *Carcinogenesis* **9**, 1918–1985. Summation of effect of uracil on two-stage and multiple models of urinary bladder carcinogenesis in F344 rats initiated by *N*-butyl-*N*-(4-hydroxybutyl)nitrosamine.

McCoy, G.D., Chen, C.B., Hecht, S.S. and McCoy, E.C. (1979) *Cancer Res.* **39**, 793–796. Enhanced metabolism and mutagenesis of nitrosopyrrolidine in liver fractions isolated from chronic ethanol-consuming hamsters.

McCoy, G.D., Tambane, P.C., Powchik, P. and Teague, C.A. (1981a) *Cancer Biochem. Biophys.* **5**, 219–227. Occurrence and distribution of ethanol metabolizing enzymes in hamster cheek pouch epithelium.

McCoy, G.D., Hecht, S.S., Katayama, S. and Wynder, E.L. (1981b) *Cancer Res.* **41**, 2849–2854. Differential effect of chronic ethanol consumption on the carcinogenicity of *N*-nitrosopyrrolidine and *N*-nitrosonornicotine in male Syrian Golden hamsters.

McCoy, G.D., Katayama, S., Young, R., Wyatt, M. and Hecht, S.S. (1982) In: *N-Nitroso Compounds: Occurrence and Biological Effects*. IACR Scientific Publication No. 41 (Bartsch, H., O'Neill, I.K., Castegnaro, N. and Okada, M. eds.). Lyon: IACR Press, pp. 635–642. Influence of chronic ethanol consumption on the metabolism and carcinogenicity of tobacco related nitrosamines.

McCoy, G.D., Hecht, S.S. and Furuya, K. (1986) *Cancer Lett.* **33**, 151–159. Effect of chronic ethanol consumption on the tumorigenicity of *N*-nitrosopyrrolidine in male Syrian golden hamsters.

McGee, H. (1984) *On Food and Cooking: The Science and Love of the Kitchen*, London: Allen and Unwin.

McGlashan, N.D., Bradshaw, E. and Harington, J.S. (1982) *Int. J. Cancer* **29**, 249–256. Cancer of the esophagus and the use of tobacco and alcoholic beverages in the Transkei.

Michoudet, C. and Baverel, G. (1987) *Febs Lett.* **216**, 113–117. Metabolism of acetaldehyde in human and baboon renal cortex.

Moller, H., Boyle, P., Maisonneuve, P., La Vecchia, C. and Jensen, O.M. (1990) *Cancer Causes Contr.* **1**, 181–188. Changing mortality from esophageal cancer in males in Denmark and other European countries, in relation to changing levels of alcohol consumption.

Morton, J.F. (1972) *Q. J. Crude Drug Res.* **12**, 1829–1841. Further association of plant tannins and human cancer.

Mufti, S.I., Slavagnini, M., Lieber, C.S. and Garro, A.J. (1988) *Biochem. Biophys. Res. Commun.* **152**, 423–431. Chronic ethanol consumption inhibits repair of dimethylnitrosamine-induced DNA alkylation.

Mufti, S.I., Becker, G. and Sipes, I.G. (1989) *Carcinogenesis* **10**, 303–309. Effect of chronic dietary ethanol consumption on the initiation and promotion of chemically-induced esophageal carcinogens in experimental rats.

Murphree, H.B., Greenberg, L.A. and Carroll, R.B. (1967) *Fed. Proc.* **26**, 1468–1473. Neuropharmacological effects of substances other than ethanol in alcoholic beverages.

Nebert, D.W., Adesnik, M., Coon, M.J., Estabrook, R.W., Gonzalez, F.J., Guengerich, F.P., Gunsalus, I.C., Johnson, E.F., Kemper, B., Levin, W., Phillips, I.R., Sato, R. and Waterman, M.R. (1987) *DNA* **6**, 1–11. The P450 gene superfamily: recommended nomenclature.

Newberne, P.M., Schrager, T. and Morarhan, S. (1983) *Fed. Proc.* **42/5**, Abstract No. 5958, 1308. Zinc deficiency, alcohol and esophageal cancer.

Nykanen, L. and Suomalainen, H. (1983) *Aroma of beer, wine and distilled alcoholic beverages.* Berlin: Academie-Verlag.

Obe, G. and Ristow, H. (1979) *Mutation Res.* **65**, 229–259. Mutagenic, carcinogenic and teratogenic effects of alcohol.

Obe, G. and Anderson, D. (1987) *Mutation Res.* **186**, 177–200. Genetic effects of ethanol.

O'Donovan, M.B. and Nevellie, L. (1966) *J. Sci. Food Agric.* **17**, 362–365. Kaffir corn malting and brewing studies. XV. The fusel oil content of Kaffir beer.

Oettle, A.G. (1967) *Natl. Cancer Inst. Monogr.* **25**, 111–131. Mortality from malignant neoplasms of the alimentary canal in whites, coloureds and Asians in South Africa, 1949–1958.

Ough, C.S. (1987) *Chem. Eng. News*, 5 January, 19–28. Chemicals used in making wine.

Pares, X. and Vallee, B.L. (1981) *Biochem. Biophys. Res. Comm.* **98**, 122–130. New human liver ADH forms with unique kinetic characteristics.

Pares, X., Farres, J. and Vallee, B.L. (1984) *Biochem. Biophys. Res. Comm.* **119**, 1047–1055. Organ specific alcohol metabolism: placental x-ADH.

Pares, X. (1991). In: *Alcoholism: A Molecular Perspective.* (T.N. Palmer ed.). New York: Plenum Press. Characterization of alcohol dehydrogenase isozymes.

Park, S.S., Ko, I.Y., Pattern, C., Yang, C.S. and Gelboin, H.V. (1986) *Biochem. Pharmacol.* **35**, 2855–2858. Monoclonal antibodies to ethanol-induced cytochrome P450 that inhibit aniline and nitrosamine metabolism.

Passmore, R. and Eastwood, M.A. (1986) *Davidson and Passmore's Human Nutrition and Dietetics.* Edinburgh: Churchill Livingstone, pp. 70–73. Alcohol.

Peng, R., Tu, Y.Y. and Yang, C.S. (1982) *Carcinogenesis* **3**, 1457–1461. The induction and competitive inhibition of a high affinity microsomal dimethylnitrosamine demethylase by ethanol.

Picheral, H. (1986) In: *Global Geocancerology, A World Geography of Human Cancers.* (Howe, G.M. ed.). Edinburgh: Churchill Livingstone, pp. 144–153. France.

Pietruszko, R. (1979) In: *Biochemistry and Pharmacology of Ethanol*, vol 1. (Majchrowicz, E. and Noble, E.P. eds.). New York: Penum Press, pp. 87–106. Nonethanolic substrates of alcohol dehydrogenase.

Postel, von W., Adam, L. and Jager, K.H. (1981) *Die Branntweinwirtschaft*, 121, 162–167. Herstellung und Zusammensetzung von Calvados.

Postel, von W., Adam, L. and Jager, K.H. (1983) *Die Branntweinwirtschaft*, 123, 414–420. Gaschromatographische Charakterisierung von Calvados.

Postel, W. and Adam, L. (1985) In: *Topics in Flavour Research*. (Berger, R., Nitz, S. and Schreier, P. eds.) Marzling-Hangenham: Eichhorn-Verlag, pp. 79–108. Quantitative determination of volatiles in distilled alcoholic beverages.

Pottern, L.M., Morris, L.E. Blot, J., Ziegler, R.G. and Fraumeni, J.F. (1981) *J. Natl. Cancer Inst.* 67, 777–783. Esophageal cancer among black men in Washington DC. I. Alcohol, tobacco and other risk factors.

Pour, P.M., Reber, H.A. and Stepan, K. (1983) *J. Natl. Cancer Inst.* 71, 1085–1087. Modification of pancreatic carcinogenesis in the hamster model. XII. Dose-related effect of ethanol.

Prakash, O. (1961) *Food and Drinks in Ancient India*. New Delhi: Munshi Ram Manohar.

Preussmann, R. and Stewart, B.W. (1984a) In: *Chemical Carcinogens*, vol. 2, ACS monograph 182 (Searle, C.E. ed.). San Diego: ACS Press, pp. 643–828. N-nitroso carcinogens.

Preussmann, R. and Eisenbrand, G. (1984b) In: *Chemical Carcinogens* vol. 2, ACS monograph 182 (Searle, C.E. ed.). San Diego: ACS Press, 829–868. N-nitroso carcinogens in the environment.

Robinson, J. (1988) *On the Demon Drink*. London: Mitchell Beazley.

Rose, A.H. (1977) *Economic Microbiology* vol. I. New York: Academic Press. Alcoholic beverages.

Rothman, K.J. (1980) *Prev. Med.* 9, 174–179. The proportion of cancer attributable to alcohol consumption.

Russell, R.M. (1980) *Am. J. Clin. Nutr.* 33, 2741–2749. Vitamin A and zinc metabolism in alcoholism.

Salo, J.A. (1983) *Scand. J. Gastroenterol.* 18, 713–721. Ethanol-induced mucosal injury in rabbit esophagus.

Sato, A., Yonekura, I., Asakawa, M., Nakahara, H., Nakajima, T., Ohta, S., Shirai, T. and Ito, N. (1986) *Jpn. J. Cancer Res.* 77, 125–130. Augmentation of ethanol-induced enhancement of dimethylnitrosamine and diethylnitrosamine metabolism by lowered carbohydrate intake.

Schmahl, D. (1976) *Cancer Lett.* 1, 215–218. Investigation on oesophageal carcinogenicity by methylphenylnitrosamine and ethyl alcohol in rats.

Schmidt, W. and De Lint, J. (1972) *Q. J. Stud. Alcohol* 33, 171–185. Causes of death in alcoholics.

Schoenberg, B.S., Bailar, J.C. and Fraumeni, J.R. (1971) *J. Natl. Cancer Inst.* 46, 63–73. Certain mortality patterns of esophageal cancer in the United States, 1930–67.

Schwarz, M., Appel, K.E., Schrank, D. and Kunz, W. (1980) *J. Cancer Res. Clin. Oncol.* 97, 233–240. Effect of ethanol on microsomal metabolism of dimethylnitrosamine.

Schweinsberg, F., Weissenberger, I., Bruckner, B., Schweinsberg, E., Burkle, V.,

Wittenberg, H. and Reinecke, H.J. (1984) In: *N-Nitroso Compounds, Occurrence, Biological Effects and Relevance to Human Cancer* (O'Neill, J.K., von Borstel, R.C., Miller, C.T., Long, J. and Bartsch, H. eds.). IARC Scientific Publication No. 57. Lyon: IARC, pp. 525–532. Effect of disulfiram on *N*-nitroso-*N*-methylbenzylamine metabolism. Biochemical aspects.

Schweinsberg, F., Danecki, S., Grotzke, J., von Karson, L. and Burke, V. (1986) *J. Cancer Res. Clin. Oncol.* **112**, 75–80. Modifying effects of disulfiram on DNA adduct formation and persistence of benzaldehyde in *N*-nitroso-*N*-methylbenzylamine-induced carcinogenesis in rats.

Segal, I., Reinach, S.G. and de Beer, M. (1988) *Br. J. Cancer* **58**, 681–686. Factors associated with esophageal cancer in Soweto, South Africa.

Seitz, H.K., Garro, A.J. and Leiber, C.S. (1981) *Eur. J. Clin. Invest.* **11**, 33–38. Enhanced pulmonary and intestinal activation of procarcinogens and mutagens after chronic ethanol consumption in the rat.

Seitz, H.K. (1985) *Drug Nutr. Interact.* **4**, 143–163. Alcohol effects in drug–nutrient interactions.

Seitz, H.K. and Simanowski, U.A. (1987) In: *Nutritional Toxicology*, vol. II (Hathcock, J.N. ed.). New York: Academic Press, pp. 63–103. Metabolic and nutritional effects of ethanol.

Shendrikova, I.A., Ermilov, V.B. and Dikum, P.P. (1984) *Cancer Lett.* **25**, 49–54. The influence of ethanol on synthesis of *N*-nitrosodimethylamine *in vivo* and *in vitro*.

Spiegelhalder, B., Eisenbrand, G. and Preussmann, R. (1982) In: *N-Nitroso Compounds: Occurrence and Biological Effects*. (Bartsch, H., O'Neill, I.K., Castegnaro, N. and Okada, M. eds.). IACR Scientific Publication No. 41. Lyon: IACR Press, pp. 443–449. Urinary excretion of *N*-nitrosamines in rats and humans.

Stocks, P. and Kay, M.N. (1933) *Ann. Eugen.* **5**, 227–280. A cooperative study of the habits, home life, dietary and family histories of 450 cancer patients and of an equal number of control patients. (Data from Registrar General's Dicennial Supplement for England and Wales 1921.)

Swann, P.F. (1982) *Banbury Report* 12, *Nitrosamines and Human Cancer*. Cold Spring Harbor: Cold Spring Harbor Laboratory, pp. 53–68. Metabolism of nitrosamines: observations on the effect of alcohol on nitrosamine metabolism and on human cancer.

Swann, P.F., Coe, A.M. and Mace, R. (1984) *Carcinogenesis* 5, 1337–1343. Ethanol and dimethyl-nitrosamine metabolism and disposition in the rat. Possible relevance to the influence of ethanol on human cancer incidence.

Swann, P.F., Graves, R.J. and Mace, R. (1987) *Mutation Res.* **186**, 261–267. Effect of ethanol on nitrosamine metabolism and distribution. Implications for the role of nitrosamines in human cancer and for the influence of alcohol consumption on cancer incidence.

Teschke, R., Hasumura, Y. and Lieber, C.S. (1975) *J. Biol. Chem.* **250**, 7397–7404. Hepatic microsomal alcohol oxidizing system. Affinity for methanol, ethanol, propanol and butanol.

Teschke, R., Hasumura, Y. and Lieber, C.S. (1976) *Arch. Biochem. Biophys.* **175**, 635–643. Hepatic ethanol metabolism: respective roles of alcohol dehydrogenase, the microsomal ethanol oxidizing system and catalase.

Tuyns, A.J. (1970) *Int. J. Cancer* **5**, 152–156. Cancer of the esophagus: further evidence of the relation to drinking habits in France.

Tuyns, A.J., Pequignot, G. and Jensen, O.M. (1977) *Bull. Cancer* **64**, 45–60. Le cancer de l'esophage en Ille-et-Vilaine en fonction des niveaux de consommation d'alcool et de tabac. Des risques qui se multiplient.

Tuyns, A.J., Pequignot, G. and Abbatucci, J.S. (1979) *Int. J. Cancer* **23**, 443–447. Oesophageal cancer and alcohol consumption: importance of type of beverage.

Tuyns, A.J. (1982) In: *Cancer of the Esophagus*, vol. 1 (Pfeiffer, C.J., ed.). Boca Raton: CRC Press, pp. 3–18. Epidemiology of esophageal cancer in France.

Tuyns, A.J. (1983a) *Int. J. Cancer* **32**, 443–444. Esophageal cancer in non-smoking drinkers and in non-drinking smokers.

Tuyns, A.J. (1983b) *Nutr. Cancer* **5**, 92–95. Sodium chloride and cancer of the digestive tract.

Tuyns, A.J., Riboli, E. and Doornbos, G. (1985) In: *Diet and Human Carcinogenesis* (Joossens, J.V., Hill, M.J. and Geboers, J. eds.). Amsterdam: Elsevier, pp. 71–79. Nutrition and cancer of the esophagus.

Tuyns, A.J., Riboli, E., Doornbos, G. and Pequigot, G. (1987) *Nutr. Cancer* **9**, 81–92. Diet and esophageal cancer in Calvados, France.

Ueng, T., Friedman, F.K., Miller, H., Park, S.S., Gelboin, H.V. and Alvares, A.P. (1987) *Biochem. Pharmacol.* **36**, 2689–2691. Studies on ethanol-inducible cytochrome P450 in rabbit liver, lungs and kidneys.

von Wartburg, J.P., Rothlisberger, M. and Eppenberger, H.M. (1961) *Helv. Med. Acta* **28**, 696–704. Inhibition of ethyl alcohol oxidation by fusel oils.

von Wartburg, J.P. (1971) In: *The Biology of Alcoholism*, vol. 1 (Kissin, B. and Begleiter, H., eds.). New York: Plenum Press, pp. 63–102. The metabolism of alcohols in normals and alcoholics: enzymes.

Waddell, W.J. and Marlowe, C. (1980) *Cancer Res.* **40**, 3518–3523. Localization of [^{14}C]nitrosonornicotine in tissues of the mouse.

Waddell, W.J. and Marlowe, C. (1983) *Science* **221**, 51–53. Inhibition by alcohols of the localization of radioactive nitrosonornicotine in sites of tumor formation.

Waddell, W.J., Marlowe, C. and Pierce, W.M. (1987) *Food Chem. Toxicol.* **25**, 527–531. Inhibition of the localization of urethane in mouse tissues by ethanol.

Warwick, G.P. and Harington, J.S. (1973) *Adv. Cancer Res.* **17**, 81–229. Some aspects of the epidemiology and etiology of esophageal cancer with particular emphasis on the Transkei, South Africa.

Webb, D.A. and Ingraham, J.L. (1963) *Adv. Appl. Microbiol.* **5**, 317–353. Fusel oil.

Wehman, H.J. and Plantholt, B.A. (1974) *Bull. Environ. Contam. Toxicol.* **11**, 267. Asbestos fibres in beverages. I. Gin.

Weinbeck, M. and Berges, W. (1981) *Clin. Gastroenterol.* **10**, 375–388. Oesophageal lesions in the alcoholic.

Weinbeck, M. and Berges, W. (1985) In: *Alcohol Related Diseases in Gastroenterology* (Seitz, H.K. and Kommerell, B. eds.). Berlin: Springer, pp. 361–375.

Weisburger, J.H., Jones, R.C., Barnes, W.S. and Pegg, A.E. (1989) *Jpn. J. Cancer Res.* **79**, 1304–1310. Mechanisms of differential strain sensitivity in gastric carcinogenesis.

Williams, A.A. (1974) *J. Inst. Brew.* **80**, 455–470. Flavour research in the cider industry.

Wilson, P. (1980) *Drinking in England and Wales*. London: HMSO (Office of Population Censuses and Surveys).

Wynder, E.L. and Bross, I.J. (1961) *Cancer* **14**, 389–413. A study of etiological factors in cancer of the esophagus.

Yang, C.G., Lipkin, M., Yang, K., Wang, C.Q., Li, J.Y., Yang, C.S., Winawer, S., Newmark, H., Blot, W.J. and Fraumeni, J.F. (1987) *J. Natl. Cancer Inst.* **79**, 1241–1246. Proliferation of esophageal epithelial cells among residents of Linxian, People's Republic of China.

Yu, M.C., Mo, C.C., Chong, W.X., Yeh, F.C. and Henderson, B.E. (1988*a*) *Cancer Res.* **48**, 1954–1959. Preserved foods and nasopharyngeal carcinoma: a case–control study in Guaigxi, China.

Yu, M.C., Garabrant, D.H., Peters, J.M. and Mack, T.M. (1988*b*) *Cancer Res.* **48**, 3843–3848. Tobacco, alcohol, diet, occupation and carcinoma of the esophagus.

Ziegler, R.G., Morris, L.E., Blot, W.J., Pottern, L.M., Hoover, R. and Fraumeni, J.F. (1981) *J. Natl. Cancer Inst.* **67**, 1199–1206. Esophageal cancer among black men in Washington DC. II. Role of nutrition.

Ziegler, R.G. (1986) *Cancer* **58**, 1942–1948. Alcohol–nutrient interactions in cancer etiology.

7

Plant products: phenolics, tannins, tea

Simple phenolics

Phenolics comprise a large complex group of compounds which occur in many fruits and vegetables, but are not found in food of animal origin. Often, as in the case of flavonoids, they occur in high concentrations, and are consumed in relatively large quantities. Many phenolics have therefore been tested for carcinogenesis, often with conflicting results. Reviews of the phenolic compounds which occur in plant foods have been published (Singleton 1981; Deshpande et al. 1984; Natori et al. 1987). As several phenolics occur in high concentrations in plant products which have been implicated in esophageal cancer, for example red wine, tea and bracken, they are very relevant to the etiology of the disease.

Simple phenolics occur as di- and tri-hydroxyphenols, usually as derivatives of cinnamic acid or benzoic acid (Fig. 7.1). One or more of the hydroxyl groups may be substituted, as with ferulic acid. Two or more monomeric phenols may condense together, as with the formation of ellagic acid from two molecules of gallic acid, and of chlorogenic acid from caffeic acid and a derivative of gallic acid (Fig. 7.2).

The flavonoids comprise a large family of phenolic plant pigments with chemical structures based on that of flavone or flavonol (Fig. 7.3). Commonly occurring derivatives consumed by man are catechin and anthocyanidin, both found more often in condensed forms as in tannins, and quercetin, which occurs mainly in the form of its glucoside, rutin (Fig. 7.4).

Occurrence

Simple phenolics have a ubiquitous distribution in the plant kingdom, and it is generally assumed that their main role is to protect the plant from disease agents, including fungi, bacteria and viruses. Thus the concentration of chlorogenic acid, the major phenolic compound in potato tubers, was shown to correlate with the resistance of the tuber to fungal diseases (Friend 1979). As the chemicals are toxic to microorganisms, it is not surprising that they should have an effect on mammalian systems. The organs of the upper alimentary tract are especially likely to be affected, as they are exposed to the highest concentrations of chemicals originating in food.

Although phenolics occur in all parts of the plant, the concentrations reached are usually higher in the leaves than elsewhere. Thus the level of kaempferol and quercetin glycosides in tea leaves (variety unspecified) can reach an astonishing 10 g/kg, and the level of quercetin in certain onions can be as high as 65 g/kg (Herrmann 1976). However, an important

Fig. 7.1. Monomeric phenols and related compounds which occur in plants.

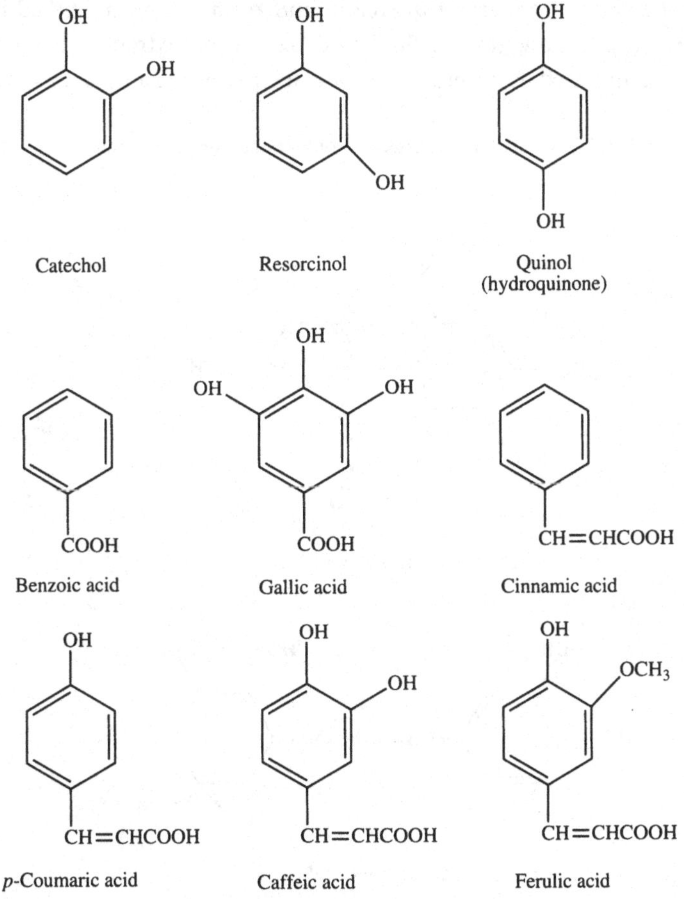

Catechol

Resorcinol

Quinol
(hydroquinone)

Benzoic acid

Gallic acid

Cinnamic acid

p-Coumaric acid

Caffeic acid

Ferulic acid

consideration is the fact that the phenolics rapidly become oxidized after the plant has been harvested, with the formation of quinones and hydroxyquinones, which then polymerize to form brown high molecular weight compounds. The concentrations of phenolics therefore decrease during storage and processing of the plant. Thus the high level of chlorogenic acid in fresh coffee beans decreases during roasting, grinding and storage.

The dietary items which have been implicated in esophageal cancer, and for which simple phenolics may be in part responsible for their carcinogenicity, are bracken fern (quercetin), alcoholic beverages, especially red wine (rutin), and tea (quercetin, kaempferol).

The mutagen quercetin occurs in many plants (for list of references see IACR 1983), including bracken fern (Pamukcu *et al.* 1980). As the leaves of this plant are a popular component of salads in Japan, a country with a high incidence of cancer of the upper alimentary tract, it has been in Japan that the carcinogenicity of quercetin and rutin has been studied in most detail. In addition, several flavonoid have been extracted from natural sources, and used as natural colouring agents. For example, in spite of the

Fig. 7.2. Dimeric phenolics commonly found in edible plants.

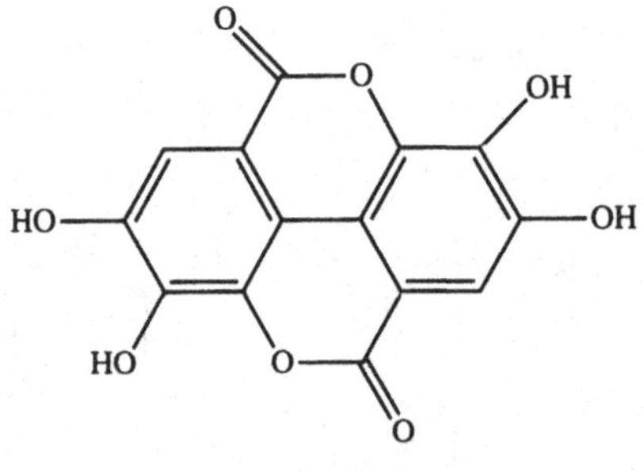

Ellagic acid

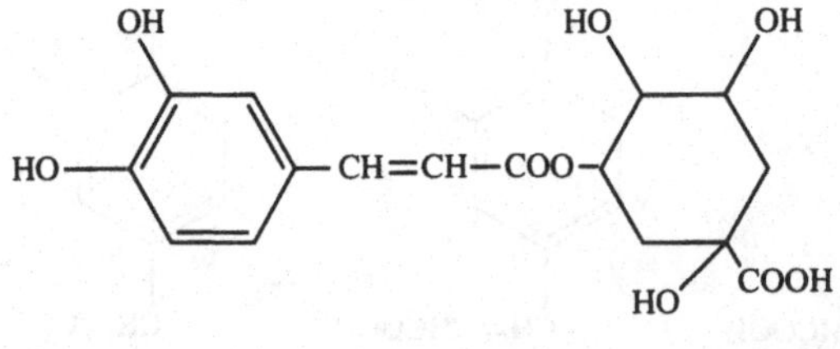

Chlorogenic acid

fact that quercetin is one of the most mutagenic flavonoids known, it has been used as a yellow dye for colouring food.

A large variety of simple phenolics occur in alcoholic beverages (for references see IACR 1988), but the concentrations do not appear to be especially high. The beverage with the greatest risk for esophageal cancer, the apple brandy calvados (see Chapter 6), does not appear to have an especially high content of phenolics, and in the case of spirits it is the fusel alcohols which occur in exceptionally high concentrations (Postel *et al.* 1981). Consumption of other beverages carries a lower risk, and it is with

Fig. 7.3. Basic flavonoid structures.

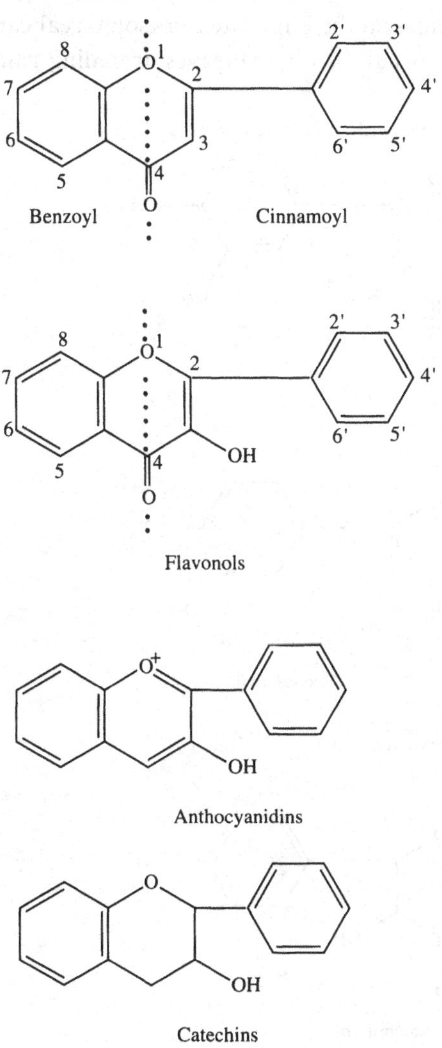

Benzoyl   Cinnamoyl

Flavonols

Anthocyanidins

Catechins

wines, especially red wines, where phenolics have been implicated in esophageal cancer (Yu *et al.* 1986). Simple phenolics occur in grapes, the levels are increased by the activity of yeast during fermentation, and also they may be extracted from the wood of the casks in which the wine is stored. Although the flavour of wines depends more on their tannin content, simple phenolics have been studied in relation to wine flavour (Singleton *et al.* 1976). The major simple phenolics in wine are caffeic and chlorogenic acids but others, for example ferulic acid, occur in appreciable amounts, the levels depending on the variety of the wine. The coloured flavonoids occur especially in red wine, where rutin has been shown to be the major pro-mutagen (Yu *et al.* 1986). It is the polymerized phenolics, however, which are more likely to be implicated in esophageal cancer.

Several simple phenolics occur also in tea leaves, including gallic acid,

Fig. 7.4. Examples of commonly occurring flavonols.

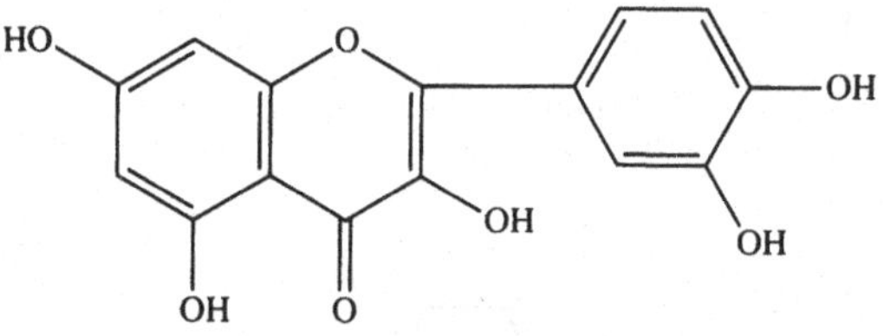

Quercetin

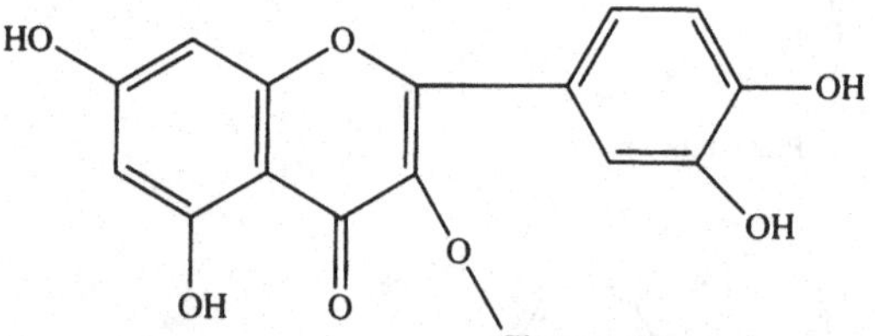

Glucose–rhamnose

Rutin
(quercetin glycoside)

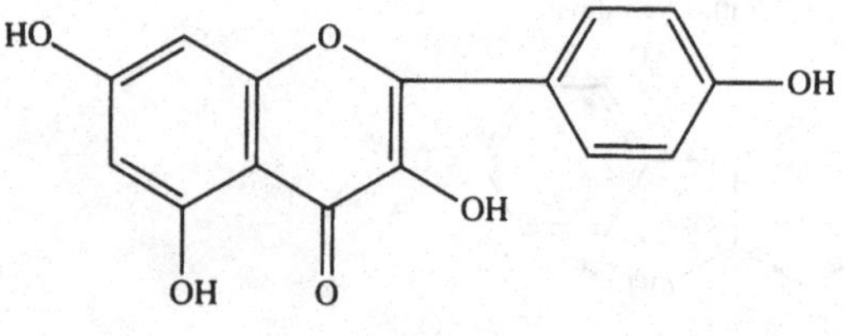

Kaempferol

chlorogenic acid and ellagic acid (Wickramasinghe 1978). However, it is the concentration of phenolics in the brewed tea rather than in the fresh leaves which is the significant factor in relation to esophageal cancer. The evidence suggests that the simple phenolics in tea may be protective rather than causative of esophageal cancer, and that, as with wine, it is the high molecular weight phenolics, the tannins, which are a cancer risk.

Carcinogenicity

The mutagenicity of quercetin was reported by Bjeldanes *et al.* (1976), and because of the widespread occurrence of flavonoids in food plants a large number of these compounds were investigated. Many were found to be potent mutagens when in the free state, but not in the form of their glycosides (Natori *et al.* 1987). Thus quercetin is a potent mutagen, while rutin, its glycoside, is only very weakly mutagenic, although its activity is increased in the presence of gut bacterial enzyme extracts. On the other hand, the clastogenic activity of quercetin is inhibited by liver homogenates. Tests for carcinogenicity could therefore depend largely on the exact nature of the animal system used, and the lack of unanimity in the results is not surprising. There is evidence both for and against the carcinogenicity of simple phenolics, and also there is evidence for a protective action against carcinogenic chemicals. Overall it is probable that the simple phenolics which occur widely in plant foods do not constitute a hazard in the amounts which are normally present, especially in view of the very effective detoxication mechanisms which exist in liver and to a smaller extent in other organs. However, the use of purified phenolics for cancer prevention is not justified at present.

An important consideration is the bioavailability of the compounds when fed in the diet. Thus simple phenolics such as caffeic acid are rapidly absorbed and excreted by animals and man, while with the more complex compound quercetin less than 1% of that consumed in the food was absorbed (Newmark 1984). In the case of chemicals which are poorly absorbed, their main action would be on the alimentary tract, with the highest concentrations reaching the mouth and esophagus.

The poor absorption of quercetin would seem to limit any carcinogenic effects to the alimentary canal. It was therefore of interest when Pamukcu *et al.* (1980) reported that quercetin fed in the diet induced intestinal and bladder cancers in Norwegian rats. Later experiments, on the other hand, found no evidence for carcinogenicity in AC1 rats (Hirono *et al.* 1981), in mice (Saito *et al.* 1980), or in hamsters (Morino *et al.* 1982). However, the possibility of the simple phenolics being carcinogenic for man, especially as regards the esophagus, arose with the discovery of the enzyme flavonol glycosidase in human saliva (Macdonald *et al.* 1983). It had been assumed that the potential mutagenic/carcinogenic activity of rutin would not be revealed until the chemical had passed down the alimentary canal as far as the colon, where it would be converted to quercetin by fecal glycosidases. The discovery of the presence of the enzyme in human saliva, however, led to the suggestion (Yu 1986) that rutin could be activated in the oral cavity and was therefore a possible carcinogen for human esophagus. It was established by Yu *et al.* (1986) that rutin is the major mutagen in red wine. There is therefore an urgent need to reassess the carcinogenicity of rutin/quercetin by determining whether the glycosylase occurs in the saliva of experimental animals and, if so, for testing the flavonoids in solution in drinking water. In this way the compounds would be free to react with proteins in the oral and esophageal mucosa, rather than with those in the food, and the situation would more closely reflect that existing during consumption of wine.

There is apparently little evidence that other simple phenolics are carcinogenic *per se*.

Effect on esophageal carcinogenicity of nitrosamines

Phenolics consumed in the diet could protect against or enhance the carcinogenicity of nitrosamines by altering their metabolic activation in the target tissue, by trapping and thereby inactivating the ultimate carcinogens formed by metabolism, or by inhibiting carcinogenesis at later stages during development or promotion.

There is evidence that two of the major simple phenolics present in tea, chlorogenic and ellagic acids, may be protective rather than carcinogenic. It was found that the chlorogenic acid reduces the cancer of the large intestine induced by methylazoxymethanol, the active principle of the Cycad nut (Mori *et al.* 1986). With reference to the esophagus, as mentioned in Chapter 5, ellagic acid fed in the diet reduced the incidence of tumors induced by NMBzA (Mandal *et al.* 1986), inhibited the metabolism and binding to DNA of *N*-nitroso-*N*-methylbenzylamine (NMBzA) in cultured rat esophagus (Mandal *et al.* 1988), and reduced the *in vivo* formation of O^6-methylguanine in esophageal DNA and the metabolism of NMBzA (Barch *et al.* 1988, 1989).

Little work has been done on the mechanism of the protective action of ellagic acid. It was shown that nitrosomethylurea-induced mutagenicity and methylation of DNA could be inhibited by ellagic acid (Dixit *et al.* 1986). The phenol reacted with double stranded DNA on the oxygen atom in guanine, preventing alkylation at this position, i.e. the site believed to be relevant in carcinogenesis, but there was less inhibition of methylation at the nitrogen-7 position. As the action of nitrosomethylurea is not dependent on its metabolic activation, the effects of NMBzA in esophagus could not be entirely due to the inhibition of metabolism described by Mandal *et al.* (1988) and by Barch *et al.* (1989).

In contrast to the possible protective action of dimeric phenols, the monomeric phenol, catechol, can have an adverse effect. In careful experiments in which animals injected with *N*-methyl-*N*-nitroso-amylamine were fed catechol in the diet, and were then killed in groups for up to 72 weeks, the catechol treatment was found to increase the number of esophageal papillomas (Mirvish *et al.* 1985). Similar experiments, in which administration of catechol in the diet was not begun until 1 week after the final injection of the nitrosamine, produced similar results (Yamaguchi *et al.* 1989). The promoting activity was related to the antioxidant nature of the catechol, rather than to the specific action of the phenol. Catechol is the most abundant phenol in cigarette smoke condensate (Mirvish *et al.* 1985), while the concentration of free catechol in plants is low.

Until the nature of the association between consumption of red wine, bracken and tea and cancer of the upper alimentary tract has been elucidated with certainty, it is impossible to say that simple phenolics are not involved. However, in view of the protective effect of consumption of fresh fruit and vegetables, it is difficult to see how compounds with a ubiquitous distribution in plants could present a significant hazard.

Tannins

Of all the naturally occurring phenolic compounds, the polymeric phenols or tannins are the most widely distributed and are the cause of most concern in animal and human nutrition. While simple phenolics, the monomeric and dimeric phenols, protect plants from microorganisms and molding, the more highly polymerized phenolics, on account of their bitter taste and astringency, are protective against browsing animals, birds and insects. Tannins react readily with proteins, and by reacting with the proteins in skin they cause it to become resistant to putrefaction, i.e. the skin is 'tanned' to form leather. Similarly, when present in food, tannins react with the proteins, inhibiting digestion, and reducing the availability of dietary protein for man and the efficiency of the feed for livestock. When tannins are consumed in solution, they react with proteins of the mucosa of the alimentary tract, causing cellular damage. Chronic damage and irritation could explain why certain food and drink items are associated with esophageal cancer. Tannins are therefore important factors in cancer etiology and in agriculture. Reviews of the subject have been published (Singleton 1981; Deshpande *et al.* 1984).

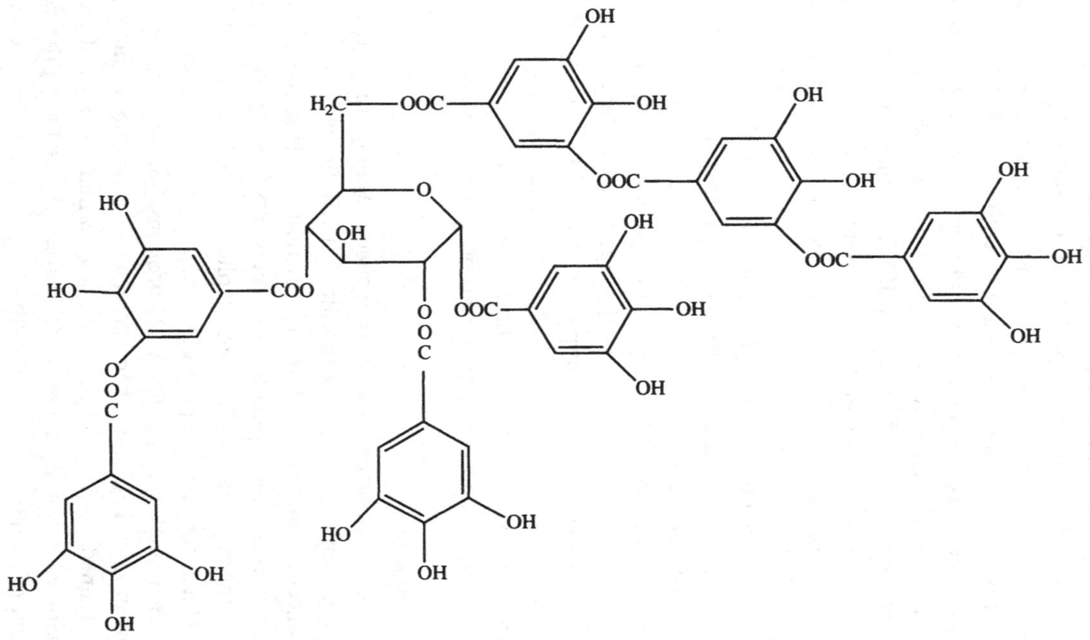

Fig. 7.5. Basic structure of a hydrolyzable tannin, gallotannin (tannic acid), composed of central glucose residue condensed with seven gallic acid residues.

Chemistry

Tannins are comprised of two groups of phenolics which differ in their chemical structure, distribution in plants, and biological properties. The hydrolyzable tannins are esters of sugars, usually glucose, with one or more phenolic carboxylic acid residues. The acid may be ellagic acid (ellagotannins) or gallic acid (gallotannins or tannic acid) (Fig. 7.5). The term tannic acid has frequently been used mistakenly as a general term for tannins, while it should more correctly refer only to hydrolyzable gallotannins (Singleton 1981). As these tannins are sugar esters, they are readily hydrolyzed by acids, bases and esterases.

The condensed tannins are polymers of various flavonoids (Figs. 7.6 and 7.7). They are also referred to as procyanidins, as on acid-catalyzed degradation they give rise to the plant pigment cyanidin. The condensed tannins are not easily hydrolyzed.

The most relevant property of the tannins with regard to esophageal cancer is the fact that polymers of more than a minimum molecular weight contain a sufficient number of hydroxyl groups to form stable cross-links with proteins. Hydrophobic binding is also involved in forming these complexes. The minimum molecular weight for protein precipitation is 350. For hydrolyzable tannins, this necessitates at least two phenolic acid residues, while for condensed tannins precipitation begins with dimeric flavonoids. Polymers with a molecular weight of more than 5000 are so insoluble in physiological solutions that they have little leather-forming capacity or astringent taste, and presumably cause less damage to the esophagus.

Occurrence

Condensed tannins are widely distributed in plant materials used for food. Most relevant in the current context is the fact that high concentrations occur in certain food items which have been associated with esophageal cancer, for example, cider, red wine, spirits and tea. Strong versions of these beverages may contain up to 1 g tannin/litre. Sorghum is another relevant food item. The high-tannin varieties are not related botanically, but can easily be distinguished on account of their brown colour.

The tannins present in human food are mainly of the condensed variety, as they occur in the fruits, seeds and leaves of higher plants. Hydrolyzable tannins are not often found in food, existing mainly in the bark and hardwood of certain trees. However, they can be leached from the wood of barrels used for storage or maturation of cider, wine and spirits.

Tannins account for the splendid colours of certain fruits. Thus apples

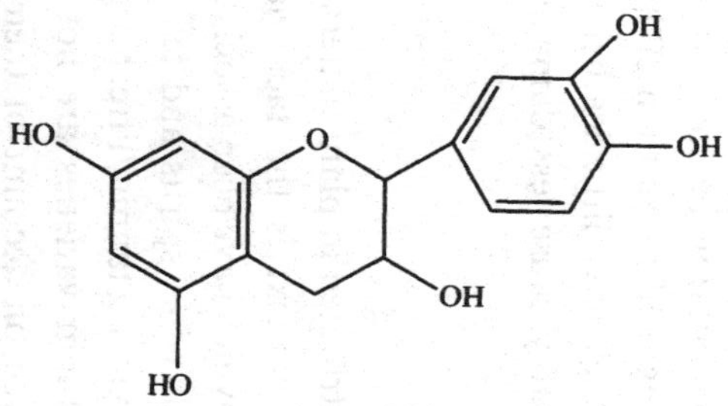

Catechin

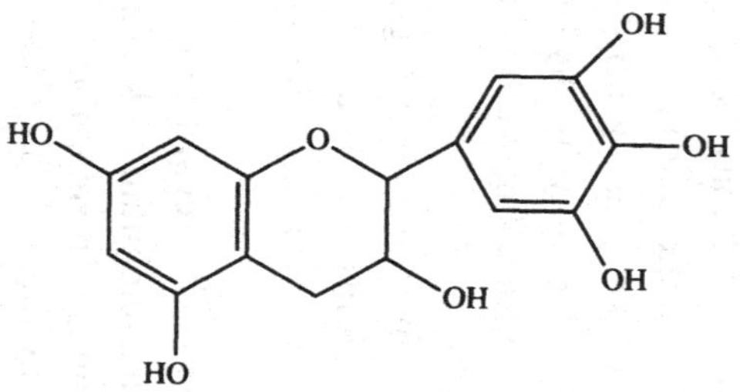

Gallocatechin

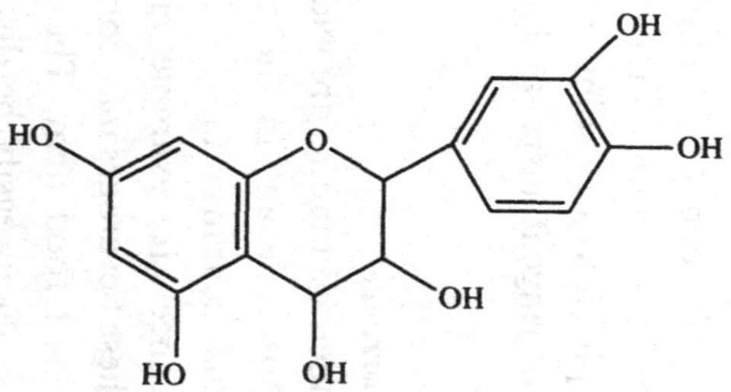

Leucocyanidin

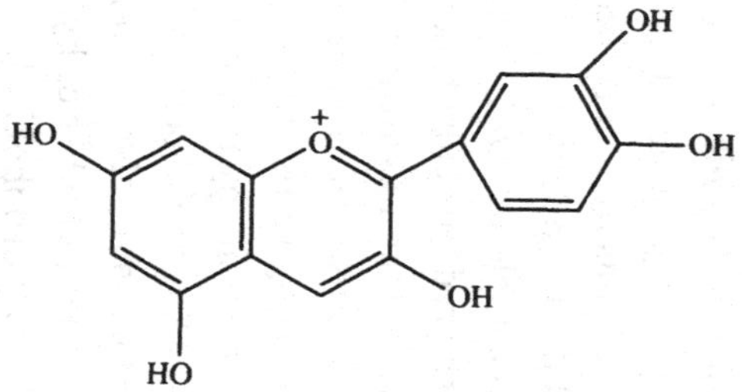

Cyanidin

Fig. 7.6. Components of condensed tannins.

used in the manufacture of cider are usually of the highly bird-resistant varieties, in which high tannin concentrations occur in the skin of the fruits. Extraction from the skin accounts for the high tannin content of cider. The tannins of red wine are also of the condensed variety, no hydrolyzable tannins having been detected (Singleton *et al.* 1969). Up to

Fig. 7.7. Basic structure of condensed tannins.

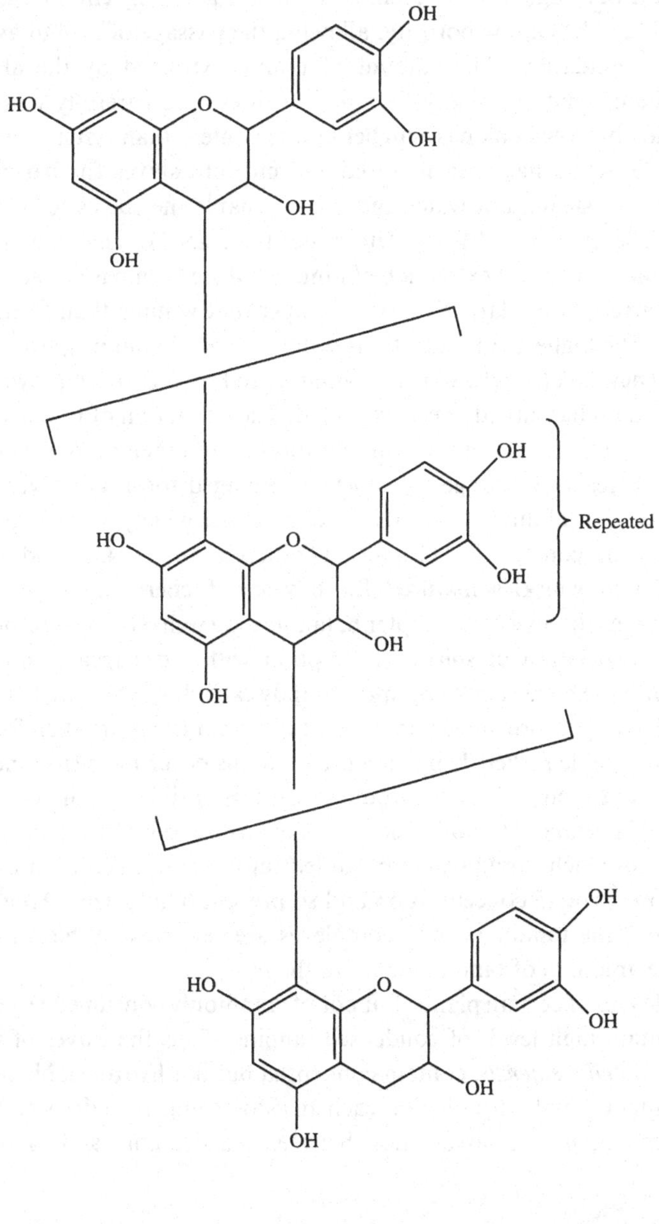

1 g/l anthocyanogenic tannins have been estimated (Singleton *et al.* 1976). With red wine, the tannins originate in the skin and pips of the grapes. If there is insufficient tannin present, the wine is flat and insipid, while if the concentration is too high the wine is harsh and rough. With white wines, the skin and pips are not included in the fermentation brew, and the tannin concentrations are therefore much lower.

In the case of spirits, tannins originate in the wood of the barrels in which the beverages are matured. Oak wood is generally employed, as this is tough and has a low porosity, allowing the passage of air but avoiding excessive oxidation. The amount of tannin extracted by the alcoholic beverage depends on many factors, and these are carefully controlled. Thus slowly grown oak has a higher tannin content than faster grown oak. When the wood has been matured and cut into staves for barrels, it is subjected to steam, hot water and fire, to enable the staves to be bent to shape. The duration of firing determines the extent of charring, and this affects the subsequent extraction of tannins. More tannin is extracted from small barrels with a larger surface area per unit volume than from larger barrels. The highest concentrations of tannins are found in spirits aged in charred new oak barrels. When previously used barrels are employed, most of the tannin has already been extracted. The extraction of tannins occurs rapidly during the first 4 years of maturation, and then more slowly for a total of 8 years of storage. Most spirits are aged for about 5 years. The tannin content of different spirits therefore varies widely, from 30 to about 500 mg/l in commercial brandies (Tolbert *et al.* 1943), and around 400 mg/l in whiskies matured for 8 years (Liebermann *et al.* 1949). However, as discussed in Chapter 6, tannins are unlikely to be responsible for the association of spirit consumption with esophageal cancer. The drink with the highest risk, the apple brandy calvados, is matured in barrels which have been previously used, and the tannin levels are therefore low.

Hydrolyzable rather than condensed tannins occur in spirits, and these tannins and their oxidation products are responsible for the colours of matured beverages. The other source of exposure to hydrolyzable tannins is beer, to which tannins may be added during manufacture in order to reduce the protein concentration and so prevent 'chill haze'. After 'chill-proofing', the tannin–protein complexes are removed by filtration, but variable amounts of tannin remain in the beer.

The leaves of certain plants, but not of commonly consumed vegetables, can contain high levels of condensed tannins. Thus the leaves of the tea plant, *Camellia sinensis*, contain condensed but not hydrolyzable tannins. The content of polyphenols can reach an astonishing 40 % dry weight, and may account for the association between tea drinking and esophageal cancer (see the section 'Human studies' below). On account of the high tannin content of oak leaves and acorns, their consumption has led to periodic losses of livestock.

Condensed tannins occur also in cereals and legumes, where bird-resistant varieties of sorghum, for example, can contain up to 7–8 % dry weight tannin. This may explain the apparent risk associated with consumption of the dark high-tannin varieties in contrast to the light low-tannin varieties (see the section 'Human studies'). No evidence was found for the presence of hydrolyzable tannins in sorghum.

Toxicity and carcinogenicity

While the tannins present in plants are beneficial to the plant in protecting it against disease or from being consumed, when the plant is harvested and used for animal feed or in the human diet the tannin content can be detrimental. In agriculture, the main concern is the lowering of the protein availability of the feed, with consequent reduction in growth rate of the animals. For man, damage to the alimentary canal is an as yet unproven but highly likely possibility.

Experimental work

During evolution, herbivores have developed the ability to tolerate low levels of tannins, while polyphenols are far more toxic to carnivores. As rodents in the wild often gnaw wood and are therefore exposed to high levels of tannins, rats and mice have evolved a protective mechanism. Tannins react most readily with proteins containing high levels of proline. In rats and mice, the submandibular and parotid salivary glands secrete proteins containing more than 40 % proline. When fed a diet with a high tannin content, the salivary glands enlarge, and the proteins secreted react with the tannins in the oral cavity and thus protect the mucosa (Mehansho *et al.* 1983, 1985*a*). This protective adaptation does not take place in hamsters, which are killed by dietary tannins at levels which have no deleterious effects on rats and mice (Mehansho *et al.* 1985*b*). Human saliva contains proline-rich proteins which give protection from low levels of dietary tannin. However, there is no evidence for enlargement of the salivary glands in people who consume high-tannin sorghums, red wine or tea.

In the early experimental tests for carcinogenicity, the techniques used were inappropriate, the tannins being administered mainly by sub-cutaneous or intravenous injection – routes very unlikely to be important in man. However, using these techniques it was shown that while hydro-lyzable and condensed tannins both produced injection-site sarcomas, only the hydrolyzable tannins were absorbed and reached the liver (Kirby 1960). Presumably the condensed tannins, being more tightly bound to the skin proteins, were not absorbed, and were less likely to reach remote sites. On the other hand, this local action would increase the likelihood of their causing damage to the mucosa of the oral cavity and esophagus after oral consumption. Evidence for hepatocarcinogenicity after oral administration of tannic acid to rats was reported (Korpassy 1959).

The astringent sensation produced by tannin solutions on the oral cavity and tongue was considered to be a result of protein precipitation and shrinkage of the tissue (Joslyn *et al.* 1964). Similar reactions could have occurred undetected in the esophagus. Gastritis, irritation and edema in the intestine as a result of chronic feeding of tannic acid and of oak tannins to experimental animals were reported (Singleton *et al.* 1969). The increased secretion of mucus by the intestine was evidently not sufficient to protect the mucosa from damage (Mitavila *et al.* 1977).

With reference to the esophagus, sloughing off of the mucosa, with edema and thickening of the crop, was found to occur in chicks fed a diet containing 5 % tannic acid (Vohra *et al.* 1966). However, it is the condensed catechin tannins which are more likely to be involved in esophageal cancer in man, and there are obvious difficulties in testing the esophageal carcinogenicity of tannins in animal experiments. Highly purified well-characterized samples of condensed tannins are not available in sufficient quantities for long-term feeding experiments. Extracts of plants with high tannin contents have been used, but other chemicals in addition to the tannins have been present in the extracts. In addition, the tannins have usually been administered in a solid diet, where they would have reacted first with proteins in the food. When given in drinking water, a situation which stimulates more closely consumption in wine, beer or tea, the tannins would come into contact with the 'bare' mucosa, and would be more likely to cause esophageal damage. Such experiments have apparently not yet been carried out.

Tannins were shown not to be mutagenic (Yu *et al.* 1987). It therefore seems probable that tannins are not initiators of carcinogenesis, reacting with DNA to produce a malignant cell, but could be co-carcinogens or promoters. On account of their reactivity with proteins, they denude the mucoproteins from the surface of the alimentary canal, and the resulting chronic irritation results in cellular damage and restorative hyperplasia. An increase in the rate of cell replication is known to increase the vulnerability of esophagus and other organs to carcinogens.

Human studies

The first evidence for hepatotoxicity of tannins appeared during World War II when, on account of its astringency, tannic acid was used in the treatment of burns. Early evidence for the esophageal carcinogenicity of tannins came from a series of fascinating field studies (Morton 1968, 1970, 1972, 1978, 1979), which accumulated persuasive circumstantial, if not statistically conclusive, evidence for the incrimination of condensed catechin tannins. Esophageal cancer was shown to be the most common type of malignant tumor for men and women in the Caribbean island of Curaçao in a 1936–60 survey, and again in 1960–5, when the crude incidence rate was 21:100000. Many factors had been studied and abandoned as possible causes of this remarkable situation. However, in Curaçao, herbal teas are widely used for self-medication and refreshment, and herb vendors do a flourishing trade with bundles of dried weeds in the herb markets. By contrast, in Aruba, an island a few kilometres distant, the use of home remedies is uncommon, the island has no herb market, and the incidence of esophageal cancer is unremarkable (Morton 1968). Extracts of the plants used in Curaçao were found to have a high content of catechin tannins.

The situation in Curaçao was followed up by comparison with plant usage in other areas of the world with high rates of esophageal cancer. In the Transkei and in India, the cancer was associated with the intake of dark sorghum, either by direct consumption or after its use in the production of beer. Dark sorghum, in contrast to the light variety, is known to have a high tannin content. In China and Japan the disease was associated with use as herbs of smartweeds (genus *Polygonum*), plants known to have skin-irritating properties on account of their high tannin content. Smartweeds were imported in large quantities into Iran, another country with a high incidence of esophageal cancer.

The high rates in certain regions of France were considered to be due to high consumption of red wines (Morton 1970). There is a regional pattern in the tannin contents of wines which are considered to be most desirable by the connoisseurs, and red Bordeaux, aged for 2–3 years in oak barrels, contains especially high levels. In northern Italy, an area with a high incidence of esophageal cancer, the wine is left standing in contact with seeds and skin of the grapes in order to increase the tannin content. In the USA, with lower cancer rates, procedures have been adopted to reduce the tannin content of wine, and the addition of dark tannins from the seeds is not permitted.

In northern France, the liquor industry is based not on grapes but on apples, and the varieties of apples used in the manufacture of cider are said to contain such high levels of tannin that they are inedible. The apple brandies prepared from the cider are aged in oak barrels (Morton 1972). In addition, perry is prepared from high-tannin pears.

As well as the herbal teas of Curaçao, manufactured black teas were also incriminated, especially when consumed in large quantities or without milk (Morton 1972). Thus in The Netherlands there is medical evidence that a high incidence of esophageal cancer existed in the eighteenth century. Around 1825, however, the increase in coffee production in the Dutch East Indies brought coffee within the reach of Dutch citizens. As coffee replaced tea as the national drink, the rate of esophageal cancer decreased. Coffee, in contrast to tea, does not contain catechin tannins, although it does contain caffeic and chlorogenic acids.

It is possible that tannin consumption in food and drink can give rise to cancer of the esophagus, but when inhaled it can cause nasopharyngeal cancer. Thus tannins inhaled in wood dust were considered to be responsible for the high rate of this form of cancer in woodworkers in the UK, France, Denmark and North Carolina (Morton 1979).

It is of interest that man is the only species which apparently enjoys the astringent sensation given by consumption of tannins. Although cattle in Curaçao and elsewhere were found to suffer from esophageal papillomas, goats in Curaçao and mountain gorillas in the Congo avoid the hazardous plants. In Wisconsin the deer do not graze on alder, and in Africa the birds do not eat the dark sorghums.

It was concluded by Morton (1978) that catechin tannins are hazardous whether consumed in commercial tea, herbal teas, dark sorghum, apple and grape products, or when extracted from oak wood. Probably the most widely consumed of these high-tannin plant products is tea.

Tea

In view of the carcinogenicity of tannins, and the fact that tea is the major source of the tannins consumed by man, tea has been for many years under suspicion as a cause of esophageal cancer. The fact that tea was being drunk in China before 350 AD, and that the 'gullet disease' has been known in China since antiquity, also suggests an association. A good deal of persuasive but not conclusive evidence has accumulated over the last few decades.

Tea is the most commonly consumed beverage world-wide after water. The drink originated in China, in mythology in about 3000 BC, but certainly around 350 AD, when the word 'T'e' appeared in a Chinese dictionary. Esophageal cancer was also described as the gullet disease in scrolls written around the same time. Previously the water used in the manufacture of tea was salted, as is still the custom in certain regions of the world, including Kashmir, another area with a high incidence of esophageal cancer. The first tea was brought to Europe by the Dutch around 1610, and had reached England by 1650 (Ukers *et al.* 1951).

The pleasant stimulating effects of tea are in part due to its caffeine content, but solutions of caffeine alone have an unpleasant bitter taste. Detailed studies of the phenolic compounds in manufactured tea have been carried out for many years (Roberts *et al.* 1959), and the distinctive taste and aroma of tea has been found to be due to interactions between caffeine and polyphenolics (Sanderson 1972). This explains why it is difficult to produce a satisfactory 'instant tea', as freeze-drying or spray-drying alters the chemical composition. The tannins present were soon found to have a deleterious effect on the mucous membrane of the mouth and alimentary canal, but at the time this was not considered to be important in view of the low concentrations which are normally present (Ukers *et al.* 1951).

Manufacture and composition

Chinese green teas and Indian black teas differ very considerably in composition. They are prepared from similar plants, strains of *Camellia sinensis*, but differ in methods of manufacture (Ukers *et al.* 1951; Sanderson 1976; Wickramasinge 1978). In the manufacture of black teas, the tea flush i.e. the three leaves at the top of the new shoot, is harvested, and a period of withering then allows partial drying of the leaves. This is followed by the rolling process, which breaks the leaf, gives it a characteristic twist, and enables endogenous enzymes (catechol oxidase and polyphenol oxidases) to come into contact with phenolic constituents. Oxidation and coupled oxidation reactions produce a range of products of molecular weight 700–40000. For example, catechin reacts with gallic acid to produce gallocatechins, which then give rise to the pigments of black tea, the thearubigins and theaflavins (Brown 1969).

Black teas are then fermented, usually on cool floors under damp cloths, and oxidation is allowed to continue until the leaves become bright red. Firing with hot air then prevents further fermentation, and also converts chlorophyll into the black pheophytin. The process also reduces the astringency of the final product, as the polyphenols in part combine with leaf protein and are inactivated (Wickramasinge 1978).

With green teas, the harvested shoots are steamed prior to maceration. This procedure inactivates the leaf enzymes, and so prevents the formation of tannins and pigments. Green teas therefore contain unoxidized phenolics which are present only in traces in black teas. Phenolics present in the tea flush include flavonols and glucosides especially quercetin, rutin and kaempferol, and phenolic acids, including gallic, chlorogenic and ellagic (Sanderson 1972).

The astringency of tea as consumed depends on the tannin content. When milk is added, proteins in the milk react with polyphenolics to form complexes. These do not precipitate, but form the familiar stable colloidal suspension. Astringency depends also on the duration of infusion, as the longer the leaves are in contact with boiling water the more extensive is the extraction of tannins. Thus a 1 minute infusion gives tea which is only slightly astringent even in the absence of milk, after a 3 minute infusion milk is necessary to prevent astringency, while a 5 minute infusion gives tea which is astringent even after the addition of milk (Sanderson *et al.* 1976).

When considering the incidence of esophageal cancer in relation to tea consumption, it is therefore very necessary to know the type of tea and details of the method of brewing used by the population under survey. Without this information the data are useless. Another source of confusion is the use of the term 'black tea', which to many people refers to tea without milk, while to others it means black as opposed to green tea.

Most of the tea made in China and Japan is of the green unfermented variety, while Indian and Ceylon teas are mainly fermented and therefore black. Indian and Ceylon teas are preferred in the UK, USA and Holland. In the USA, however, the use of tea bags is popular, and tea is often brewed for about 1 min. In the UK the use of tea pots is more popular, tea is brewed for 3–5 minutes, and larger quantities of tea are used per serving. Institutional teas, prepared for example in restaurants and canteens, also tend to be brewed for longer periods. UK tea is therefore more likely to be hazardous than that consumed in the USA.

Association with cancer

For many years the UK has had the reputation of having the highest consumption of tea world-wide (Ukers *et al.* 1951). In the 1900s, Russia came second, but by 1939 the UK consumption at 9 lb per capita per year was far above Russia's 0.2 lb per capita per year. With USA annual consumption at 0.7 lb per capita and France at 0.07 lb per capita, tea consumption obviously is not correlated with the incidence of esophageal cancer. However, it was noted that Ireland, with an exceptionally high incidence of esophageal cancer, especially in women, has a high consumption of tea (Bokuchava 1960).

Some of the first attempts to study tea consumption in relation to esophageal cancer were carried out by Morton (1968, 1970, 1972, 1978,

1979) as discussed in the previous section relating to tannins. An early study in Japan (Segi 1975) showed that the mortality rate from esophageal cancer for males correlated closely with the consumption of tea gruels. To prepare the gruel, tea leaves are packed in pouches, water and rice are added, and the mixture is boiled. The gruel is eaten usually at burning hot temperatures. It was suggested that the high temperature of the gruel, its tannin content, and especially the increased reactivity of tannins at high temperature, could be involved. Other surveys have linked tea consumption with cancer of the pancreas (Kinlen *et al.* 1984), of the rectum (Heilbron *et al.* 1986), and of the stomach, lungs and kidneys (Kinlen *et al.* 1988), but as yet there appears to be no statistically validated epidemiological link with cancer of the esophagus.

Many surveys investigating the causes of esophageal cancer in high-incidence areas have included tea consumption in their observations, but in none is the incriminating evidence conclusive (IARC 1991). Thus bread and tea were found to be almost the sole components of the diet in high-incidence areas of Iran, but the cause could be the presence of a carcinogen in bread or tea, silica fibres in the flour, or the lack of fruit, vegetables or animal protein (Nadim *et al.* 1986). High tea consumption was linked to esophageal cancer in the Caspian littoral region of Iran by Ghaderian (1987), and in Bombay by Notani (1987). In China, however, tea did not appear to be a risk factor in the high-incidence areas (Li 1989). Here the population was found to have a low intake of any type of fluid, and it was pointed out that high rates of esophageal cancer often occurred in arid regions of the world where fluid intake was likely to be low.

The importance of temperature

An important question which has arisen in many of these surveys is the relevance of the temperature at which the tea is consumed. In high-risk populations the beverage is often drunk while 'burning hot'. The heat could damage the esophagus by direct thermal injury (Yioris *et al.* 1984), or by increasing the reactivity of tannins in the tea. In view of the early onset of precursor lesions, the incidence of chronic esophagitis was studied among high-risk adolescents, selected on the basis of having a first-degree relative with esophageal cancer (Wahreindorf *et al.* 1989). It was found that the occurrence of chronic esophagitis correlated with consumption of very hot tea, but also with infrequent consumption of fresh fruit and of any dietary staple other than maize.

Studies specifically designed to test the importance of temperature were carried out among drinkers of Paraguayan or Brazilian tea, or maté. This tea is prepared from the dried leaves of the shrub, *Ilex paraguayensis.*

Natives climb the trees and cut off the leafy branches. The leaves are then allowed to wither and dried slowly, during which time fermentation takes place, with condensation of phenolics and production of tannins. To brew the tea, leaves are placed in a hollow gourd, boiling water and possibly sugar, milk or lemon juice are added, and the liquid is drunk through a tube of metal or reed. The tea therefore does not come into contact with the oral cavity but reaches the posterior part of the tongue directly and is swallowed. Maté can therefore be consumed at temperatures which could not be tolerated if it was drunk in the usual way. Areas of South America where the tea is consumed show a high incidence of esophageal cancer.

An initial case–control study carried out in Uruguay suggested that maté was a risk factor (Vassallo *et al.* 1985). A detailed survey in southern Brazil, on the other hand, revealed the main risk factors to be consumption of alcohol, mainly distilled cane spirits, tobacco smoking, and rural residence, while maté caused only a relatively small increase in risk (Victora *et al.* 1987). Maté drinkers, however, were more likely to develop esophagitis than were non-maté drinkers (Munoz *et al.* 1987), and it is possible that for this reason maté increased the effect of alcohol and tobacco smoking. Further work in Uruguay confirmed the initial observation of a strong association between esophageal cancer and the amount of maté consumed (De Stefani *et al.* 1990). Further work aimed at clarifying the importance of the high temperature at which maté is drunk is being carried out in Paraguay, where the habit of maté drinking is widespread but the beverage is consumed cold, and the incidence of esophageal cancer is lower than in Brazil and Uruguay.

Experimental studies

Surprisingly there are apparently no reports of work in which the carcinogenicity of tea infusions given in the drinking water have been tested in experimental animals. Probably the use of hamsters would be more appropriate than that of rats, as tannin exposure in hamsters does not produce an adaptive increase in size of the salivary glands. Tannin-containing fractions of the tea plant *Camellia sinensis* were found to produce injection-site tumors when given subcutaneously to rats (Kapadia *et al.* 1976), but this type of tumor is not good evidence for carcinogenicity, especially in relation to the esophagus.

Black and green teas were found to be strongly mutagenic in the Ames *Salmonella* test (Nagao *et al.* 1979), the mutagenicity of one cup of tea being greater than that of the smoke condensate of one cigarette. The activity was shown to be due to a variety of constituents, including quercetin, kaempferol (Uyeta *et al.* 1981), hydrogen peroxide, methylglyoxal, caffeic acid and chlorogenic acid (Ariza *et al*. 1988). As already mentioned, the tannins, the components more likely to be implicated in esophageal cancer, have been shown not to be mutagenic (Yu 1987).

In view of the complex composition of tea infusions, and of the nature of the evidence incriminating tea as an esophageal carcinogen, it is not surprising that evidence exists also for a protective effect. Thus it has been shown that extracts of black, green and persimmon teas can exert anti-mutagenic effects (Nakamura *et al*. 1986). In keeping with this it was shown recently (Han *et al*. 1989) that treatment of rats with tea given in the drinking water reduced the esophageal carcinogenicity caused by intubation of *N*-nitrosomethylbenzylamine, or of its precursors, methyl-benzylamine and nitrite. The mechanisms involved in this interesting observation have not yet been elucidated.

In summary, as concluded by the IARC report (1991), there is inadequate evidence for the carcinogenicity in humans of tea drinking, or for the carcinogenicity of tea in experimental animals. With reference to maté, IARC concluded that there was limited evidence for the car-cinogenicity of hot maté drinking, and that hot maté drinking is probably carcinogenic to humans. A plausible concept is that nitrosamines, in view of the ubiquitous human exposure, are responsible for the initiation of esophageal cancer. As DNA damage is repaired only very slowly in the esophagus (Craddock *et al*. 1986), the potentially malignant initiated cells could lie quiescent until stimulated to replicate. Damage to the esophagus, caused by consumption of the tannins in tea or maté, especially when swallowed at high temperature, could damage the mucosa, induce restorative hyperplasia, and thereby act as a potent potentiating factor.

References

Ariza, R.R., Dorado, G., Barbancho, M. and Pueyo, C. (1988) *Mutation Res.* **201**, 89–96. Studies of the causes of direct-acting mutagenicity in coffee and tea using the ara test in *Salmonella typhimurium*.

Barch, D.H. and Fox, C. C. (1988) *Cancer Res.* **48**, 7088–7092. Selective inhibition of *N*-methylbenzylnitrosamine-induced formation of esophageal O^6-methy-lguanine by dietary ellagic acid.

Barch, D.H. and Fox, C.C. (1989) *Cancer Lett.* **44**, 39–44. Dietary ellagic acid reduces the esophageal microsomal metabolism of methylbenzylnitrosamine.

Bjeldanes, L.F. and Chang, G.W. (1977) *Science* **197**, 577–578. Mutagenic activity of quercetin and related compounds.

Bokuchava, M.A. and Skolbeleva, N.I. (1980) *Crit. Rev. Food Sci. Nutr.* **12**, 303–370. The biochemistry and technology of tea manufacture.

Brown, A.G., Eyton, W.B., Holmes, A. and Ollis, W.D. (1969) *Nature* **221**, 742–744. Identification of the arubgins as polymeric proanthocyanidins.

Craddock, V.M. and Henderson, A.R. (1986) *J. Cancer Res. Clin. Oncol.* **111**,

192   *Phenolics, tannins, tea*

229–236. Effect of *N*-nitrosamines carcinogenic for oesophagus on O^6-alkyl-guanine-DNA-methyl transferase in rat oesophagus and liver.

Deshpande, S.S., Sathe, S.K. and Salunkhe, D.K. (1984) In: *Nutritional and Toxicological Aspects of Food Safety* (Friedman, M. ed.). New York: Plenum Press, pp. 457–495. Chemistry and safety of plant polyphenols.

DeStefani, E., Munoz, N., Esteve, J., Vassallo, A., Victora, C.G. and Teuchmann, S. (1990) *Cancer Res.* 50, 426–431. Maté drinking, alcohol, tobacco, diet and esophageal cancer in Uruguay.

Dixit, R. and Gold, B. (1986) *Proc. Natl. Acad. Sci.* 83, 8039–8034. Inhibition of nitrosomethylurea-induced mutagenicity and DNA methylation by ellagic acid.

Friend, J. (1979) In: *Biochemistry of Plant Phenolics. Recent advances in photochemistry*, vol. 12. New York: Plenum Press, pp. 557–588. Phenolic substances and plant disease.

Ghadirian, P. (1987) *Nutr. Cancer* 9, 147–157. Food habits of the people of the Caspian littoral of Iran in relation to esophageal cancer.

Han, C. and Xu, Y. (1989) IARC 10th international meeting on N-nitroso compounds, mycotoxins and tobacco smoke: relevance to human cancer, 69. The anticarcinogenic affect of Chinese tea by inhibiting the occurrence of esophageal tumor induced by *N*-nitrosomethylbenzylamine and blocking *N*-nitrosomethylbenzylamine formation.

Heilbrun, L.K., Nomura, A. and Stemmermann, G.N. (1986) *Br. J. Cancer* 54, 677–683. Black tea consumption and cancer risk: a prospective study.

Herrmann, K. (1976) *J. Food Technol.* 11, 433–448. Flavonols and flavones in food plants; a review.

Hirono, I., Ueno, I., Hosaka, S., Takanashi, H., Matushima, T., Sugimura, T. and Natori, S. (1981) *Cancer Lett.* 13, 15–21. Carcinogenicity examination of quercetin and rutin in AC1 rats.

International Agency for Research on Cancer (1983) *IARC monographs on the evaluation of carcinogenic risks to humans* 31, 213–229. Quercetin.

International Agency for Research on Cancer (1988) *IARC monographs on the evaluation of carcinogenic risks to humans* 44. Alcohol drinking.

International Agency for Research on Cancer (1991) *IARC monographs on the evaluation of carcinogenic risks to humans* 51, Coffee, tea, maté, methylxanthines and methylglyoxal.

Joslyn, M.A. and Goldstein, J.L. (1964) *Adv. Food Res.* 13, 179–217. Astringency of fruits and fruit products in relation to phenolic content.

Kapadea, G.J., Paul, B.D., Chung, E.B., Ghosh, B. and Pradhan, S.N. (1976) *J. Natl. Cancer Inst.* 57, 207–209. Carcinogenicity of *Camellia sinensis* (tea) and some tannin-containing folk medicinal herbs administered subcutaneously to rats.

Kinlen, L.J., Willows, A.N., Goldblatt, P. and Yudkin, J. (1988) *Br. J. Cancer* 58, 397–401. Tea consumption and cancer.

Kinlen, L.J. and McPherson, K. (1984) *Br. J. Cancer* 49, 93–96. Pancreas cancer and coffee and tea consumption: a case–control study.

Kirby, K.S. (1960) *Br. J. Cancer* 14, 147–150. Induction of cancer by tannin extracts.

Korpassy, B. (1959) *Cancer Res.* 19, 501–504. Hepatocarcinogenicity of tannic acid.

Li, J.Y., Ershow, A.G., Chen, Z.J., Wacholder, S., Li, G.Y., Guo, W., Li, B. and Blot, W.J. (1989) *Int. J. Cancer* **43**, 755–761. A case–control study of cancer of the esophagus and gastric cardia in Linxian.

Liebermann, A.J. and Scherl, B. (1949) *Ind. Eng. Chem.* **41**, 534–543. Changes in whisky while maturing.

Macdonald, I.A., Mader, J.A. and Bussard, R.G. (1983) *Mutation Res.* **122**, 95–102. The role of rutin and quercitrin in stimulating flavonol glycosidase activity by cultured cell-free microbial preparations of human feces and saliva.

Mandal, S., Shivapurkar, N., Superczynski, M. and Stoner, G.D. (1986) *Proc. Am. Assoc. Cancer Res.* Abstract no. 489. Inhibition of nitrosomethylbenzylamine-induced esophageal tumors in rats by ellagic acid.

Mandal, S., Shivapurkar, N.M., Galati, A.J. and Stoner, G.D. (1988) *Carcinogenesis* **9**, 1313–1316. Inhibition of nitrosomethylbenzylamine metabolism and DNA binding in cultured rat esophagus by ellagic acid.

Mehansho, H., Hagerman, A., Clements, S., Butler, L., Rogler, J. and Carlson, D.M. (1983) *Proc. Natl. Acad. Sci.* **80**, 3948–3952. Modulation of proline-rich protein biosynthesis in rat parotid glands by sorghums with high tannin levels.

Mehansho, H., Clements, S., Sheares, B., Smith, S. and Carlson, D.M. (1985*a*) *J. Biol. Chem.* **260**, 4418–4423. Induction of parotid-rich glycoprotein synthesis in mouse salivary glands by isoproterenol and by tannins.

Mehansho, H., Rogler, J., Butler, L. and Carlson, D.M. (1985*b*) *Fed. Proc.* **44**, Abstract no. 8463. An unusual growth-inhibiting effect of tannins on hamsters.

Mirvish, S.S., Salmasi, S., Lawson, T.A., Pour, P. and Sutherland, D. (1985) *J Natl. Cancer Inst.* **74**, 1283–1290. Test of catechol, tannic acid, *Bidens pilosa*, croton oil, and phorbol for cocarcinogenesis of esophageal tumors induced in rats by methyl-*n*-amylnitrosamine.

Mitavila, S., Lacombe, C., Carrera, G. and Derache, R. (1977) *J. Nutr.* **107**, 2113–2121. Tannic acid and oxidized tannic acid on the functional state of rat intestinal epithelium.

Mori, H., Tanaka, T., Shima, H., Kuniyasu, T. and Takahashi, M. (1986) *Cancer Lett.* **30**, 49–54. Inhibitory effect of chlorogenic acid on methylazoxymethanol-acetate-induced carcinogenesis in large intestine and liver of hamsters.

Morino, K., Matsukura, N., Kawachi, T., Ohgaki, H., Sugimura, T. and Hirono, I. (1982) *Carcinogenesis* 3, 93–97. Carcinogenicity test of quercetin and rutin in golden hamsters by oral administration.

Morton, J.F. (1968) *Cancer Res.* **28**, 2268–2271. Plants associated with esophageal cancer cases in Curaçao.

Morton, J.F. (1970) *Econ. Bot.* **24**, 217–226. Tentative correlations of plant usage and esophageal cancer zones.

Morton, J.F. (1972) *Q. J. Crude Drug Res.* **12**, 1829–1841. Further association of plant tannins and human cancer.

Morton, J.F. (1978) *Econ. Bot.* **32**, 11–118. Economic botany in epidemiology.

Morton, J.F. (1979) *Recent Adv. Phytochem.* **14**, 53–73. Search for carcinogenic principles.

Munoz, N., Victora, C.G., Crespi, M., Saul, C., Braga, N.M. and Correa, P. (1987) *Int. J. Cancer* **39**, 708–709. Hot maté drinking and precancerous lesions of the oesophagus: an endoscopic survey in Southern Brazil.

194   *Phenolics, tannins, tea*

Nadim, A. and Nasseri, K. (1986) In: *Global Geocancerology* (Howe, G.M. ed.). Edinburgh: Churchill Livingstone, pp. 241–252. Iran.

Nagao, M., Takahashi, Y., Yamanaka, H. and Sugimura, T. (1979) *Mutation Res.* **68**, 101–106. Mutagens in coffee and tea.

Nakamura, Y., Shimoi, Y., Hara, Y. and Tomita, I. (1986) *Toxicol. Lett.* Suppl. **31**, P14–40. Crude extracts of tea may reduce carcinogenesis: catechins and *L*-ascorbic acid, as major ingredients of tea leaves, exert desmutagenic/antimutagenic and antipromotic effects.

Natori, S. and Ueno, I. (1987) In: *Bioactive Molecules*, vol. 2. Naturally occurring carcinogens of plant origin: toxicology, pathology and biochemistry (ed. Hirono, I). Amsterdam: Elsevier, pp. 53–84. Flavonoids: chemistry and distribution in plants.

Newmark, H.L. (1984) Nutr. Cancer **6**, 58–69. A hypothesis for dietary components as blocking agents of chemical carcinogenesis: plant phenolics and pyrrole pigments.

Notani, P.N. and Jayant, K. (1987) *Nutr. Cancer* **10**, 103–113. Role of diet in upper aerodigestive tract cancers.

Pamukcu, A.M., Yalciner, S., Hatcher, J.F. and Bryan, G.T. (1980) *Cancer Res.* **40**, 3468–3472. Quercetin, a rat intestinal and bladder carcinogen present in bracken fern (*Pteridium aquilinum*).

Postel, Von. W., Adam, L. and Jager, K.H. (1981) *Die Branntweinwirtschaft* 162–167. Herstellung und Zusammensetzung von Calvados.

Roberts, E.A.H. and Myers, M. (1959) *J. Sci Food Agric.* **10**, 167–172. The phenolic substances of manufactured tea. IV. Enzymic oxidations of individual substrates.

Saito, D., Shirai, A., Matsushima, T., Sugimura, T. and Hirono, I. (1980) Teratogenesis Carcinog. Mutagen. **1**, 213–221. Test for carcinogenicity of quercetin, a widely distributed mutagen in food.

Sanderson, G.W. (1972) *Recent Adv. Phytochem.* **5**, 247–316. Chemistry of tea and tea manufacturing.

Sanderson, G.W., Ranadive, A.S., Eisenberg, L.S., Farrell, F.J., Simons, R., Manley, C.H. and Coggon, P. (1976) In: *Phenolic, Sulfur and Nitrogen Compounds in Food Flavors.* ACS Symposium No. 26 (Charalambous, G. and Katz, I. eds.). Washington, D.C.: pp. 14–46. Contribution of polyphenolic compounds to the taste of tea.

Segi, M. (1975) *Gan No Rinsho* **66**, 199–202. Tea-gruel as a possible factor for cancer of the esophagus.

Singleton, V.L. and Kratzer, F.H. (1969) *J. Agric. Food Chem.* **17**, 497–512. Toxicity and related physiological activity of phenolic substances of plant origin.

Singleton, V.L. and Esau, P. (1969) *Phenolic Substances in Grapes and Wine, and their Significance.* Adv. Food Res. Suppl. 1. New York: Academic Press.

Singleton, V.L. and Noble, A.C. (1976) In: *Phenolic, Sulfur, and Nitrogen Compounds in Food Flavors.* ACS Symposium No. 26 (Charalambous, G. and Katz, I. eds.). Washington, DC.: ACS, pp. 47–70. Wine flavor and phenolic substances.

Singleton, V.L. (1981) *Adv. Food Res.* **27**, 149–242. Naturally occurring food toxicants: phenolic substances of plant origin common in foods.

Tolbert, N.E., Amerine, M.A. and Guymon, J.F. (1943) *Food Res.* **8**, 231–236. Studies with brandy. II. Tannin.

Ukers, W.H. and Prescott, S.C. (1951) In: *The Chemistry and Technology of Food and Food Products* (Jacobs, M.B. ed.). New York: Interscience, pp. 1656–1705. Coffee and tea.

Uyeta, M., Taue, S. and Mazaki, M. (1981) *Mutation Res.* **88**, 233–240. Mutagenicity of hydrolysates of tea infusions.

Vassallo, A., Correa, P., de Stefani, E., Cendan, M., Zavala, D., Chen, V., Carzoglio, J. and Deneo-Pelligrini, H. (1985) *J. Natl. Cancer Inst.* **75**, 1005–1009. Esophageal cancer in Uruguay: a case–control study.

Victora, C.G., Munoz, N., Day, N.E., Barcelos, L.B., Peccin, D.A. and Braga, N.M. (1987) *Int. J. Cancer* **39**, 710–716. Hot beverages and oesophageal cancer in Southern Brazil: a case–control study.

Vohra, P., Kratzer, F.H. and Joslyn, M.A. (1966) *Poultry Sci.* **45**, 135–142. The growth-depressing and toxic effects of tannins to chicks.

Wahrendorf, J., Chang-Claude, J., Liang, Q.S., Rei, Y.G., Munoz, N., Crespi, M., Raedsch, R., Thurnham, D. and Correa, P. (1989) *Lancet* **i**, 1239. Precursor lesions of oesophageal cancer in young people in a high-risk population in China.

Wickramasinghe, R.L. (1978) *Adv. Food Res.* **24**, 229–286. Tea.

Yamaguchi, S., Hirose, M., Fukushima, S., Hasegawa, R. and Ito, N. (1989) *Cancer Res.* **49**, 6015–6018. Modification by catechol and resorcinol of upper digestive tract carcinogenesis in rats treated with methyl-N-amylnitrosamine.

Yioris, N., Ivankovic, S. and Lehnert, T. (1984) *Oncology* **41**, 36–38. Effect of thermal injury on oral administration of N-methyl-N'-nitro-N-nitroso-guanidine on the development of esophageal tumors in Wistar rats.

Yu, C-L., Swaminathan, B., Butler, L.G. and Pratt, D.E. (1986) *Mutation Res.* **170**, 103–113. Isolation and identification of rutin as the major mutagen of red wine.

Yu, C-L. and Swaminathan, B. (1987) *Food Chem. Toxicol* **25**, 135–139. Mutagenicity of proanthocyanidins.

8

Plant products: opium, silica, bracken, dihydrosafrole

Opium

Opium usage is common in many regions of Asia, including localities where there is a high incidence of esophageal cancer. Consumption is especially high in countries where alcohol is forbidden for religious reasons, and opium is used as a substitute. The crude opium is smoked, and the smoked residues remaining in the pipe (opium dross or sukhteh) and refined pyrolysis products (shireh) are eaten. The pipe scrapings are much less expensive than opium or shireh, and are therefore used mostly by the poorer people, who also have the higher incidence of esophageal cancer. In addition to being used for pleasure, opium is used for the treatment of disease, for insomnia, as a painkiller, and to quiet crying babies.

With reference to esophageal cancer, opium usage has been studied mainly in north-east Iran. Although the use of opium in Iran was made illegal in 1955, the fact that morphine metabolites were detected in the urine of 50 % of the population over the age of 35 indicated that opium use continued to be very common in men and women in the areas studied (Joint Iran-IARC Study Group 1977).

Clinical studies of patients with esophageal cancer led to the suggestion that opium addiction was associated with the disease (Dowlatshahi et al. 1977). Black particles of burnt opium were often found in the esophageal mucosa of the patients. A Joint Iran–IARC Study Group (1977) also found evidence that the distribution of esophageal cancer in north-east Iran paralleled the use of opium. Later studies revealed a correlation in different regions between the incidence of esophageal cancer and the levels of urinary morphine metabolites (Ghadirian et al. 1985). Unfortunately these studies had to be abandoned on account of civil disturbances related to the Islamic revolution.

The evidence implicating opium in the etiology of esophageal cancer was not supported in other work. Thus surveys in Turkoman villages with a high incidence of esophageal cancer showed high levels of esophagitis in adults of all ages, but the levels were not higher in opium addicts than in the remainder of the population. If these lesions are a pre-malignant condition, this implies that opium may not be an important factor (Crespi *et al.* 1979). Surveys by Mahboubi *et al.* (1980) also led to the opinion that opium use in high-risk areas was no greater than elsewhere in Iran, and case–control studies implied that opium use did not explain the very high risk in certain areas. In addition, it was pointed out that the esophageal cancer rate was high in neighbouring Turkenistan, although opium had been scarce in that region for 60 years. It was concluded that the role of opium, if any, was very weak. The apparently conflicting results may be due in part to the fact that esophageal cancer would be related more to the consumption of sukhteh, which is swallowed, than to the opium, which is smoked.

Mechanism of carcinogenicity

Mutagenicity
One way in which opium could cause cancer is by direct genotoxic activity. The major alkaloid present in opium is morphine, but others include codeine, thebaine, papaverine, noscapine, narceine and sanguinarine (Malaveille *et al.* 1982). Morphine itself is not mutagenic, and this is in agreement with the fact that crude opium has not been shown to be a mutagen. The pyrolysis products which are consumed, however – the pipe residues or sukhteh, and the purified pyrolysis products, or shireh – were both found to be mutagenic in bacterial systems (Hewer *et al.* 1978). Morphine has a decomposition point of 250 °C, and its pyrolysis products have been studied after heating in air at 300–600 °C. Although the temperature in an opium pipe may be as high as 800–900 °C (Friesen *et al.* 1987), presumably some morphine must remain after the opium has been smoked under pipe conditions, or the pipe residues would not give the opioid sensations for which they are used.

The mutagenic pyrolysis products were shown to be heterocyclic aromatic amines and primary aromatic amines (Malaveille *et al.* 1982). Codeine on pyrolysis yielded products with only 1 % of the mutagenic activity of those produced by morphine.

The most abundant mutagens in opium pyrolysate have been characterized (Friesen *et al.* 1985, 1987). These previously unknown compounds all contained the phenanthrene ring and nitrogen. The most mutagenic component of the mixture is illustrated in Fig. 8.1. Opium and morphine pyrolysates transformed Syrian hamster embryo cells in culture, but carcinogenicity tests using intact animals were limited by the small amounts of pure samples which were available.

Further evidence for genotoxicity was given also by the discovery that opium pyrolysates induced sister chromatid exchange in human peripheral lymphocytes (Perry *et al.* 1983). The possibility that the aromatic amines are direct-acting carcinogens therefore merits further study.

Effect on esophageal motility
Opioid peptides, the enkephalins, occur in high concentrations in the myenteric plexus and lower esophageal sphincter, and enkephalin-containing processes have been found especially in the muscularis mucosa of the lower esophagus (Uddman *et al.* 1980; Rattan *et al.* 1983). The effect of morphine on motility of the esophagus was therefore studied, and it was shown that the alkaloid inhibits relaxation of the lower esophageal sphincter in man (Dowlatshahi *et al.* 1985). Papaverine, another alkaloid present in opium, had a direct inhibitory effect on esophageal peristalsis. Therefore opium, as a result of inhibition of relaxation of the sphincter and inhibition of peristalsis, would impede the passage of the contents of the esophagus into the stomach. The stasis caused by achalasia is known to result in inflammation of the lower end of the esophagus, and to be associated with risk of esophageal cancer (see the section Motility diseases in Chapter 3).

In contrast to this possible cancer-promoting activity, opioids have been shown to have inhibitory effects on cell growth (Maneckjee *et al.* 1990). The action of opium on cell replication in the esophagus merits study.

Effect on carcinogen metabolism
Opium dross can reduce the activity of hepatic mono-oxygenases in rodents (Ghadirian *et al.* 1985). The possibility exists that it could inhibit metabolism of nitrosamines in liver, so that the exposure of the esophagus to these carcinogens would be increased.

Conclusion
The evidence suggests that opium is very likely to be involved in the etiology of esophageal cancer in certain regions of the world, but it may well not be the only or even the major cause, even in areas where its use is extensive. In the high-risk regions of north-east Iran, the population consumes a very limited diet of bread and tea, and many families never eat fresh fruit and vegetables (Nadin *et al.* 1986). As a result, these people

could well be deficient in micronutrients, including riboflavin and zinc, each of which has been especially implicated in esophageal cancer. In addition, the bread of the region often contains biogenic silica fibres which cause damage to the esophagus (see next section). Opium is more likely to be effective in an esophagus already made especially vulnerable by other factors. The very high-risk cancer areas could therefore occur where several risk factors happen to co-exist.

Silica

It has been known for 200 years that Protozoa can make glass. Silica is the hardest material laid down in biological systems and for this reason it is made use of sporadically throughout the plant kingdom, but especially in primitive plants. It is used for strengthening and support in the cell walls of algae, protozoans and sponges, where microscopic examination has revealed the formation of intricate complex regular structures. More relevant to esophageal cancer, it is used in the form of sharp fibers and laminae as a protection against predators. While dicotyledonous plants use mainly chemical defense mechanisms, for example the bitter-tasting tannins (Chapter 7), monocotyledons are more primitive plants, and lack the complex biochemical systems involved. Instead, daggers of silica fibers make consumption of the plant a painful process.

Biogenic silica is especially important in grasses, which are a major food source only for grazing animals. Hence grasses and grazing animals have had an intimate evolutionary history since their simultaneous appearance in the Eocene. One hazard associated with consumption of plants containing silica fibers is mechanical abrasion of the dentine enamel.

Fig. 8.1. Pyrolysis of morphine to produce the hydroxyphenanthrene derivative with the highest mutagenicity in the *Salmonella typhimurium* TA 98 assay.

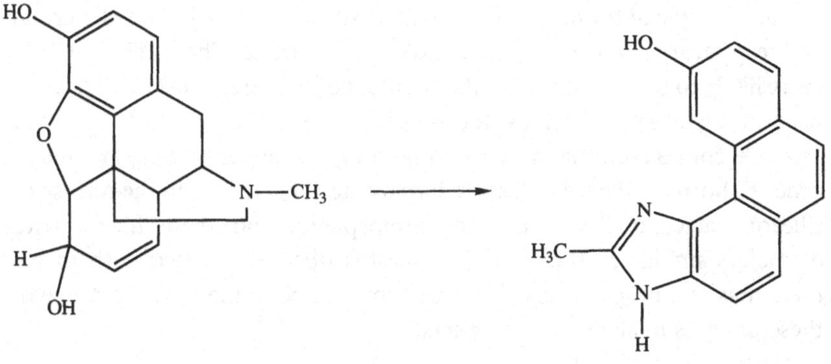

Morphine

2-Methyl-3H-phenanthrol[3,4-*d*]
imidazol-10-ol

Cattle, which tend to pull off tufts of grass, suffer less in this way than do sheep, which prefer to nibble. Animals responded to the silica in grass by developing hypsodont dentine, which is less affected by mechanical abrasion. The grasses responded by increasing their silica content. Thus plants exposed to the higher levels of herbivory, i.e. those growing on short-grass plains, have higher levels of leaf silica than those from locations with lower herbivore exposure. Both plants and animals make daily adaptations to the hazard presented by the other. Herbivores can discriminate between high- and low-silica plants, and will preferentially feed on the latter. Grasses have an inducible defense against herbivores, as is shown by the fact that blade silica is increased when the plants are defoliated (McNaughton *et al.* 1983). Man, however, has developed no means of defense, and apparently does not detect a hazard when, as often happens in certain regions of the world, plants with a high content of silica are eaten. One result is the penetration into the esophageal mucosa of sharp-pointed silica fibers.

Silicates absorbed from the soil are converted by the plant first into monosilicic acid, $Si(OH)_4$, which may precipitate as a form of opal. The acid is then polymerized to form the hydrated oxide, $SiO_2 \cdot nH_2O$, a form of glass. The shape of the particles is adapted to the site where they are found. They may take the form of sharp fibers, as in the hairs which occur on seeds of cereals and leaves of nettles. The hairs are hollow but are reinforced at the tip by a high concentration of silica. In bracken, *Pteridium aquilinum*, silica occurs in the form of laminae 500 μm long, 6 μm in width. Both the sharp-pointed fibers and the sharp-edged sheets have a high penetrating ability. This causes injury first to the nose and mouth of animals attempting to eat the grain (Bhatt *et al.* 1984). Injury is inflicted on man when these plants are handled or consumed, and trauma at the site of exposure causes a variety of health problems (Newman 1986).

One example of the hazard presented by silica is the conjunctival, dermal and respiratory diseases of grain handlers in Australia. These afflictions are more likely to be caused by the silica content of the cereal dust, with its high penetrating ability, than by the density of nondescript dust. Another example comes from the practice of igniting whole fields of sugar cane in order to burn off the leaves before harvesting. This results in the release of siliceous acicular fibers into the atmosphere, and these fibers, with diameters similar to those of the asbestos fibers associated with meso-theliomas and lung cancers, have been implicated in the high incidence of these diseases in sugar-cane workers.

Link with esophageal cancer

In cattle, there is good suggestive evidence associating the consumption of bracken, a plant with a high content of silica, with esophageal cancer in Brazil, Turkey and Scotland (Jarrett 1973; see following section). Bracken, however, is known to contain in addition several chemical carcinogens, and silica is more likely to act as a promoter of the carcinogenicity of these compounds than as the sole cause of esophageal cancer. Therefore it is difficult to obtain conclusive evidence for the role of silica in animals or in man, as additional risk factors are always present in the populations under study.

With reference to human cancer, silica has been implicated in each of the three areas of the world which have exceptionally high cancer rates: the Transkei, north-east Iran and northern China. In the Transkei, a variety of plants eaten by the Bantu contain high levels of silica. In north-east Iran and in northern China, it is the silica consumed in cereals which has been implicated.

The Transkei

As mentioned above, silica was known to occur in monocotyledonous species, notably the grasses, but it had not until recently been located extensively in dicotyledons. However, on account of their ability to promote esophageal cancer (Mirvish *et al.* 1985), certain plants consumed by the Bantu were examined, and herbaceous species of dicotyledons were found to contain high levels of biogenic silica (Parry *et al.* 1986). The plants included species of *Sonchus*, *Amaranthus*, *Bidens* and *Solanium*. The silica was found to occur in epidermal outgrowths or microhairs. As the plants are consumed as a porridge with maize and spinach, and the sharp fibers are not destroyed by cooking, they could well penetrate the esophageal mucosa during the passage of a bolus of food. Examination of the mucosa of esophageal cancer patients in the Transkei would be of much interest.

North-eastern Iran

In both north-east Iran and northern China, silica consumed in the cereals has been implicated in esophageal cancer. While in north-east Iran contamination of the wheat by grasses is the route of exposure, in northern China silica fibres are present in the millet bran which is consumed, and their presence in food is not due to the presence of a contaminant.

Consumption of bread containing silica is probably one of several factors which combine together to cause a high rate of esophageal cancer in the north-east littoral region of Iran. The staple diet of the region is bread and tea, but contamination of these major items by environmental carcinogens, including polycyclic aromatic hydrocarbons, nitrosamines and aflatoxin, was not considered to be important (Mahboubi *et al*. 1980). A significant factor seems to be that, in contrast to neighbouring regions with a low cancer incidence, people of the Caspian littoral eat bread instead of rice. The wholemeal flour from which the bread is made was found to contain seeds of the Mediterranean grass *Phalaris canariensis* (canary grass). This led to the contamination of the flour with silica fibers, up to levels of 3000 fibers per gram (O'Neill *et al*. 1980). Apparently the grass grows in the fields with the wheat, and the fruits are broken off and milled with the flour. When baked, this flour produces hard scratchy bread which damages the esophagus (Fig. 8.2).

Additional risk factors, however, suggest that the scratchy bread is not the only item responsible for the high cancer rate. The adults of the region drink 20–40 cups of very hot tea per day, and this could well be a contributory cause (see Chapter 7). Another risk factor arises from the semi-arid conditions of the region, and the traditional nomadic way of life of many of its inhabitants. These circumstances limit the cultivation of fruit and vegetables, and while a few families buy these items in neighbouring cities, 95 % of the families do not eat vegetables at all. Fruit consumption is limited to figs and pomegranates (Ghadirian 1987). The diet therefore lacks the protective effect of these foods.

Dietary deficiencies are another factor which may well increase the vulnerability of the esophagus to carcinogens. The intake of several vitamins and minerals is known to be low, while the need for a good diet for women is increased by the high birth rate. The average number of pregnancies is eight, women who have more than seven pregnancies often becoming anemic, with vitamin and iron deficiency. One more factor which may well contribute to esophageal cancer is the use of opium, but here again the evidence is not conclusive (see previous section). Certain factors implicated in esophageal cancer elsewhere in the world, for example alcohol and tobacco use, were not thought to be relevant in Iran. In addition, one of the major occupations, carpet manufacture, did not appear to be a hazard (Mahboubi *et al*. 1980). It has been suggested that, because horsemen of the region ride extensively under very windy conditions, a considerable amount of desert sand is swallowed, and that this could damage the esophagus. However, the mineral silica in sand would have been worn to a smooth finish, in contrast to the sharp fibers and laminae of biogenic silica, and would be unlikely to damage the mucosa.

The explanation of the exceptional cancer rate in north-east Iran is most likely to be the fact that low consumption of fruit and vegetables, high

Fig. 8.2. Minute sharply pointed silica hairs on seeds of canary grass, *Phalaris canariensis*, which contaminates cereals grown in north-east Iran and elsewhere. Their presence in 'scratchy bread' can damage the esophagus (from Bhatt *et al.* 1984, with permission from International Union Against Cancer).

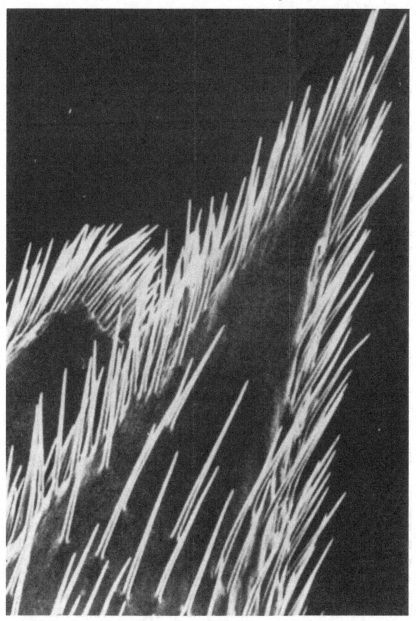

consumption of hot tea and scratchy bread and opium use, combine together in this region to give a high risk.

Northern China

A somewhat different situation is responsible for the consumption of silica in northern China. In this region millet, *Setaria italica*, rather than wheat is grown, and silica occurs in the millet bran itself and not in a contaminant. A significant fact is that in the Linxian region, where there is a notoriously high rate of esophageal cancer, but apparently not elsewhere, the bran as well as the grain is consumed by man. Fibers and sheets of silica occur in the bran, as they are present in the inflorescence bracts which surround the grain. In the Linxian region, bran is mixed with persimmon fruit to form a cake and, as the bran can contain up to 30% silica, there is a high level of silica in the cakes. At one time these cakes formed a major part of the diet, but although still eaten, their popularity has declined.

Sharply pointed fragments of silica have been detected in the esophagus of cancer patients. These fibers were found lodged both in the esophageal tumors and in the surrounding mucosa. The fibers were studied after acid extraction from the mucosa, and also by *in situ* examination (O'Neill *et al.* 1982). The length of the extracted fibers was 180–415 μm, the silica being present at levels of about 0.4 mg/g tissue. Energy-dispersive X-ray analysis of freeze-fractured samples of esophagus showed the silica fragments to be distributed throughout the depth of the mucosa. Studies of acid extracts of esophagus of domestic chickens in Linxian, animals which also have a high incidence of esophageal cancer, were found to contain a similarly high content of silica.

Experimental studies

Little experimental work has been carried out to test the implications of the epidemiological surveys. Pioneering experiments with fibers from *Phalaris canariensis* showed that the isolated fibers, free of organic material, promoted carcinogenesis when applied with light pressure to mouse skin which had been initiated with a polycyclic hydrocarbon (Bhatt *et al.* 1984). In an interesting study of various likely promoting agents and esophageal cancer if was shown that feeding the plant *Bidens pilosa* to rats increased the incidence of esophageal carcinomas which had been induced by methyl *n*-amylnitrosamine (Mirvish *et al.* 1985). As mentioned previously, this plant has a high content of silica fibers (Parry *et al.* 1986). Further experiments in which high-silica foods are fed in the diet to animals in which esophageal cancer has been induced by nitrosamine treatment would be of much interest.

Mechanism of action

Silica lodged in the esophagus could act as a nidus for nitrosating bacteria, which then produce nitrosamines carcinogenic for the esophagus *in situ*. In addition, fibers could act as a nidus for viruses, and infection by viruses has been implicated in esophageal cancer in cattle (referred to above) and in man (Chapter 11).

It seems more likely, however, that silica fibers would act by a promoting mechanism, mediated by a stimulation of cell replication. Fibers or sheets of silica lodged in the esophagus would cause continuous trauma to the mucous membrane, resulting in restorative hyperplasia and replication of basal cells. In addition, fibers of a critical length act in a similar way to asbestos fibers, and stimulate cell growth. Glass fibers 100–250 μm in length were found to stimulate division of cells in culture. A fiber 250 μm long is the ideal length for certain cells to stretch out along the surface and to replicate. Many fibers of 70–200 μm were found in the grass weed *Phalaris canariensis* which grows with wheat in the fields in Turkoma and elsewhere. These fibers had a mean diameter of 15 μm and were sharply pointed, with a tip diameter of 0.5 μm. By acting as a site for anchorage, they would stimulate cell replication (Stoker *et al.* 1968; O'Neill *et al.* 1990).

Concluding remarks

The current evidence suggests that silica is very probably one of several factors which promote esophageal cancer, especially in the high-risk areas of the world. In combination with dietary deficiencies, consumption of large volumes of very hot tea, and lack of the protective effects of fresh fruit and vegetables, it could help to cause the exceptionally high cancer rates. The nature of a genotoxic carcinogen in bracken is described in the following section. The identity of the initiating esophageal carcinogen in people of the Transkei, north-east Iran and northern China, assuming that such a factor exists, is still unknown.

Bracken

Bracken (*Pteridium aquilinum*) is an exceptionally successful plant, and grows in all continents with the exception of Antarctica. It is cultivated in Japan, New Zealand, Canada and the north-eastern United States for human consumption (Woo *et al.* 1988), in spite of the fact that it has been known for a long time to cause illness in grazing animals. Significantly, it has been shown to cause cancer of the esophagus and stomach in cattle (Jarrett 1972, 1973). Bracken itself is eaten by man on a large scale only in Japan. However, a carcinogen is known to be able to pass from cows grazing on bracken into the milk, and people who drink locally produced milk in regions where cattle consume bracken have a risk of developing cancer of the alimentary tract. This may explain why human esophageal cancer rates are especially high in regions where bracken contaminates the pastures, as in highland areas in Scotland, and in certain regions in Wales where 7% of the country is covered with bracken, the coverage in the north reaching 20%. In addition, as a carcinogen is leached by rain from the plant, it could reach the water supply. More recently, bracken spores were found to be a hazard. Esophageal cancer resulting from bracken exposure is therefore a very real possibility.

The association of bracken exposure with esophageal and gastric cancer has been studied only in regions with an exceptionally high incidence of these diseases in animals or in man. A great deal of effort has been expended in an attempt to identify the chemicals in bracken which are responsible for these diseases, but for reasons described below, this has proved to be unusually difficult. The epidemiological studies and experimental work will be briefly described in this section. Detailed reviews have been published (Evans 1984, 1987).

Epidemiological studies

With animals

Evidence for an association between bracken consumption and esophageal cancer came first with the report of squamous cell carcinoma of the esophagus and of the squamous region of the stomach among giant forest hogs free-living in a bracken-infested forest in the Nasampoli valley of Kenya, and that a high incidence of esophageal cancer existed in the cattle of the area (Plowright *et al.* 1971). The high rate of esophageal cancer in cattle in Kenya, Turkey and Brazil was confirmed, and bracken fern was incriminated as the source of the carcinogen (Jarrett 1973). Similarly, a high incidence of the disease in cattle was found in western Scotland in those regions where bracken occurs in the grazing, while no cases were found in other regions studied. An additional factor was a constant association of the tumors with papillomas caused by the papova group of viruses. This suggests that the carcinomas arise in pre-existing virus-induced papillomas. The cancer cases occurred in farms which had previously experienced outbreaks of acute bracken poisoning. There was therefore good evidence that bracken, in association with viral infection, caused esophageal cancer in cattle.

With man

Bracken is consumed extensively in Japan where, to satisfy the demand, large quantities are imported from Siberia. The ferns are collected before the fronds have unfurled, and they are used mainly in mixed salads. Bracken is regarded as a delicacy, and is prepared in a variety of ways. Before consumption, the astringent taste is usually removed by boiling the bracken in water containing wood ash or sodium carbonate, although it may be boiled only in water. Alternatively, the fresh bracken may be pickled in salt, and then immersed in boiling water before use. When treated with alkali in boiling water, the processed bracken contains much less carcinogen than the fresh fern, but not all the carcinogenic activity is removed (Hirono *et al.* 1972). To enable bracken to be eaten throughout the year, it is now canned, dried or vacuum packed, but the carcinogenic activity of the commercially available products has apparently not been tested.

For the reasons presented above, the risk of consumption of bracken is difficult to evaluate. However, at least one valuable epidemiological survey has been carried out. Bracken is consumed most extensively in the mountainous area of central Japan. Here it was found (Hirayama 1979*a*, *b*; Hirono 1981) that the risk of esophageal cancer was higher in people who ate bracken every day or hot tea gruel (chagaya) every day, and that it was especially high when both food items were consumed.

The most obvious indirect route of exposure is via milk and dairy products. Until recently in the UK, and currently in certain areas, dairy cattle graze on lowland terrain infested with bracken, and on marginal upland pastures. Experimental work showed that a carcinogen passes into the milk. With the inception of the Milk Marketing Board in 1932, the gradual increase in the practise of selling to dairies and the consequent bulking of samples would have reduced exposure. In the past, however, this must have presented a hazard, and exposure from milk consumption may explain why regions in which cattle are known to have grazed on bracken-infested pastures, as in North Wales and certain regions of Scotland, there is an especially high incidence of esophageal and gastric cancer. The long latent period between exposure and esophageal cancer implies that customs of 10–20 years ago can be the cause of present-day cancers.

Another possible route of exposure is via the drinking water in those regions where the catchment area is bracken-infested. Leachates obtained by repeated cold water washing of fronds are known to cause a variety of tumors in mice (Evans 1984). Bracken also has a very extensive underground system of perennial rhizomes, which can also be leached by drainage water. With the use of large reservoirs the dilution factor obviates the effect of water-soluble carcinogens, but water from wells and springs still represents a hazard.

More recently it has been discovered that exposure to the bracken carcinogen could be via inhalation of the spores. These are shed annually from July to September, a single frond producing as much as a gram of spores annually. The spores are shot out by the catapult mechanism of the sporangium in hot dry weather, they become air-borne, and can travel in turbulent air currents for long distances, possibly up to 800 km. The spores can be inhaled in the same way as pollen grains and mold spores, and because of their small size (31–32 μm diameter) they are first trapped on the mucosa of the respiratory tract, and finally reach the stomach. As the spores have a low water content (8 % compared with 80 % for the remainder of the plant) a concentration effect could cause the spores to have a high carcinogen content. Experimental evidence (Evans 1984) to be discussed later shows that tumors can be induced by treatment of animals with bracken spores.

Experimental studies: carcinogenicity

As epidemiological studies had given good evidence for an association of tumors at various sites, especially the esophagus, in cattle feeding on bracken, experiments were carried out to investigate the carcinogenicity of bracken in laboratory animals.

In a pioneering experiment, dried frond was incorporated into the diet of rats (Evans *et al.* 1965). Bracken consumption by horses causes 'bracken staggers', and this has been shown to be due to the presence of a thiaminase in the bracken. Therefore thiamine was injected into the experimental rats to prevent thiamine deficiency. Within a year, the animals had succumbed to multiple adenomas of the intestinal mucosa. Similar results were obtained by Hirono *et al.* (1972) in experiments comparing the carcinogenicity of processed and unprocessed fronds. The induction of bladder tumors in rats depends on the dosing regime. Mice developed leukemias, pulmonary adenomas and squamous carcinomas of the forestomach. Esophageal cancer was not induced, although the squamous epithelium of the forestomach is very similar in histological appearance to that of the esophagus. Squamous metaplasia was induced in the urinary bladder of guinea pigs.

In summary, esophageal cancer has not yet been induced in experimental animals by feeding bracken preparations, in spite of the fact that consumption of bracken by cattle is associated with a high incidence of the disease. The explanation could be species differences in susceptibility, or to the fact that the appropriate conditions for induction in small animals have not yet been tested.

Identification of toxic and carcinogenic chemicals in bracken

In spite of intensive efforts, the identity of the carcinogens present in bracken remained elusive for many years. Symptoms of acute bracken poisoning in cattle are similar to those of radiomimetic compounds, i.e. destruction of bone marrow leading to thrombocytopenia, leukopenia, aplastic anemia, intestinal ulceration, hematuria, and anemia resulting from blood loss. It therefore seemed reasonable to suppose that the long-term effects of a low dose of bracken toxin might also be radiomimetic and therefore possibly carcinogenic. However, although the malignancies occurred on farms which had previously experienced outbreaks of acute bracken poisoning, there was no conclusive evidence that the acute toxic factor(s) is identical to the carcinogenic chemical(s). Therefore acute toxic effects, which are relatively rapid to detect, could not be used as a measure of the carcinogen content of bracken extracts.

The only reliable way to identify an esophageal carcinogen for cattle is to isolate a suspected chemical from bracken, to feed it to the animal for more than a year, and to examine the esophagus for malignancy. A reasonable number of cattle are needed, and therefore a large amount of the highly purified suspected compound must be prepared from bracken samples, all of which should be collected at the same time of year from a single region of pasture. The investigations are therefore lengthy and expensive.

An additional complicating factor is the probability that bracken contains several different chemicals which are involved in causing cancer at different sites and in different species of animal. Promoters and modulating factors are also known to be present, which would have variable effects in different organs and in the different species studied. For example, the silica which occurs in bracken would be likely to promote cancer of the esophagus, but probably not of the urinary bladder.

In spite of these problems, valuable work has been carried out in an attempt to identify the carcinogens. It was found that the carcinogenicity of fresh ferns is similar to those dried at 70–90 °C. The carcinogens must therefore be relatively stable to heat (Hirono 1981). Among the chemicals which have been studied are tannins, silica, shikimic acid, quercetin, and other compounds isolated from *Pteridium aquilinium* (Fig. 8.3).

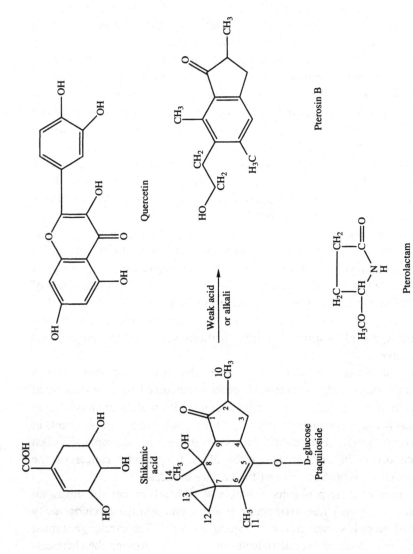

Fig. 8.3. Structure of chemicals which have been considered as toxic and carcinogenic factors in bracken fern.

Tannins

Bracken was known to contain a high concentration of tannins (see Chapter 7), and initial evidence suggested that this complex group of compounds was responsible for bladder cancer (Wang *et al.* 1976; Pamukcu *et al.* 1980*a*). However, as discussed previously (Chapter 7), tannins are more likely to act in a promoting capacity rather than as initiating genotoxic carcinogens, and the findings of positive carcinogenicity by Wang *et al.* (1976) and Pamukcu *et al.* (1980) could not be confirmed by other workers.

Silica

A factor which is very likely to be involved in esophageal cancer, although probably not in cancer of the stomach or urinary bladder, is silica. The effect of the occurrence of this compound in bracken has been discussed in the previous section.

Shikimic acid

Shikimic acid (2,3,5-trihydroxy-1-cyclohexane-1-carboxylic acid) is synthesized by the plant from glucose, and is a metabolic intermediate in the biosynthesis of aromatic ring compounds, including phenylalanine, tyrosine, tryptophan and safrole. The chemical was isolated from bracken, and was considered as a candidate for carcinogenicity. Preparations from bracken, however, were carcinogenic in mice only in fractions which had a higher malignant potential than that which could have been due to the shikimic acid content, and oral administration of shikimic acid to rats failed to induce tumors (Evans 1984). In view of these results, and the fact that the chemical occurs widely in many edible plants, it is unlikely to be responsible for the carcinogenicity of bracken.

Quercetin

As discussed in Chapter 7, flavonoids occur widely in many edible plants, and have been tested for mutagenicity and carcinogenicity. The major part of the flavonoid content of bracken is composed of the glycosides of kaempferol (astragalin) and quercetin (isoquercetrin), while the free aglycones do not occur in bracken (Evans 1984). Kaempferol and quercetin are mutagenic in the *Salmonella* test system, but the glycosides show mutagenicity only after treatment with glycosidases, and therefore activity is dependent on the action of intestinal microflora. Although early work suggested carcinogenicity associated with bracken-derived quercetin (Pamukcu *et al.* 1980), later work failed to confirm these results (Hirono *et al.* 1987).

Additional compounds
A review of the attempts at and eventually the successful identification of one of the bracken carcinogens is given by Hirono *et al.* (1987). Pterolactam (5-methoxy-2-pyrrolidone; Fig. 8.3) was isolated from bracken, and was found not to be carcinogenic. Similarly, the indanones pterosin and pteroside were isolated from fronds and rhizomes, but no evidence was obtained for carcinogenicity.

A chemical which, after treatment with alkali, was responsible for more than 50 % of the mutagenicity of bracken was extracted by van der Hoeven *et al.* (1983). This chemical they called aquilide A, and its chemical structure and that of the mutagen to which it gave rise were determined.

A compound was then extracted with boiling water from dried powdered bracken (Hirono *et al.* 1987). The extract was fractionated by a succession of procedures, and the presence of the active principle was followed by determination of carcinogenic activity in each fraction. Eventually, from 3 kg of bracken powder, 0.6 g of a pure compound was isolated. This product was characterized as ptaquiloside, a glucoside composed of D-glucose and a norsesquiterpene (Fig. 8.3). Ptaquiloside was identical to the aquiloside of van der Hoeven *et al.* (1983). In agreement with carcinogenicity tests with bracken, ptaquiloside was unstable in acid and alkaline solutions at room temperature, yielding the aromatic sesquiterpenes, pterosins and pterosides.

The biological properties of ptaquiloside were tested by intragastric administration to rats. The animals developed hematuria and mammary cancers, i.e. cancers of the type which had been induced in Sprague–Dawley rats fed bracken. Multiple ileal carcinomas and squamous metaplasia of the urinary bladder were also induced. The question of acute bracken poisoning was tested by giving a 6-month-old calf a daily drench of ptaquiloside. Examination of blood samples showed an increasing leukocyte and granulocyte count for 17 days, which was followed by a period of fluctuating concentrations, and finally by a decrease in the levels. There was a slow depression in the thrombocyte levels. When the animal was examined by autopsy 86 days after the start of the experiment, destruction of bone marrow of the sternum was obvious. These results strongly suggest that ptaquiloside was one of the carcinogenic and toxic factors in bracken fern.

In summary, the present situation seems to be that bracken is very probably a contributory cause of esophageal cancer in Japan. Here, although the people continue to eat bracken, the marketing of safe products in which the carcinogens have been destroyed is an obvious possibility. Other aspects of human exposure which require further investigation are the extent of exposure and the hazard presented by inhalation of bracken spores, and from the contamination of water supplies.

With reference to experimental work, the metabolism of ptaquiloside and the possible formation of DNA adducts should be studied. If ptaquiloside does not mimic all the various carcinogenic activities of bracken in different animal species, the painstaking search for additional carcinogens and toxic factors in bracken fronds should be pursued.

Dihydrosafrole

Safrole and chemically related compounds are present in many edible plants, for example citrus fruits, carrots and parsley, in herbal teas and folk medicines, and more especially in spices, including ginger, black pepper, mace, nutmeg and cinnamon. The group of compounds are extracted in the essential oils, an odorous heterogeneous mixture of safrole-related compounds, aldehydes, ketones, esters and terpenes. They are extracted by steam distillation and solvent extraction, and are soluble in alcohol but only to a limited extent in water. Safrole is a component of many essential oils, but especially the oil prepared from the bark and roots of the sassafras tree (*Sassafras albidum*), of which it comprises 70–80%. Sassafras oil has been widely used as a flavouring agent, for example in root beer, chewing gum and toothpaste. In addition, several synthetic safrole derivatives have been used as flavorings and fragrances, and in pesticides and cosmetics. Among these is dihydrosafrole.

Safrole itself and several related compounds have been found to be carcinogenic, mainly for the liver, but of special interest here is the esophageal carcinogenicity of dihydrosafrole (Long *et al.* 1963). Although dihydrosafrole has so far not been shown to occur naturally, it has been prepared industrially for use as a flavouring agent. Safrole is a derivative of allylbenzene (3,4-methylenedioxy-1-allylbenzene). In dihydrosafrole (3,4-methylenedioxy-1-propylbenzene) the allyl side chain is saturated (Figs. 8.4 and 8.5).

Biological properties

The hepatic toxicity which follows ingestion of large amounts of sassafras oil by humans has been known for over a hundred years, but its carcinogenic properties in rats and mice were not reported until 1960. Detailed reviews of the toxicity, carcinogenicity and metabolism of safrole and related compounds have been presented (Enomoto 1987; Woo *et al.* 1988). Safrole and more especially dihydrosafrole have a low toxicity. Thus the LD_{50} for safrole for rats was 1950 mg/kg, and for mice 2350 mg/kg,

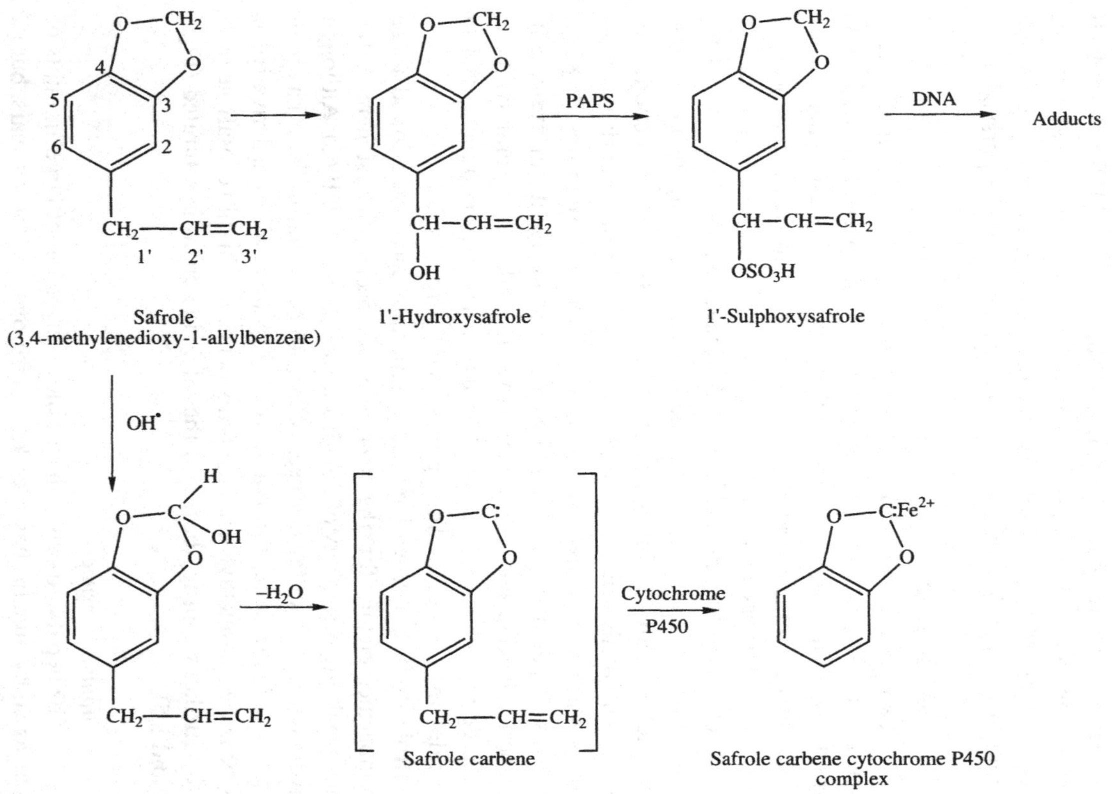

Fig. 8.4. Metabolism of safrole.

and for dihydrosafrole the corresponding toxicities were 2260 mg/kg (rats) and 3700 mg/kg (mice) (Hagen *et al.* 1965). The acute toxic effects of safrole and its congeners are probably a result of inhibition of P450 enzymes. Later effects caused by treatment at 250–750 mg/kg per day produced liver enlargement, due to an increase in the volume of cytoplasm. This probably resulted from an induction of microsomal P450 enzymes, which followed the acute inhibition. Other consequences included bile duct hyperplasia and depression of the central nervous system.

Carcinogenicity

Safrole was found to be carcinogenic in 1961 (Abbot *et al.* 1961; Homberger *et al.* 1961). When fed at high concentrations in the diet to rats, a low incidence of liver tumors was induced. In contrast, dihydrosafrole fed to Osborne Mendel rats for 2 years was not carcinogenic for liver, but induced tumors in the esophagus (Long *et al.* 1963; Hagen *et al.* 1965, 1967). A proportion of the tumors were carcinomas. Dihydrosafrole, however, was a very weak carcinogen, and required prolonged insult at high levels of exposure before tumors were induced in the esophagus. Thus, a dose level of 1000 ppm was ineffective, and 250 ppm was necessary to induce an incidence of malignant tumors of 5% of the animals. This is in striking contrast to the esophageal carcinogenicity of certain nitrosamines, some of which have been reported to occur in food. For example, *N*-nitroso-*N*-methylbenzylamine fed at 1 ppm induced a 100% incidence of esophageal carcinomas (Druckey *et al.* 1967). When fed to mice, dihydrosafrole was carcinogenic for the forestomach and liver (Innes *et al.* 1969; Reuber 1979). There is evidence that dogs fed dihydrosafrole for 2 years developed hyperplasia of the esophagus (FDA unpublished data, cited in Reuber 1979).

Fig. 8.5. Metabolism of dihydrosafrole.

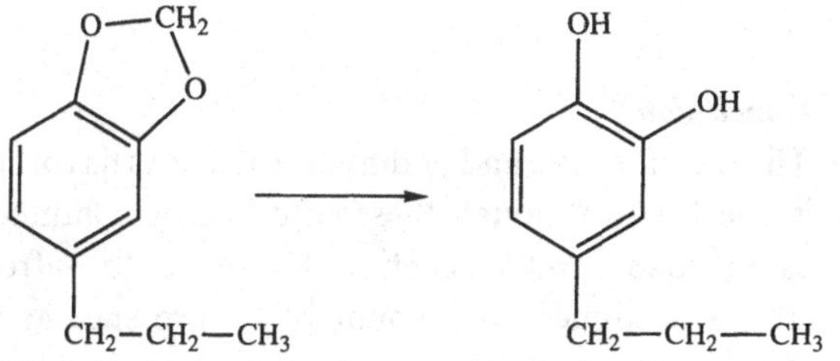

Dihydrosafrole
(3,4-methylenedioxy-1-propylbenzene)

3,4-Dihydroxy-1-propylbenzene

Metabolism

Extensive studies of the metabolism of allylbenzene compounds have been carried out by the Millers and their colleagues at Wisconsin (Miller *et al.* 1979, 1982). Safrole follows three metabolic routes: $1'$-hydroxylation of the allyl side chain, epoxidation of the double bond of the allyl side chain, and oxidative demethylenation of the methylene dioxy group (Fig. 8.4). *In vitro* experiments showed that $1'$-hydroxysafrole reacts with $3'$-phosphoadenoside-$5'$-phosphosulfate (PAPS) in the presence of sulfotransferase, an enzyme present in the cytosol of mouse and rat liver, and it is the sulfate thus formed which is considered to be the major ultimate carcinogen (Wislocki *et al.* 1976). Use of labelled compounds has given evidence for covalent binding of the activated carcinogen to DNA (Phillips *et al.* 1981). The N^2-atom of guanine and the N^6-atom of adenine are involved.

In contrast to safrole, the major metabolic route of dihydrosafrole is demethylenation (Fig. 8.5), with the formation of 4(1-propyl)catechol (Klungsohr *et al.* 1982). As the saturated compound cannot undergo a similar activation to form the sulfate as does safrole, it is probable that some other ultimate carcinogen is formed. Thus, if different enzyme systems are responsible for the activation of safrole and dihydrosafrole, this may be the reason why in rats dihydrosafrole is carcinogenic for the esophagus and safrole for the liver.

In addition to the reaction of activated safrole with DNA described above, there is suggestive evidence that safrole is carcinogenic on account of an epigenic mechanism (Ioannides *et al.* 1981). Hydroxylation of the methylenedioxy group could give rise to a carbene intermediate, which would react with the heme of cytochrome P450. This could damage the endoplasmic reticulum with consequent degranulation of ribosomes – an event which has often been associated with carcinogenicity. A reaction of this type could be responsible for the carcinogenicity of dihydrosafrole.

Neither safrole nor dihydrosafrole was found to be active in the Ames *Salmonella* test for mutagenicity.

Conclusion

The use of safrole and of dihydrosafrole as flavoring agents is now banned in the USA, although these carcinogens continue to be used as fragrances in soaps and cosmetics. Exposure to safrole but not to dihydrosafrole continues on account of its presence at low levels in a variety of edible plants and in spices. Exposure of dihydrosafrole may occur as a result of its continued use as a fragrance in products which are not consumed in the diet, and from its occurrence as an intermediate in the manufacture of the insecticide piperonyl butoxide. But in view of the low levels of exposure to dihydrosafrole, and of the very high doses needed to induce esophageal cancer, at least in rats, it is unlikely that dihydrosafrole is important at present as a human esophageal carcinogen. Exposure in the past, however, could account for some of the present-day cancers, and the levels of dihydrosafrole present in consumer products should be kept under review.

References

Abbott, D.D., Packman, E.W., Wagner, B.M. and Harrison, J.W.E. (1961) *Pharmacologist* 3, 62. Chronic oral toxicity of oil of sassafras and safrole.

Bhatt, T., Coombs, M. and O'Neill, C. (1984) *Int J. Cancer* 34, 519–528. Biogenic silica promotes carcinogenesis in mouse skin.

Crespi, M., Munoz, N., Garsii, A., Aramesh, B., Amiri, G., Mojtakai, A. and Casale, V. (1979) *Lancet* ii, 217–222. Oesophageal lesions in Northern Iran: a pre-malignant condition

Dowlatshahi, D., Mobarhan, S. and Daneshbod, A. (1977) *Digestion* 16, 237. Clinical studies of carcinoma of the esophagus in Northern Iran.

Dowlatshahi, K. and Miller, R.J. (1985) *Cancer Res.* 45, 1906–1907. Role of opium in esophagal cancer: a hypothesis.

Druckrey, H., Preussmann, R., Ivankovic, S. and Schmahl, D. (1967) *Z. Krebsforsch* 69, 103–201. Organope carcinogene Wirkungen bei 65 verschiedenen *N*-nitroso-Verbindungen an BD-Ratten.

Enomoto, M. (1987) In: *Bioactive Molecules*, vol. 2, *Naturally Occurring Carcinogens of Plant Origin* (Hirono, I. ed). Amsterdam: Elsevier, pp. 139–159. Safrole.

Evans, I.A. and Mason, J. (1965) *Nature* 208, 913–914. Carcinogenic activity of bracken.

Evans, I.A., Widdop, B., Jones, R.S., Barber, G.D., Leach, H., Jones, D.L. and Mainwaring-Burton, R. (1971) *Biochem. J.* 124, 28–29. The possible human hazard of the naturally occurring bracken carcinogen.

Evans, I.A. and Osman, M.A. (1974) *Nature* 250, 348–349. Carcinogenicity of bracken and shikimic acid.

Evans, I.A. (1984) In: *Chemical Carcinogens*. ACS Monograph 182 (Searle, C.E. ed.). Washington DC: ACS, pp. 1171–1204. Bracken carcinogenicity.

Evans, I.A. (1987) In: *Reviews on Environmental Health*. International Quarterly Scientific Reviews, vol. VII, no. 3 & 4. (James, D.V. ed.). Israel: Freund, pp. 1–41. Bracken carcinogenicity.

Friesen, M., O'Neill, I.K., Malaveille, C., Garren, L., Hautejeuille, A., Cabral, J.R.P., Galendo, D., Lasne, C., Sala, M., Chouroulinkov, I., Mohr, U., Turusov, U., Daly, N.E. and Bartsch, H. (1985) *Mutation Res.* 150, 177–191. Characterization and identification of 6 mutagens in opium pyrolysates implicated in oesophageal cancer in Iran.

Friesen, M., O'Neill, I.K., Malaveille, C., Garren, L., Hautejeuille, A. and Bartsch, H. (1987) *Carcinogenesis* 83, 1423–1432. Substituted hydroxyphenanthrenes in opium pyrolysates implicated in esophageal cancer in Iran: structures and *in vitro* metabolic activation of a novel class of mutagens.

Ghadirian, P., Stein, G.F., Gorodetzky, C., Roberfroid, M.B., Mahon, G.A.T., Bartsch, H. and Day, N.E. (1985) *Int. J. Cancer* **35**, 593–597. Oesophageal cancer studies in the Caspian littoral of Iran: some residual results, including opium use as a risk factor.

Ghadirian, P. (1987) *Nutr. Cancer* **9**, 147–157. Food habits of the people of the Caspian littoral of Iran in relation to esophageal cancer.

Hagen, E.C., Jenner, P.M., Jones, W.I., Fitzhugh, O.G., Long, E.L., Brouwer, J.G. and Webb, W.K. (1965) *Toxicol. Appl. Pharmacol.* **7**, 18–24. Toxic properties of compounds related to safrole.

Hagen, E.C., Hansen, W.H., Fitzhugh, O.G., Jenner, P.M., Jones, W.I., Taylor, J.M., Long, E.L., Nelson, A.A. and Brouwer, J.B. (1967) *Food Cos. Toxicol.* **5**, 141–157. Food flavourings and compounds of related structure. II. Subacute and chronic toxicity.

Hewer, T., Rose, E., Ghadirian, P., Castegnaro, M., Bartsch, H., Malaveille, C. and Day, N. (1978) *Lancet* **ii**, 494–496. Ingested mutagens from opium and tobacco pyrolysis products and cancer of the esophagus.

Hirayama, T. (1979a) In: *Naturally Occurring Carcinogen-Mutagens and Modulators of Carcinogenesis* (Miller, E.C., Miller, J.A., Hirono, I., Sugimura, T. and Takayama, S. eds.). Baltimore: University Park Press, pp. 359–380. Epidemiological evaluation of the role of naturally occurring carcinogens and modulators of carcinogenesis.

Hirayama, T. (1979b) *Nutr. Cancer* **1**, 67–81. Diet and Cancer.

Hirono, I., Shibuya, C., Shimizu, M. and Fushimi, K. (1972) *J. Natl. Cancer Inst.* **48**, 1245–1250. Carcinogenic activity of processed bracken used as human food.

Hirono, I. (1981) *CRC Crit. Rev. Toxicol.* **8**, 235–277. Naturally occurring products of plant origin.

Hirono, I. and Yamada, K. (1987) In: *Bioactive Molecules*, vol. 2 (Hirono, I. ed.). Amsterdam: Elsevier, pp. 87–120. Bracken fern.

Homburger, F., Kelly, T., Friedler, G. and Russfield, A.B. (1961) *Med. Expt.* **4**, 1–11. Toxic and possible carcinogenic effects of 4-allyl-1,2-methylene dioxybenzene (safrole) in rats on deficient diets.

Innes, J.R.M., Ulland, B.M., Valerio, M.G., Petrucelli, L., Fishbein, I., Hart, E.R., Pallotta, A.J., Bates, R.R., Falk, H.L., Gart, J.J., Klein, M., Mitchell, I. and Peters, J. (1969) *J. Natl. Cancer Inst.* **42**, 1101–1114. Bioassay of pesticides and industrial chemicals for tumorigenicity in mice: a preliminary note.

Ioannides, C., Delaforce, M. and Parke, D.V. (1981) *Food Cosmet. Toxicol.* **19**, 657–666. Safrole: its metabolism, carcinogenicity and interactions with cytochrome P450.

Jarrett, W.F.H. (1973) *Br. J. Cancer* **28**, 93. Esophageal and stomach cancer in cattle: a candidate viral and carcinogenic model system and its possible relevance to man.

Jarrett, W.F.H., McNeil, P.E., Grimshaw, W.T.R., Selman, I.E. and McIntyre, W.I.M. (1978) *Nature* **274**, 215–217. High incidence area of cattle cancer with a possible interaction between an environmental carcinogen and a papilloma virus.

Jarrett, W.F.H. (1982) *Proc. R. Soc. Edinb.* **81B**, 79–83. Bracken and cancer.

Joint Iran International Agency for Research on Cancer Study Group (1977) *J. Natl. Cancer Inst.* **54**, 1127–1138. Esophageal cancer studies in the Caspian littoral of Iran: results of population studies – a prodrome.

Klungsoyr, J. and Scheline, R.R. (1982) *Biomed. Mass Spectrom.* **9**, 323–329. Metabolism of isosafrole and dihydrosafrole in the rat.

Long, E.L. and Jenner, P.M. (1963) *Fed. Proc.* **22**, 275. Esophageal tumors produced in rats by the feeding of dihydrosafrole.

Mahboubi, E.O. and Aramesh, B. (1980) *Prev. Med.* **9**, 613–621. Epidemiology of esophageal cancer in Iran, with reference to nutritional and cultural aspects.

Malaveille, C., Friesen, M., Camu, A.-M., Garren, L., Haukfeuille, A., Bereziat, J.-C., Ghadirian, P., Day, N.E. and Bartsch, H. (1982) *Carcinogenesis* **3**, 557–585. Mutagens produced by the pyrolysis of opium and its alkaloids as possible risk factors in cancer of the bladder and esophagus.

Maneckjee, R., Biswas, R. and Vonderhaar, B.K. (1990) *Cancer Res.* **50**, 2234–2238. Binding of opioids to human MCF-7 breast cancer cells and their effects on growth.

McNaughton, S.J. and Tarrants, J.L. (1983) *Proc. Natl. Acad. Sci.* **80**, 790–791. Grass leaf silicification: natural selection for an inducible defense against hervibores.

Miller, J.A., Swanson, A.B. and Miller, C. (1979) In: *Naturally Occurring Carcinogens: Mutagens and Modulators of Carcinogenesis*. Proceedings of the 9th International Symposium of The Princess Takamatsu Cancer Research Fund, Tokyo, 1979. (Miller, E.C., Miller, J.A., Hirono, I., Sugimura, T., Takayama, S. eds.). Tokyo: Japan Scientific Societies Press, pp. 111–125. The metabolic activation of safrole and related naturally occurring alkenylbenzenes in relation to carcinogenesis by these agents.

Miller, J.A., Miller, E.C. and Phillips, D.H. (1982) In: *Carcinogens and Mutagens in the Environment*, vol. 1. (Stich, H.F. ed). Boca Raton: CRC Press, pp. 83–96. The metabolic activation and carcinogenicity of alkenylbenzenes that occur naturally in many spices.

Mirvish, S.S., Salamasi, S., Lawson, T.A., Poser, P. and Sutherland, D. (1985) *J. Natl. Cancer Inst.* **74**, 1283–1289. Test of catechol, tannic acid, *Bidens pilosa*, croton oil, and phorbol for co-carcinogenesis of esophageal tumors induced in rats by *N*-methyl-*N*-*n*-amylnitrosamine.

Nadim, A. and Nassen, K. (1986) In: *Global Geocancerology* (Howe, M.G. ed.). Edinburgh: Churchill Livingstone, pp. 241–252. Iran.

Newman, R. (1986) *Nutr. Cancer* **8**, 217–221. Association of biogenic silica with disease.

O'Neill, C.H., Hodges, G.M., Riddle, P.N., Jordan, P.W. and Newman, R.H. (1980) *Int. J. Cancer*, **26**, 617–628. A fine fibrous silica contaminant of flour in the high oesophageal cancer area of North-East Iran.

O'Neill, C., Clarke, G., Hodges, G., Jordan, P., Newman, R., Pan, Q., Liu, F., Ge, M., Chang, Y. and Toulson, E. (1982) *Lancet* **i**, 1202–1206. Silica fragments from millet in mucosa surrounding oesophageal tumours in patients in Northern China.

O'Neill, C., Jordan, P. and Riddle, P. (1990) *J. Cell. Sci.* **95**, 577–586. Narrow linear strips of adhesive substratum are powerful inducers of both growth and total focal contact area.

220   *Opium, silica, bracken, dihydrosafrole*

Pamukcu, A.M., Wang, C.Y., Hatcher, J. and Bryan, G.T. (1980a) *J. Natl. Cancer Inst.* **65**, 131–136. Carcinogenicity of tannin and tannin-free extracts of bracken fern (*Pteridium aquilinum*).

Pamukcu, A.M., Yalciner, S., Hatcher, J.F. and Bryan, G.T. (1980b) *Cancer Res.* **40**, 3468–3472. Quercetin, a rat intestinal and bladder carcinogen present in bracken fern (*Pteridium aquilinum*).

Parry, D.W., O'Neill, C.H. and Hodson, M.J. (1986) *Ann. Bot.* **58**, 641–647. Opaline silica deposits in the leaves of *Bidens pilosa* L. and their possible significance in cancer.

Perry, P.E., Thomson, E.J., Vijayalaxmi, Evans, H.E., Day, N.E. and Bartsch, H. (1983) *Carcinogenesis* **4**, 227–230. Induction of SCE by opium pyrolysates in CHO cells and human peripheral blood lymphocytes.

Phillips, D.H., Miller, J.A., Miller, E.C. and Adams, B. (1981) *Cancer Res.* **41**, 2664–2672. The N^2-atom of guanine and the N^6-atom of adenine residues as sites for covalent binding of metabolically activated 1'-hydroxysafrole to mouse liver DNA *in vivo*.

Plowright, W., Linsell, C.A. and Peers, F.G. (1971) *Br. J. Cancer* **25**, 72–80. A focus of rumenal cancer in Kenyan cattle.

Rattan, S. and Goyal, R.K. (1983) *J. Pharmacol. Exp. Ther.* **224**, 391–397. Identification and localization of opioid receptors in the opossum lower esophageal sphincter.

Reuber, M.D. (1979) *Digestion* **19**, 42–47. Neoplasms of the fore-stomach in mice ingesting dihydrosafrole.

Stoker, M., O'Neill, C., Berryman, S. and Waxman, V. (1968) *Int. J. Cancer* **3**, 683–693. Anchorage and growth regulation in normal and virus-transformed cells.

Uddman, R., Alumets, J., Hakanson, R. and Sundler, R. (1980) *Gastroenterology* **78**, 732–737. Peptidergic (enkephalin) innervation of the mammalian esophagus.

Van der Hoeven, J.C.M., Lagerweij, W.J., Posthumus, M.A., van Veldhuizen, A. and Holterman, H.A.J. (1983) *Carcinogenesis* **4**, 1587–1590. Aquilide A, a new mutagenic compound isolated from bracken from (*Pteridium aquilinum* (L) Kuhn).

Wang, C.Y., Chiu, C.W., Pamukcu, A.M. and Bryan, G.T. (1976) *J. Natl. Cancer Inst.* **56**, 33–36. Identification of carcinogenic tannin isolated from bracken fern (*Pteridium aquilinum*).

Wislocki, P.G., Borchert, P., Miller, J.A. and Miller, E.C. (1976) *Cancer Res.* **36**, 1686–1695. The metabolic activation of the carcinogen 1'-hydroxysafrole *in vivo* and *in vitro* and the electrophilic reactivities of possible ultimate carcinogens.

Woo, Y.T., Lai, D.Y., Arcos, J.C. and Argus, M.F. (1988) In: *Chemical Induction of Cancer*, vol. IIIC. New York: Academic Press, pp. 159–177. Bracken fern toxins.

Woo, Y.T., Lai, D.Y., Arcos, J.C. and Argus, M.F. (1988) In: *Chemical Induction of Cancer*, vol. IIIC. New York: Academic Press, pp. 267–319. Safrole, estragol and related compounds.

9

Molds and mycotoxins

Introduction

Molds are usually considered to be a hazard mainly in hot humid climates, where their presence is readily apparent. These regions are not the locations of the world where the incidence of esophageal cancer is especially high. The mold most likely to be implicated in esophageal cancer, however – *Fusarium* – is found growing most often under cooler conditions. It is therefore generally a field fungus rather than a storage fungus.

The ability to grow under cold conditions gives *Fusaria* an advantage over other molds, and surprisingly it flourishes on vegetation growing under snow. This led to the tragic events which made *Fusarium* notorious as a human hazard. In Russia, after the First World War, when labour was not available for harvesting the cereals in autumn, crops were left to overwinter in the fields under the snow. In the following spring when they were harvested and used for making bread, outbreaks of alimentary toxic aleukia were widespread. The disease was shown to be due to infection of the corn with *Fusarium* species (Joffe 1974, 1978), and among the symptoms, to be described in more detail later, were hemorrhagic necrotic lesions in the esophagus. It is regrettable that the survivors of these disasters were not followed up and examined for evidence of carcinogenicity of the mold. However, crude extracts of *Fusarium* isolated from the toxic grain associated with the disease caused hyperkeratosis and basal cell hyperplasia of the esophageal squamous epithelium when fed to rats.

The hazard presented by *Fusarium* mycotoxins has sprung into the limelight recently and has been a major cause of concern for many people, including politicians, around the world. Toxic 'yellow rain' fell from the sky and contaminated trees in north Thailand. This rain contained trichothecenes, one of the major toxins produced by *Fusarium*, and controversy arose as to whether the toxin originated in the droppings from bees which had fed on infected pollen, or whether it was the result of biological warfare (Seeley 1985).

The fungi (Eumycetes) are a group of plants which have no root, stem, leaf or chlorophyll. Fungi are comprised of the mushrooms (Basidiomycetes), yeasts (Ascomycetes) and molds (Phycomycetes). It is mainly the molds which are regarded as a cancer hazard, and general concern is limited to a small number of species. Thus *Aspergillus* and its toxin, aflatoxin, gained notoriety as a liver carcinogen, but there is no epidemiological or experimental evidence for an association between liver and esophageal cancer. For example, while liver cancer is endemic in Mozambique, esophageal cancer is rare, and in South Africa liver cancer is predominant in the hot, humid lower altitudes where the more aggressive mold *Aspergillus* flourishes, while esophageal cancer predominates in higher, more temperate regions where *Fusarium* can thrive.

There has been a steady accumulation of evidence linking consumption of *Fusarium*-contaminated food with esophageal cancer in the three regions of the world with the highest incidence of the disease, i.e. China, Iran and South Africa.

Properties of molds implicated in esophageal cancer

Reviews of the characteristics of *Fusarium* species and their mycotoxins have been published (Wyllie *et al.* 1977; Ueno 1983). Different species of mycotoxins tend to infect different types of plants, and the toxicoses produced in farm animals depend on the species of *Fusarium* and the species of animal. An additional complication is that while most species of the mold can produce the same toxins, they are formed in different proportions. Identification of the species of *Fusarium* and of the toxins most likely to be implicated in esophageal cancer is therefore difficult.

The taxonomy of *Fusarium* was confused until around 1940, because even when grown from monospore cultures the mold develops with a variable morphology. Beginning in the 1940s, a taxonomy was developed based on constant morphological and physiological properties, for example the pathogenicity for crop plants. This system reduced the number of species to nine. *F. poae* and *F. sporotrichioides* were isolated from overwintered millet in the former USSR, and these species were responsible for the outbreaks of alimentary toxic aleukia in man. *F. tricinctum* is found in corn, wheat, and in fescue hay in the USA, and the toxicoses produced in farm animals result in serious economic problems. *F. equiseti*, *F. moniliforme* and *F. graminearum* cause hyper-estrogenism and emesis in swine in the USA. *F. solani* has been responsible for corneal damage in man in Florida. *F. moniliforme* is a very prevalent species found in corn in America which causes a variety of toxicoses in addition to the effect on swine mentioned above, including necrosis of the brain in horses, and is the species most often linked to cancer of the esophagus in man. People handling infected vegetation are at risk of exposure to the mycotoxins, in addition to those who consume the produce.

On account of the ability of *Fusarium* to grow under cool conditions, it is found mainly in temperate northern regions of the world, and at high altitudes elsewhere. *Fusarium* infects many growing plants, where it causes wilts, blights and rots, and the mold grows also on dead and dying plants. It therefore contaminates many foods and feeds, although it has been studied most extensively on corn. Ear and stalk rot in corn have caused serious loss of crops world-wide. *Fusarium* spp. cause scab in wheat and barley, stalk rot in sorghum (Black *et al.* 1987), endosepsis in figs, crown rot in asparagus, 'pokkah-boeng' or top rot in sugar cane, and stunting in rice. The mold has been detected in grape juice in Germany (Schwenke 1988), and it can cause dry rot in potatoes. In fact the name of the mold, *Fusarium*, originated in work carried out on rotten potatoes in Germany around 1840, from the Lower German word '*Fusel*' applied to bad consumables, as in bad brandy and other spirits giving fusel oils, bad coffee and tobacco (Littel *et al.* 1978). Later, contamination was detected on potatoes grown in Iran where, on account of the low socioeconomic conditions, rotten potatoes may be consumed (Desjardins *et al.* 1947; Steyn *et al.* 1978). More recently, however, rotten potatoes have become a problem in more developed countries, as automatic potato-graders can damage the surface of the potato, and the resulting rupture of the skin allows the fungus a site of access. *Fusarium* grows also on silage, and can cause skin and mucosal irritation and inflammation of the gastrointestinal tract of animals given infected feed. The most widespread cause of concern, however, is contamination of cereals and their industrially made products, for example beer (see the section Epidemiology and carcinogenicity below).

In view of the widespread occurrence of *Fusarium* species, it is important to determine the level and nature of the mycotoxins present in the food before an attempt can be made to link consumption with esophageal cancer.

Properties of mycotoxins implicated in esophageal cancer

The method most often used to prepare *Fusarium* mycotoxins for chemical study is to grow the mold on cereals at room temperature where, in the absence of competition from more aggressive molds, there is maximum growth of mycelia. The temperature is then lowered to about

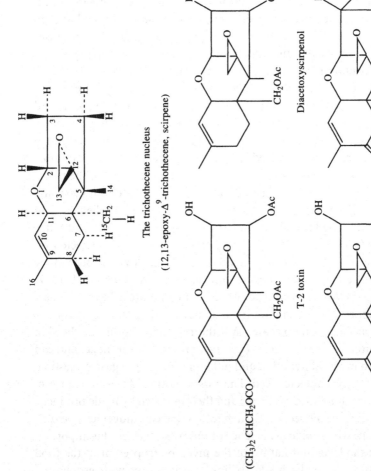

The trichothecene nucleus
(12,13-epoxy-Δ^9-trichothecene, scirpene)

Diacetoxyscirpenol

Fusarenone-X

T-2 toxin

Deoxynivalenol

Fig. 9.1. Trichothecenes implicated in esophageal cancer. OAc, acetate.

8 °C, and with a humidity above 20% there is maximum production of mycotoxins. Storage of the mold induces mutation, and the relative proportions of the various mycotoxins can alter.

The most common groups of toxins isolated from *Fusarium* are the zearalenones, trichothecenes and fusarins. The zearalenones belong to a group of natural products, resorcylates, based on 6-(10-hydroxy-6-oxo-trans-1-undecenyl)β-resorcyclic acid lactone. These toxins are non-steroidal estrogens, and can cause hyper-estrogenism, a syndrome detected mainly in swine. The trichothecenes are all derivatives of 12,13-epoxy-trichothec-9-ene (scirpene), the most obvious effect on farm animals of these toxins being hemorrhage throughout the alimentary canal. When zearalenones and trichothecenes occur together, certain symptoms may predominate, or one toxin may synergize the action of the other. It is the trichothecenes rather than the zearalenones which are implicated in esophageal cancer.

The absence of a conjugated unsaturation system in the trichothecenes explains why they have no ultraviolet absorption spectrum (Fig. 9.1). There is no simple chemical method of identification and assay, a fact which has slowed down study of this important group of toxins. The bioassay most often used for trichothecene-like activity is application to the shaved skin of the rat, a rapid assay which is based on the extent of local irritation, inflammation, desquamation, subepidermal hemorrhage and necrosis. In addition an *in vivo* assay is used, in which oral administration causes necrosis in the mouth, erosion of the mucosa of the stomach and intestines, rectal hemorrhage, and necrosis.

Trichothecenes are formed by a complex biosynthetic pathway from mevalonic acid. They are produced by eight species of *Fusarium*, and approximately 37 naturally occurring derivatives of scirpene have been characterized. These are divided into three groups: A, those with a

Fig. 9.2. Fusarin C.

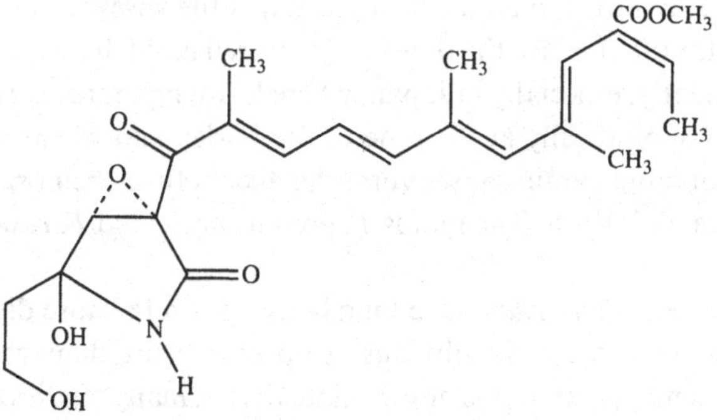

functional group other than a ketone at C-8; B, those with a ketone at C-8; C, with an epoxide group between carbons 7 and 8. The majority of the toxic trichothecenes belong to groups A and B. The most often studied in group A are T-2 toxin and diacetoxyscirpenol (DS), and in group B deoxynivalenol (vomitoxin) and fusarenone X (Fig. 9.1). All the naturally occurring trichothecenes have at least one hydroxyl or ester group at C-3, 4, 7, 8 or 15, and they are therefore all alcohols or esters. All those with an ester group are hydrolyzed by treatment with a base to give the parent alcohol, T-2 toxin giving T-2 tetraol and DS giving scirpentriol, in each case with a reduction of biological activity. On account of the stereochemistry of the trichothecenes, the epoxide group is shielded from nucleophilic attack, although the ring can be opened by prolonged boiling, by strong acid, or by reductive cleavage. Destruction of the epoxide group inactivates the toxins. Thus the trichothecenes are chemically stable and can be stored, although the levels in infected plants may decrease as the toxins can be decomposed by bacteria.

A toxin which has been isolated from corn infected with *F. moniliforme*, and which is especially important on account of its mutagenicity, is fusarin C. The molecular structure was determined by Gaddamidi *et al.* (1985), mainly by analysis of nuclear magnetic resonance data, and is shown in Fig. 9.2. In contrast to the trichothecenes, fusarin C is destroyed by heat, and is unlikely to survive in cooked food.

Toxicoses in livestock and experimental animals

The first report of a red mold which presented a health hazard must be that recorded in the Bible in Leviticus 14:34-36, where the Mosaic prescription of how to deal with a 'plague' known to attack the walls of dwelling houses is described. If red patches were found to spread over the walls, the stones should be removed and cast into an unclean place without the city. The red patches could have been *Fusarium roseum* or other *Fusarium* species, and in view of the problems involved in inactivating *Fusarium* toxins, removal to an unclean place was the wisest procedure to adopt (Schoental 1980). Since the time of Moses, red mold disease has been described frequently, especially in Japan, where low temperatures and high humidity occur sporadically at the time of the barley and wheat harvest. Consumption of moldy grain causes vomiting, feed refusal, hemorrhage of tissues, diarrhea and death. The molds *F. graminearum* and *F. roseum* are responsible.

Molds of the genus *Fusarium* have long been known to cause disease in animals and in man, the most obvious symptoms being damage to the mouth and alimentary canal. It is unfortunate that in many studies the fact that the animal has an esophagus has been ignored. Only more recently has damage to the esophagus become evident, and *Fusarium* species have been implicated in esophageal cancer. The mycotoxins most likely to be responsible are the trichothecenes. Reviews of the subject include those by Rodricks *et al.* (1977), Wyllie *et al.* (1977), Ueno (1983) and Schoental (1985).

When it had become apparent that *Fusarium* is a highly toxic genus of mold, attempts were made to identify the toxins responsible. The trichothecene diacetoxyscirpenol first isolated from plants infected with *F. equiseti* by Brian *et al.* (1961), was found to be the most toxic of the trichothecenes. It was suggested that DS was not important in causing disease of plants parasitized by *Fusarium*, but that it may cause toxicoses in animals fed infected grain. The high toxicity of DS was confirmed by Ueno (1970), who found DS to be more acutely toxic than Fusarenone-X, nivalenol, or butenolide, another chemical which has been identified in *Fusarium*. Although more extensive studies have been carried out on the closely related T-2 toxin, it is probable that exposure to DS is more frequent (Mirocha 1976).

Infection of corn has often been a problem in the mid-west of the United States, especially when wet weather has preceded harvest, as in 1965 and 1972. Corn infected with *F. roseum* and other *Fusarium* species causes three main symptoms when fed to swine: hyper-estrogenism, due to zearalenone; emesis, caused by low concentrations of T-2 toxin; and feed refusal, caused by vomitoxin, at that time thought to be DS but later identified as deoxynivalenol (Mirocha 1976).

Fusarium causes a wide range of diseases in different species of animal, from lameness in water buffalo in India due to consumption of moldy rice straw (Wyllie 1978), to the death of lactating cows in the mid-west of the United States as a result of eating grain infected by T-2 toxin produced by *F. tritinctum* (Hsu *et al.* 1972). Feeding culture material prepared from maize infected with *F. moniliforme* caused pulmonary edema in pigs, nephrosis and hepatitis in sheep, congestive heart failure and hepatic cirrohsis in baboons, leukoencephalomalacia in horses, and cardiac thrombosis and hepatic cirrhosis in rats (Kriek *et al.* 1981). The reason why the major symptom recorded in pigs was pulmonary edema, while most studies have stressed emesis, feed refusal and hyper-estrogenism, is probably due to the variable toxigenic potential of different isolates of *F. moniliforme* (Kriek *et al.* 1981).

The fact that consumption of *Fusarium* toxins can damage the esophagus was clearly recognized only when by chance a species of animal was afflicted in which the esophagus is the organ most vulnerable to the toxin.

In October 1973 ducks, geese, horses and swine on five different farms in British Columbia, Canada, showed upper alimentary distress. Barley infected with *Fusarium* was found to be the cause of disease in each case. Many of the geese vomited, rejected the remainder of the feed, and eventually died. The only visible lesions were severe necrosis in the esophagus, proventriculum and gizzard. The proventriculum and esophagus showed complete degeneration of the mucous membranes, and clumps of bacteria occurred throughout (Greenway *et al.* 1975). The explanation of the especially high vulnerability of the esophagus of geese in comparison with that of ducks and chickens appears to be that geese, in contrast to other birds, have no crop. Food therefore remains for a longer period in the esophagus, resulting in an increase in exposure to the toxins. Necrotic oral lesions were induced in broiler chicks fed DS or T-2 toxin (Chi *et al.* 1978).

The nature of the acute effects of trichothecene exposure suggested that chronic treatment might cause cancer. Thus replicating cells were found to be especially vulnerable to this group of toxins. The epidermis and hair follicles of guinea pigs underwent degeneration and necrosis (Ueno 1970), and radiomimetic effects, including degeneration of actively dividing cells in the thymus, bone marrow, small intestine, testis and ovary were described in mice (Ueno 1977). Administration of T-2 toxin by a variety of routes to rats caused necrosis of lymphoid tissue and of dividing cells in the gastrointestinal tract (Brennecke *et al.* 1982). It was suggested that endotoxins produced as a consequence of the resulting overgrowth of bacteria in the gut might add to the toxicity of the mycotoxin. Significant in the present context, DS was shown to cause lesions and erosions in the buccal cavity and esophagus of swine (Ueno 1983), an important effect which, in spite of many studies, had not been revealed by previous work. While hematopoietic tissue may recover from the hypoplastic effect of trichothecenes, lymphoid tissue remained atropic (Schiefer *et al.* 1985; van Rensburg *et al.* 1987). The outcome of the effect of chronic treatment on the esophagus took longer to unravel.

Epidemiology and carcinogenicity

Food which has become infected by molds is more likely to be consumed by agricultural animals than by man, with the result that animals are more likely to be exposed to levels of mycotoxins sufficiently high to produce acute toxic effects. The possibility therefore existed that certain toxins, T-2 toxin for example, might be stored in edible animal tissues, and so be consumed by man in food of animal origin (Stoloff 1982). However, in cases where their metabolism has been studied, trichothecenes were shown to be cleared from the animal in the form of polar metabolites. Milk is the product most likely to be contaminated with T-2 toxin, but experiments with a pregnant Holstein cow and with a crossbred sow showed that, at the levels of T-2 toxin likely to be encountered in nature, only very low levels would be present in the milk (Robison *et al.* 1979). Work involving treatment of a lactating Jersey cow with tritium-labelled toxin suggested that approximately 0.2% of the dose passed into the milk (Yoshizawa *et al.* 1981). The main source of exposure to mycotoxins for man is consumption of contaminated cereals, fruit or vegetables.

High concentrations of *Fusarium* mycotoxins have been detected in corn grown in the USA, Canada, Germany, France, India and Scotland (Ueno 1985). Conditions in the UK are more favourable for *Fusarium* than for some of its competitors, including *Aspergillus*, and *Fusarium* species were detected in the majority of samples of wheat taken over the period studied (MAFF 1987). The presence of *Fusarium* species does not necessarily imply the presence of *Fusarium* mycotoxins, and it has been claimed that the great majority of samples of UK-grown cereals contained only low levels of mycotoxins (Gilbert *et al.* 1983; Patterson 1983; MAFF 1987). The levels recorded, however, vary greatly with the period studied, presumably depending on the weather conditions at the time of harvest. Thus high levels of deoxynivalenol were recorded in a high proportion of the samples of barley (20–100 μg/kg) and wheat (101–500 μg/kg) (MAFF 1987). Another important factor is that samples were taken only from the main growing areas in the UK, i.e. from the regions where production of mycotoxins is least likely to occur. The contamination in wetter low-growth regions, which are roughly those with a high incidence of esophageal cancer in women (Chapter 4), would be of much interest. Levels of contamination as high as those detected in China have been recorded in UK-grown cereals (Tanaka 1986).

Bread manufacture in the UK usually involves the blending of imported and home-grown wheat, and a proportion of imported wheat is contaminated with deoxynivalenol, although the levels are no higher than in bad years for UK wheat. Imported maize, used mainly in the manufacture of breakfast cereals and in the brewing industry, can also be contaminated with deoxynivalenol. While with bread manufacture the toxins in the cereal are present in the bread, in the processing of other products it is claimed that the toxins do not pass into the fractions designated for human consumption but into those used for animal feed.

Obviously contamination with molds can occur also during domestic storage, and the only realistic way of determining human exposure is to study the samples of food actually consumed. A survey of this type is urgently needed, before the possibility of an association of a mycotoxin with a human disease can be assessed.

Fusarium moniliforme (*F. vertecellioides*) is one of the most prevalent fungi growing on vegetables in Linxian County in the Honan province of China, and also on corn grown in the former USSR grain belt and in southern Africa, i.e. in the three regions of the world which have an exceptionally high incidence of esophageal cancer. The consumption of moldy food has long been associated with cancer of the esophagus in China, but possibly the first evidence that damage to the esophagus had been caused by mycotoxins was provided by the outbreaks of alimentary toxic aleukia in the former USSR.

Former USSR

It is only under exceptional circumstances that the level of exposure to mycotoxins in man is sufficient to cause acute toxic symptoms. The Republics of the former USSR, Turkomania and Uzbekistan, suffer from a high incidence of esophageal cancer, and it is in these grain-growing regions that the outbreaks of alimentary toxic aleukia occurred (Tuyns 1970). The disease was caused by consumption of bread prepared from overwintered grain, when toxigenic species of *Fusarium* had grown on the corn under the snow. For 3–9 days after consumption of bread baked from contaminated grain, the main symptom of the disease was acute damage to the alimentary tract, the esophagus being especially badly affected. During the following 2 weeks to 2 months the patients appeared to recover, but leukopenia and thrombocytopenia developed. This loss of immune protection often resulted in death from opportunistic infections (Joffee 1978).

China

Moldy and fermented foods are popular items in the Linxian district of China, where the rate of esophageal cancer has been exceptionally high since antiquity. Pickled vegetables, for example, are a regular part of the diet (Yang 1980; Li *et al.* 1980). The pickles are prepared in autumn, when the leaves of Chinese cabbage, soya beans and other vegetables are chopped, pressed, covered with water in ceramic containers, and allowed to ferment for several months. During this time they become covered with a white mold. The vegetables, their juices and the mold are eaten either directly or after cooking, sometimes throughout the year. A survey carried out in 1973 (Li *et al.* 1980; Yang 1980) of communes in a high- and a low-incidence area showed that the incidence of esophageal cancer varied with the extent of consumption of pickled vegetables. The incidence varied also with the consumption of a fermented food, laozao, prepared by mixing vegetables with a paste made from fish and crustaceans which had been fermented for 1–2 years. Corn, dried sweet potatoes and dried turnips were often found to be moldy in the high cancer incidence regions, and bread was often eaten when 4–5 days old.

Many studies have been carried out in an attempt to discover the cause of the hazard associated with the moldy food consumed in China. Extracts of pickled vegetables were found to be mutagenic. When fed to rats, extracts produced a variety of tumors, and also epithelial dysplasia in the esophagus and forestomach (Li *et al.* 1984). Treatment with corn meal which had been inoculated with *Fusarium moniliforme* induced epithelial hyperplasia in the esophagus, while feeding meal infected with *Aspergillus flavus* did not. It was concluded that moldy foods could induce hyperplasia and dysplasia in the esophagus, but there was no evidence at that time of carcinogenicity.

When corn bread was allowed to become moldy, breakdown of protein followed by secondary reactions resulted in an increase in the level of secondary amines. There was also an increase in the reduction of nitrate to nitrite. The growth of the mold therefore resulted in an increase in the concentration of the precursors of nitrosamines (Li *et al.* 1986). A high proportion of the amines formed were especially hazardous for the esophagus, as they resulted from the methylation of primary amines, with the formation of asymmetric methyl-alkyl-amines, which in turn would give rise to asymmetric nitrosamines (Ji *et al.* 1986). Members of this group of nitroso compounds are more potent esophageal carcinogens than the symmetric nitrosamines. Although other molds catalyzed these reactions, the increase in the formation of amines and nitrite was greatest in the presence of *F. moniliforme*.

In addition catalyzing reactions giving rise to the precursors of nitrosamines, *Fusarium* also catalyzed the nitrosation reactions, the presence of the mold resulting in an increase in the level of nitrosamines formed. This catalysis may have resulted simply from the increase in the acidity of the infected bread caused by metabolites of the mold.

The significance of these results was shown that by the fact that, when rats had been fed moldy bread, nitrosamines could be detected in the stomach. This did not occur when the animals were fed fresh bread. There is therefore good evidence for the view that the molds which infect Chinese pickled vegetables and corn bread can cause cancer by catalyzing the formation of nitrosamines (Cheng *et al.* 1982).

A comparative study of two staple foods, corn and wheat, showed contamination with *Fusarium* mycotoxins to be considerably higher in high cancer incidence regions (Luo *et al.* 1990). The proportion of kernels infected and the levels of contamination by trichothecenes in corn were higher than in wheat, but both cereals showed more contamination in Linxian than in Shangqiu. Thus in corn the incidence of contamination with deoxynivalenol was 2.4 times and with 15-acetyldeoxynivalenol 16.3 times higher in Linxian, and the mean levels were 5.8 times and 2.6 times higher respectively. The evidence incriminating moldy food as a cause of esophageal cancer is therefore very strong, but not yet conclusive.

South Africa

Consumption of maize has been associated with esophageal cancer (Franceschi *et al.* 1990), the explanation generally given being that maize is less nutritious than other grains. Hence when this cereal constitutes the staple diet, the development of deficiency in certain micronutrients may ensue (Darby *et al.* 1977). There is much independent evidence suggesting that micronutrient deficiency is associated with esophageal cancer (Chapter 10). However, in the case of maize, it has been pointed out that the incidence of esophageal cancer in man is highest in the south-west of the republic of Transkei, and relatively low in the north-east, while corn is the main dietary staple in both areas (Marasas 1981). It was the consumption of moldy maize, rather than the fact that maize was the major food item in the diet, which was associated with esophageal cancer. The most prevalent fungus associated with maize throughout the world is *Fusarium moniliforme*, and in keeping with this the levels of contamination by the *Fusarium* mycotoxins deoxynivalenol and zearalenone were higher in the regions with a higher incidence of esophageal cancer (Marasas *et al.* 1979).

Animal studies

In spite of the suggestive epidemiological evidence, extracts of culture material of *F. moniliforme* have not been shown to cause esophageal cancer in experimental animals. Pioneering studies on the chronic effects of treatment of laboratory animals were carried out by Schoental *et al.* (1974). *Fusarium* strains from the original alimentary toxic aleukia episode in the former USSR were grown on wheat for 40 days, extracts of the cultures were prepared, and rats were administered the toxic preparations by various routes. High doses of the toxins caused damage to lymphoid tissue, and hemorrhage in the gastrointestinal tract (Schoental *et al.* 1974). Treatment of weanling rats, using a short 'stomach' tube, caused ulceration, keratinization and desquamation of the esophagus. During chronic treatment at a lower dose level, the initial damage to the esophagus was repaired by regeneration, with basal cell hyperplasia of the squamous epithelium. Both the increase in cell replication in the esophagus and the concomitant immune suppression would promote the action of esophageal carcinogens. Treatment of Porton Wistar rats with T-2 toxin resulted in the appearance of malignant tumors in the stomach, duodenum, pancreas and brain, with hyperkeratosis, hyperplasia and submucosal edema in the esophagus (Schoental *et al.* 1979). The absence of organ specificity in the distribution of the malignancies suggested that the carcinogenicity was more likely to have been a result of immunosuppression than of the action of a specific carcinogen.

Similar results were obtained when maize which had become naturally contaminated by fungi was studied (Purchase *et al.* 1975). Food was collected from the stores of esophageal cancer patients in South Africa, and used to prepare meals according to local customs. When fed to rats these preparations induced first atrophy and then hyperplasia in the esophagus, and esophageal papillomas were present in two rats which survived for 2 years.

As the major mutagen present in maize, fusarin C, is destroyed by heat, the effect of feeding both freeze-dried and oven-dried material was studied (Marasas *et al.* 1984). Hepatocellular carcinoma developed in 80% of the animals, but again only basal cell hyperplasia with no evidence of malignancy occurred in the esophagus. As maize does not supply a good nutritional balance of amino acids, it was suggested that maize has two actions: first it provides a deficient diet, and secondly one of the mycotoxins produced is carcinogenic for the esophagus. Animals were therefore fed a semi-purified diet low in nutrients, in addition to the extracts prepared from cultures of *Fusarium*, but although esophageal papillomas developed, there was no sign of malignancy (Jasiewicz *et al.* 1987). The development of hepatocellular carcinoma was confirmed, but again no esophageal cancers were detected (Wilson *et al.* 1985).

The fact that fusarin C is mutagenic to bacteria and induces clastogenic effects in mammalian cells suggested that it could be carcinogenic. The ability of the toxin to initiate cancer was therefore studied by treatment of mouse skin, using a phorbol ester as a promoting agent, and for liver cancer, using phenobarbital as promoter (Gelderblom *et al.* 1986). No skin or liver cancers were induced. However, it is unfortunate that the fusarin C was given by intraperitoneal injection, so that its possible effect on esophagus could not be studied.

The conclusion from these limited experiments is that the mycotoxins do not initiate esophageal cancer, but possibly act by promoting the action of environmental esophageal carcinogens by increasing the rate of basal cell replication (Craddock *et al.* 1987*a*, 1988), or by causing immunosuppression (La Farge *et al.* 1981). Evidence for a cancer promoting potential of *F. moniliforme* in liver was provided by experiments in which the mold was fed in the diet to animals which had received an initiating treatment with diethylnitrosamine (Gelderblom *et al.* 1988).

Fungal esophagitis

When corn infected with *Fusarium* species is consumed, it is the mycotoxins which were produced by the mold while growing on the cereal which present a cancer hazard, and not the mold itself. However, other fungi when consumed are able to invade the esophageal mucosa, and numerous mycelia and spores penetrate into the epithelium. When established, the mold causes inflammation and hyperplasia in the basal cells, thus increasing the vulnerability of the esophagus to carcinogens. The mold most often responsible for fungal esophagitis is *Candida*. This genus, in common with *Fusarium*, can reduce nitrate to nitrite, and can catalyze the formation of nitrosamines (Hsia 1978). Obviously, when formed *in situ*, the carcinogenic nitrosamines would be especially hazardous.

A high incidence of fungal infection in regions of China where there is a high rate of esophageal cancer has been demonstrated (Hsia 1983*b*). Esophageal biopsies and cytological smears taken from inhabitants of the notorious Linxian region showed a high incidence of fungal infections, and these were associated with hyperplasia and dysplasia. The majority of the invading fungi were *Candida* species, although the staple foods were most often contaminated by fungi of the *Fusarium* genus. The infections occurred mainly in the middle third of the esophagus, which is the location of about 73 % of the carcinomas. Foci of cancerous lesions were found intermingled with those of fungal esophagitis. In addition, *Candida albicans* was shown to be able to nitrosate methylbenzylamine, a possible food constituent, to form the potent esophageal carcinogen nitroso-methylbenzylamine (Hsia 1978, 1981).

The high level of infection of populations living in high cancer incidence regions was confirmed by determination of serum titers of anti-*Candida* antibody (Hsia 1983*b*). The percentage of people studied who lacked the antibody was 20 % in Linxian and 59 % in Beijing. Similar investigations showed that 50 % of the patients with dysplasia and early carcinoma had fungal invasion of the mucosa, and 50 % of the fungi were identified as *Candida* species (Xia 1984).

Experimental work on fungal esophagitis has been limited. It had been suggested that treatment of patients with broad-spectrum antibiotics resulted in an increased susceptibility to *Candida* infection. In order to test the validity of this impression, rats were inoculated orally with a suspension of *Candida*, and were given tetracycline in the drinking water (Russell *et al.* 1972). This treatment was found to cause an increased rate of *Candida* infection, presumably as a result of the eradication of competing bacteria. The infection caused hyperplasia, inflammatory changes in the tongue, and loss of papillary structure. Unfortunately the esophagus was not examined.

Obviously experimental work should be carried out to determine whether *Candida* infection causes esophageal cancer in laboratory animals, and also whether it enhances the effect of esophageal carcinogens. Both these possibilities could well apply to certain regions of the world in which there is a high incidence of esophageal cancer.

Esophageal cell culture studies

Successful methods for the culture of rat esophagus with the aim of using the technique for the study of esophageal carcinogens have been developed (Stoner *et al.* 1981; Hillman *et al.* 1980). Use of a chemically defined medium allowed growth of explants in which normal morphology was maintained for 28 days, with a constant uptake of [^{3}H]thymidine into the nuclei of the basal cells, and a constant incorporation of [^{3}H]leucine into protein. These methods were used to study the effect of T2 toxin on cultured fetal human esophagus (Hsia *et al.* 1983*a*; Xia 1984). The presence of the mycotoxin at a relatively high concentration, 4 ng/ml for 6 days, resulted in necrosis of the esophageal epithelium, but a lower dose, 0.2–1.2 ng/ml, was mitogenic, causing focal basal cell hyperplasia and dysplasia. The high level of toxin therefore caused damage similar to that seen *in vivo* in cases of alimentary toxic aleukia, while with the lower dose the picture was similar to that found in pre-malignant human esophageal carcinoma. Similar results were obtained when adult human esophageal material was used (Hsia *et al.* 1983*b*). There is therefore a good basis for studying the metabolism and chemical effects of T2 toxin and other mycotoxins in esophageal cell cultures.

Mechanisms involved in association of mycotoxins with esophageal cancer

Mutagenicity of Fusarium *mycotoxins*

Although the degree of correlation between the mutagenicity and carcinogenicity of chemicals is far from perfect, nevertheless potent mutagens should be regarded as possible carcinogenic hazards. *Fusarium* is one of the most common fungi infecting food consumed by animals and man, is implicated in causing esophageal cancer, and *Fusarium* toxins have been investigated for mutagenicity. Extracts of *Fusarium moniliforme* grown on a variety of natural hosts are mutagenic in the Salmonella typhimurium assay. Thus when a total of 33 isolates of *F. moniliforme* from various food and feed crops were grown on corn, 64% were found to be mutagenic in the TA 100 assay (Bjeldans *et al.* 1979). The activity of a proportion of the extracts was increased by including liver S9 fraction in the assay.

The identity of the mutagens in *F. moniliforme* extracts has not yet been completely established. Several trichothecenes have been tested, but none has yet been found to be a potent mutagen. Thus T-2 toxin and fusarenon X were not mutagenic in the Salmonella typhimurium system, either with or without the inclusion of a liver S9 fraction in the assay (Ueno *et al.* 1978). Similarly 2-deoxynivalenol, or vomitoxin, and mono-, di-, and tri-acetoxyscirpenol were not mutagenic (Wehner *et al.* 1978). The inactivity of 2-deoxynivalenol was confirmed in a hepatocyte-mediated mutation assay using V79 Chinese hamster lung cells (Rogers *et al.* 1983).

The major mutagen present in extracts of *F. moniliforme* is Fusarin C, whether the mold is derived from corn grown in North America, the Transkei, or China. Thus Wiebe *et al.* (1981) used *F. moniliforme* isolated from corn grown in North America for the extraction and purification of a mutagenic toxin. 2.5 kg molded corn yielded 1 g Fusarin C. The molecular formula was $C_{23}H_{29}NO_7$. Gelderblom *et al.* (1983), using corn grown in the Transkei, confirmed the molecular formula of the mutagen, but its chemical nature remained unknown. *F. moniliforme* from corn grown in the notorious cancer regions in China also contained Fusarin C, the mutagenicity of which was increased by metabolic activation (Cheng *et al.* 1985). The chemical nature of the mutagen was determined by Lu *et al.* (1988). In spite of the presence of an epoxide group (Fig. 2), the most pure preparations required metabolic activation for mutagenicity. Activation was associated with the microsomal fraction of liver S9 preparations, the activation being increased by induction with Aroclor or phenobarbital.

Extracts of *F. moniliforme*, and preparations of Fusarin C, have not been shown to cause esophageal cancer (see previous section), in spite of the epidemiological association of consumption of infected food with the disease. It is therefore very probable that non-genotoxic mechanisms are responsible.

Metabolism of trichothecenes
The metabolic fate of the trichothecenes, and especially of the potentially genotoxic epoxide group, determine the role of the toxins in carcinogenesis. The absence of mutagenicity implied that metabolism of the mycotoxins, at least by the liver S9 fraction, did not give rise to intermediates which would react with DNA, and at first the evidence

supported the idea that the toxins were rapidly converted into polar metabolites and excreted. Initial *in vivo* experiments with rats and mice suggested rapid elimination of the toxins in the urine, and a metabolic pathway by which this was achieved was proposed by Yoshizawa *et al.* (1980). In liver homogenates, T-2 toxin underwent deacetylation first at the C-3 position to form HT-2, then further deacetylation at the C-15 position, and finally at position C-8 with the formation of T2-tetrol (Fig. 9.3). While with liver deacetylation was complete, strips of stomach and small intestines produced additional minor metabolites. Experiments with a lactating cow confirmed the presence of deacetylated T-2 toxin in the plasma, milk and excreta, while reaction with the 4-(p-nitrobenzyl)-pyridine/tetraethylenepentamine reagent indicated the presence of a metabolite with an intact 12,13-epoxide ring (Yoshizawa *et al.* 1981).

Rapid elimination of polar metabolites did not explain the biological effects of the trichothecenes, especially the acute toxicity in the gastro-intestinal tract. To relate the localization of injury to the presence of T-2 toxin, mice were intubated with the toxin, killed at successive intervals of time, when the organs were examined for the presence of T-2 toxin by use of a specific antibody which was visualized by an immunoperoxidase reaction (Lee *et al.* 1984). The toxin appeared in the esophagus within 5 minutes of dosing, and remained in superficial and in deeper squamous cells for 24 hours. In the gastrointestinal tract, the reaction for T-2 toxin was strong in the stomach and duodenum, and but weak in the jejunum, and could not be detected in the ileum. The toxin was not detected in the liver, presumably on account of its rapid conversion by esterases into HT-2. These results show that the presence of T-2 toxin for a considerable period, as in the esophagus and upper gastrointestinal tract, correlates with the appearance of cellular damage.

Similar experiments designed to localize T-2 toxin were carried out in swine by use of the tritium-labelled compound (Corley *et al.* 1986). Although the toxin was given by intravenous injection, the major part of

Fig. 9.3. Metabolites of T-2 toxin (Yoshizawa *et al.* 1980). OAc, acetate.

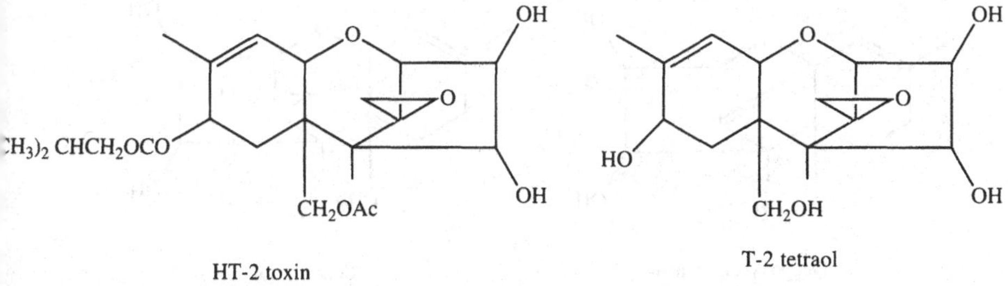

HT-2 toxin

T-2 tetraol

the dose was again located in the gastrointestinal tract. The suggestion was that the toxin was taken up by the liver, and passed via the bile to the gastro-intestinal tract.

The fate of the epoxide group is of major importance. It was suggested that, as T-2 toxin does not compete with substrates for epoxide hydrolase, and as the epoxide group is stereochemically protected from reaction, it would be stable *in vivo* (Bieger *et al.* 1985). The first evidence that de-epoxidation occurred came from experiments not with T-2 toxin but with diacetoxyscirpenol (Sakamoto *et al.* 1986). After oral administration to rats, the parent compound was not detected in the urine or feces, but deacetylation occurred with concomitant disappearance of the epoxide group, and the formation of the intermediates shown in Fig. 9.4. Mass and nuclear resonance spectroscopy of urinary and fecal metabolites identified the compounds and showed that they represented approximately 50% of the dose.

Although consumption of contaminated grain leads to hemorrhagic damage in the bovine alimentary canal, it was found that T-2 toxin, diacetoxyscirpenol and deoxynivalenol are metabolized by deacetylation and loss of the epoxide group by microorganisms present in the rumen (Swanson *et al.* 1987). Presumably removal of the toxin by the micro-organisms would offer some protection to the lower alimentary canal, but this would not apply to the esophagus.

Fig. 9.4. Metabolites of diacetoxyscirpenol (Sakamoto *et al.* 1986). OAc, acetate.

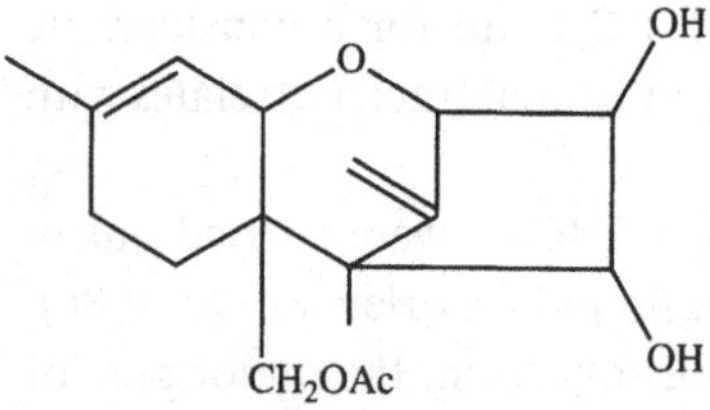

15-Acetoxydeepoxyscirpenol

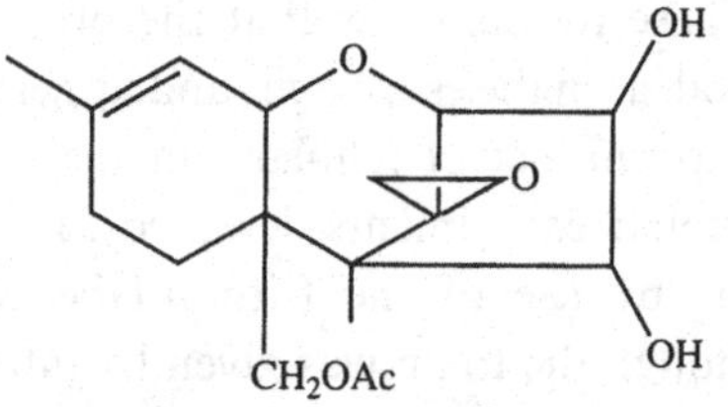

15-Monoacetoxyscirpenol

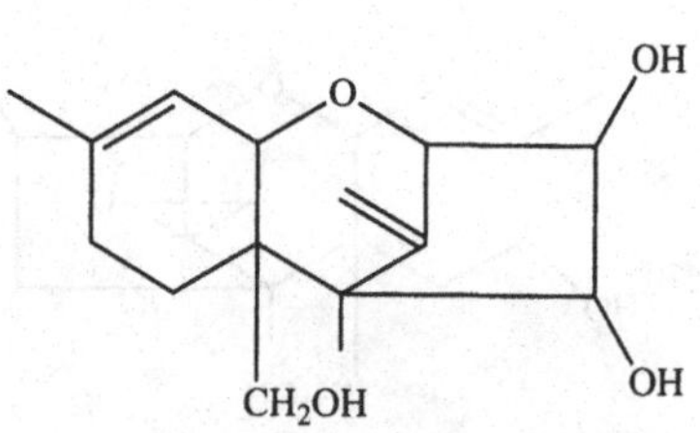

Deepoxyscirpentriol

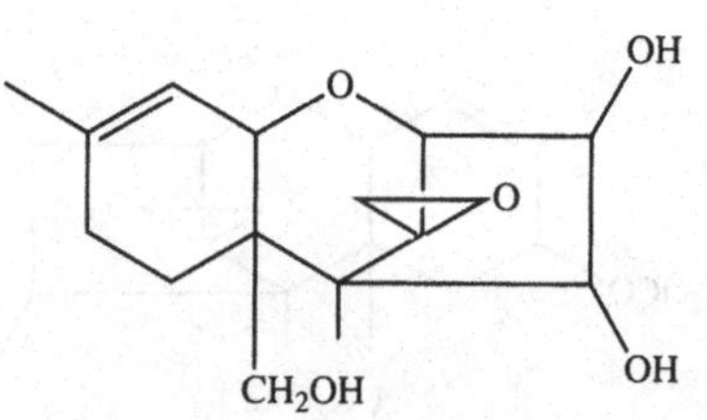

Scirpentriol

The epoxide group is shielded by the ring system of the trichothecene nucleus, and is broken only after intramolecular ring rearrangement by dramatic treatment with reducing (lithium aluminium hydroxide), oxidizing (hydrogen peroxide) or hydrolytic (50 % sulfuric acid) reagents *in vitro* with the formation of an apotrichothecene ring system (Ueno 1983; Wyllie *et al.* 1977). *In vivo* the epoxide is presumably labilized by enzymic action. Whichever side of the oxygen atom is attacked by the epoxidase, a carbon residue would acquire a positive charge and the metabolite thus formed would react as an electrophilic reagent. In theory it could alkylate nucleic acids or proteins, but as yet there is no evidence for the occurrence of these reactions. It would be of much interest to test for DNA adducts especially, using the very sensitive techniques now available.

The effect of trichothecenes on cell biochemistry, DNA damage and repair, and cell replication

The trichothecenes are not potent mutagens, and feeding experiments have not shown extracts of cultures of *Fusarium moniliforme* to induce esophageal cancer. It is therefore probable that the association of the disease with consumption of contaminated food is not mediated by the presence of a primary initiating carcinogen in the mold, but that its action is brought about by promoting the effect of carcinogens derived from another source. Although the trichothecenes cause immunosuppression, the organ specificity of their association with cancer suggests that this is not the entire explanation. An important fact is that esophageal hyperplasia was induced when oven-dried culture material was fed to rats (Marasas *et al.* 1984), as this implies that the trichothecenes rather than fusarin C are the relevant mycotoxins, and that they may promote cancer by causing an increase in cell replication.

The effect of the toxins on the cell biochemistry must in some way bring about the hyperplastic response. One of the most dramatic effects of trichothecenes is their inhibition of protein synthesis, these toxins being among the most potent low molecular weight inhibitors known. Of the mycotoxins tested, only trichothecenes inhibited the incorporation of amino acids in the reticulocyte assay (Ueno *et al.* 1973*a*), a property which was used as a method for assay of the toxins. Of the fourteen trichothecenes studied, diacetoxyscirpenol, T-2 toxin and HT-2 toxin were the most potent inhibitors (Ueno *et al.* 1973*b*). The different trichothecenes appear to act by a variety of routes, some inhibiting protein synthesis irreversibly at the initiation stage, others having a reversible effect at the elongation stage (Liao *et al.* 1976). Another important far-reaching effect of trichothecenes, which must be involved in their effects on macromolecular synthesis, is their inhibition of sulfhydryl enzymes (Ueno *et al.* 1975). A detailed study of the effect of the toxins on protein synthesis or on sulfhydryl-dependent enzymes *in vivo* has not yet been carried out, and their effect on these reactions in the esophagus would be of much interest. While feeding experiments showed that T-2 toxin reduced the protein content of liver and intestinal mucosa (Suneja *et al.* 1983), this was not shown to be due to inhibition of protein synthesis.

Many of the acute toxic effects of the trichothecenes are probably dependent on the inhibition of protein synthesis. For example, there is evidence that this is the cause of the cardiac lesions induced in mice by deoxynivalenol (Robbana-Barnat *et al.* 1987). As a result of the potent inhibition of protein synthesis brought about by diacetoxyscirpenol, an attempt was made to use the compound, under the name of anguidine, in cancer chemotherapy. The toxicity of the drug rapidly caused this possibility to be abandoned.

Evidence that the toxins cause damage to the DNA molecule came from measurements of unscheduled DNA synthesis. Mice were injected with T-2 toxin then killed at intervals, the DNA being isolated from various organs and subjected to analysis by alkaline elution from cellulose ester filters (Lafarge *et al.* 1981). Single-strand breaks were not observed in liver, but were significant in spleen. The DNA lesions had apparently been repaired 24 hours later. Further evidence that the trichothecenes do not inhibit repair enzymes was given by experiments with diacetoxyscirpenol (Craddock *et al.* 1987*b*). Acute or chronic treatment did not inhibit O^6-methylguanine–methyl-DNA transferase in esophagus.

While it is possible that damage to DNA is responsible for the association of the consumption of infected food with esophageal cancer, the stimulating effect on basal cell replication is very likely to be involved. The effect on DNA synthesis and cell replication, however, depends on the organ concerned, and may reflect the variable nature of the metabolism of the toxin in different organs. As might be expected, trichothecenes were not found to inhibit DNA synthesis either *in vivo* or *in vitro* in those organs in which it was not especially toxic, as in liver (Lafarge *et al.* 1981), but DNA synthesis was inhibited in tissues in which the toxins are known to cause a rapid inhibition of cell replication *in vivo*, as in lymphoid tissue (Lafarge *et al.* 1981; Cooray *et al.* 1984).

A single dose of DS, given by gavage to rats, caused an increase in cell replication in the basal cells of the esophagus and also in the squamous and glandular stomach (Craddock *et al.* 1987). An increased incorporation of tritiated thymidine in DNA and induction of ornithine decarboxylase were demonstrated in squamous stomach. The increase in cell replication did not appear to result from cell damage and restorative hyperplasia but, as with the cell culture studies mentioned previously, suggested that DS had a direct mitotic action. When fed in the diet, DS caused hyperplasia in the squamous stomach in a limited number of animals which survived for 9 months, but there was no evidence of hyperplasia in the esophagus (Craddock *et al.* 1988). However, as suggested also by the cell culture studies, the levels of toxin which cause either damage or mitosis may be restricted to a narrow range. This may be the explanation of the fact that simultaneous treatment of animals with DS and with *N*-methyl-*N*-benzylnitrosamine did not increase evidence of esophageal cancer (Craddock *et al.* 1986). The mechanism by which trichothecenes stimulate mitosis is completely unknown, and merits investigation. However, it is relevant that in many systems an increase in the rate of cell replication enhances their vulnerability to carcinogens. Although definitive proof of an association between consumption of *Fusarium* mycotoxins and esophageal cancer has not been established (IACR 1983*a,b*), compelling evidence shows that the toxins are one of the factors which can be involved.

References

Agrelo, C.E. and Schoental, R. (1980) *Toxicol. Lett.* 5, 155–160. Synthesis of DNA in human fibroblasts treated with T-2 toxin and HT-2 toxin (the trichothecene metabolites of *Fusarium* species) and the effects of hydroxyurea.

Bieger, A.R. and Dose, K.P. (1985) In: *Trichothecenes and other Mycotoxins* (Lacey, J. ed.). New York: Wiley, pp. 331–336. Resistance to metabolic conversion of the epoxide group in trichothecenes.

Bjeldanes, L.F. and Thomson, S.V. (1979) *Appl. Environ. Microbiol.* 37, 1118–1121. Mutagenicity of *Fusarium moniliforme* isolates in the *Salmonella typhimurium* assay.

Black, R.M. Clarke, R.J. and Read, R.W. (1987) *J. Chromatogr.* 388, 365–378. Detection of trace levels of trichothecene mycotoxins in environmental residues and foodstuffs using gas chromatography with mass spectroscopy or electron-capture detection.

Bradlaw, J.A., Swentzel, K.C., Alterman, E. and Hauswrith, J.W. (1985) *Food Them. Toxicol.* 23, 1063–1067. Evaluation of purified 4-deoxynivalenol (vomitoxin) for unscheduled DNA synthesis in the primary rat hepatocyte-DNA repair assay.

Brennecke, L.H. and Neufeld, H.A. (1982) *Fed. Proc.* 41, 924. Pathological effects and LD_{50} doses of T2 toxin in rats by intramuscular, subcutaneous and intraperitoneal routes of administration.

Brian, P.W., Dawkins, A.W., Grove, J.F., Hemming, H.G., Lowe, D. and Norris, G.L.F. (1961) *J. Exp. Bot.* 12, 1–12. Phytotoxic compounds produced by *Fusarium equiseti*.

Cheng, S.J., Sala, M., Li, M.H. and Chouroulinkov, I. (1982) *Carcinogenesis* 7, 167–174. Esophageal cancer in Linxian County, China: a possible etiology and mechanism.

242   *Molds and mycotoxins*

Cheng, S.J., Jiang, Y.Z. and Lo, H.Z. (1985) *Carcinogenesis* **6**, 903–905. A mutagenic metabolite produced by *Fusarium moniliforme* isolated from Linxian Country, China.

Chi, M.S. and Mirocha, C.J. (1978) *Poultry Sci.* **57**, 807–808. Necrotic oral lesions in chicken fed diacetoxyscirpenol, T-2 toxin, and crotocin.

Cooray, R. (1984) *Food Cosmet. Toxicol.* **22**, 529–534. Effects of some mycotoxins on mitogen-induced blastogenesis and SCE frequency in human lymphocytes.

Corley, R.A., Swanson, S.P., Gullo, G.J., Johnson, L., Beasley, V.R. and Buck, W.B. (1986) *J. Agric. Food. Chem.* **34**, 868–875. Deposition of T-2 toxin, a trichothecene mycotoxin, in intravenously dosed swine.

Craddock, V.M., Sparrow, S. and Henderson, A.R. (1986) *Cancer Lett.* **31**, 197–204. The effect of trichothecene mycotoxin diacetoxyscirpenol on nitrosamine-induced esophageal cancer in the rat.

Craddock, V.M., Hill, R.J. and Henderson, A.R. (1987a) *Cancer Lett.* **37**, 199–209. Stimulation of DNA replication in rat esophagus and stomach by the trichothecene mycotoxin diacetoxyscirpenol.

Craddock, V.M. and Henderson, A.R. (1987b) *Cancer Lett.* **37**, 81–86. Effect of the esophageal carcinogen methylbenzylnitrosamine and of a putative potentiating factor, a trichothecene mycotoxin, on O^6-methylguanine–DNA methyltransferase in rat esophagus and liver.

Craddock, V.M., Hill, R.J. and Henderson, A.R. (1988) *Cancer Lett.* **41**, 287–294. Acute and chronic effects of diacetoxyscirpenol on cell replication in rat esophagus and stomach.

Darby, W.J., McNutt, K.W. and Todhunter, E.N. (1977) *Nutr. Rev.* **33**, 289–297. Niacin.

Desjardins, A.E. and Plattner, R.D. (1989) *J. Agric. Food Chem.* **39**, 388–392. Trichothecene toxin production by strains of *Gibberella pilicaris* (*Fusarium sambuanum*) in liquid culture and in potato tubers.

Franceschi, S., Bidoli, E., Baron, A.E. and La Vecchia, C. (1990) *J. Natl. Cancer Inst.* **82**, 1407–1411. Maize and cancers of the oral cavity, pharynx and esophagus in north-eastern Italy.

Gaddamidi, V., Bjeldanes, L.F. and Shoolery, N. (1985) *J. Agric. Food. Chem.* **33**, 652–654. Fusarin C: structure determination by natural abundance $^{13}C-^{13}C$ coupling and deuterium-induced ^{13}C shifts.

Gelderblom, W.C.A., Thiel, P.G., van der Merive, K.J., Marassas, W.F.O. and Spies, H.S.C. (1983) *Toxicon* **21**, 467–473. A mutagen produced by *Fusarium moniliforme*.

Gelderblom, W.C.A., Thiel, P.G., Jaskiewicz, K. and Marasas, W.F.O. (1986) *Carcinogenesis* **7**, 1899–1901. Investigations on the carcinogenicity of Fusarin C – a mutagenic metabolite of *Fusarium moniliforme*.

Gelderblom, W.C.A., Marasas, W.F.O., Jaskiewicz, K., Combrinck, S. and van Schalkwyk, D.J. (1988) *Carcinogenesis* **9**, 1405–1409. Cancer promoting potential of different strains of *Fusarium moniliforme* in a short-term cancer initiation/promotion assay.

Gilbert, J., Shepherd, M.J. and Startin, J.R. (1983) *J. Sci. Food Agric.* **34**, 86–92. A survey of the occurrence of the trichothecene mycotoxin deoxynivalenol (vomitoxin) in UK-grown barley and in imported maize by combined gas chromatography–mass spectrometry.

Greenway, J.A. and Puls, R. (1976) *Can. J. Comp. Med.* **40**, 12–15. Fusariotoxicosis from barley in British Columbia.

Hillman, E.A., Vocci, M.J., Schurch, W., Harris, C.C. and Trump, B.F. (1989) In: *Methods in Cell Biology*, vol. 21B, Harris, C.C., Trump, B.F. and Stoner, G.D. (eds.). New York: Academic Press, pp. 331–348. Human esophageal organ culture studies.

Hsia, C.C. and Tsao, I.Y. (1978) *Natl. Med. J. China* **58**, 392–396. Fungal invasions in esophageal tissue and its possible relation to esophageal carcinoma. (In Chinese. Quoted in Hsia *et al.* 1983*a*).

Hsia, C.C., Sun, T.T., Wang, Y.Y., Anderson, L.M., Armstrong, D. and Good, R.A. (1981) *Proc. Natl. Acad. Sci.* **78**, 1878–1881. Enhancement of formation of the esophageal carcinogen methylbenzylnitrosamine from its precursors by *Candida albicans*.

Hsia, C.C., Tzian, B.L. and Harris, C.C. (1983*a*) *Carcinogenesis* **4**, 1101–1107. Proliferative and cytotoxic effects of *Fusarium* T2 toxin on cultured human fetal esophagus.

Hsia, C. (1983*b*) In: *Human Carcinogenesis* (Harris, C.C. and Autrup, H.N. eds.). New York: Academic Press, pp. 883–911. Possible roles of fungal infection and mycotoxin in human esophageal carcinogenesis.

Hsu, I.C., Smalley, E.B., Strong, F.M. and Ribelin, W.E. (1972) *Appl. Microbiol.* **24**, 684–690. Identification of T-2 toxin in mouldy corn associated with a lethal toxicosis in dairy cattle.

International Agency for Cancer Research (1983) Monograph No. 31, 265–278. Trichothecenes, T2.

International Agency for Cancer Research (1983) Monograph No. 31, 153–161. Trichothecenes, Fusarenon X.

Jasiewicz, K., van Rensburg, S.J., Marasas, W.F. and Golderblom, W.C. (1987) *J. Natl. Cancer Inst.* **78**, 321–325. Carcinogenicity of *Fusarium moniliforme* culture material in rats.

Ji, C., Li, M.H., Li, J.L. and Lu, S.J. (1986) *Carcinogenesis* **7**, 301–303. Synthesis of nitrosomethylisoamylamine from isoamylamine and sodium nitrite by fungi.

Joffe, A.Z. (1974) In: *Mycotoxins* (Purchase, I.F.H. ed.). Amsterdam: Elsevier, pp. 229–262. Toxicity of *Fusarium poae* and *F. sporotrichioides* and its relation to alimentary toxic aleukia.

Joffe, A.Z. (1978) In: *Mycotoxic Fungi, Mycotoxins, Mycotoxicoses: An Encyclopedic Handbook*. (Wyllie, T.D. and Morehouse, L.G. eds.). New York: Marcel Dekker, pp. 21–86. *Fusarium poae* and *F. sporotrichioides* as principal causal agents of alimentary toxic aleukia.

Kriek, N.P.J., Kellerman, T.S. and Marasas, W.F.O. (1981) *Onderstepoort J. Vet. Res.* **48**, 129–131. A comparative study of the toxicity of *Fusarium verticillioides* to horse, primates, pigs, sheep and fungi.

Krupp, C.A., Swanson, S.P. and Buck, W.B. (1986) *J. Agric. Food Chem.* **34**, 865–868. *In vitro* metabolism of T-2 toxin by rat liver microsomes.

Lacey, J. (1985) *Trichothecenes and Other Mycotoxins*. New York: Wiley.

Lacey, J. (1988) *J. Stored Prod. Res.* **24**, 39–50. The microbiology of cereal grains from areas of Iran with a high incidence of esophageal cancer.

La Farge-Frayssinet, C., Decloitre, F., Mousset, S., Martin, M. and Frayssinet, C. (1981) *Mutation Res.* **88**, 115–123. Induction of DNA single-strand breaks by

T-2 toxin, a trichothecene metabolite of *Fusarium*. Effect on lymphoid organs and liver.

Lee, S.C., Berry, J.T. and Chu, F.S. (1984) *Toxicol. Appl. Pharmacol.* **72**, 228–235. Immunoperoxidase localization of T-2 toxin.

Li, M., Li, P. and Li, B. (1980) *Adv. Cancer Res.* **33**, 173–249. Recent progress in research on esophageal cancer in China.

Li, M.H. and Cheng, S.J. (1984) In: *Carcinoma of the Esophagus and Gastric Cardia* (Huang, G.J. and K'ai, W.Y. eds.). Berlin: Springer, pp. 26–51. Etiology of carcinoma of the esophagus.

Liao, L.L., Grollman, A.P. and Horwitz, S.B. (1976) *Biochem. Biophys. Acta* **454**, 273–284. Mechanism of action of the 12,13-epoxytrichothecene, anguidine, an inhibitor of protein synthesis.

Lindenfelser, L.A., Lillehoj, E.B. and Burmister, H.R. (1974) *J. Natl. Cancer Inst.* **52**, 113–116. Aflatoxin and trichothecene toxins: skin tumor induction and synergistic acute toxicants in white mice.

Littel, W., Fowler, H.W. and Coulson, J. (1978) *The Shorter Oxford English Dictionary*, 3rd edn. Oxford: Clarendon Press.

Lu, S.J., Ronai, Z.A., Li, M.H. and Jeffrey, A.M. (1988) *Carcinogenesis* **9**, 1523–1527. *Fusarium moniliforme* metabolites: genotoxicity of culture extracts.

Luo, Y., Yoshizawa, T. and Katayama, T. (1990) *Appl. Environ. Microbiol.* **56**, 3723–3726. Comparative study on the natural occurrence of Fusarium mycotoxins (trichothecenes and zearalenone) in corn and wheat from high- and low-risk areas for human esophageal cancer in China.

MAFF (Ministry of Agriculture, Fisheries and Food) (1987) Food Surveillance Paper No. 18. London: HMSO. Mycotoxins.

Marasas, W.F.O., van Rensburg, S.J. and Mirocha, C.J. (1979) *J. Agric. Food Chem.* **27**, 1108–1112. Incidence of *Fusarium* species and the mycotoxins deoxynivalenol and zearalenone in corn produced in esophageal cancer areas in Transkei.

Marasas, W.F.O., Wehner, F.C., van Rensburg, S.J. and van Schalkwyk, D. (1981) *Phytopathology* **71**, 792–796. Mycoflora of corn produced in human esophageal areas in Transkei, South Africa.

Marasas, W.F.O., Kreik, N.P.J., Fincham, J.E. and van Rensburg, S.J. (1984) *Int. J. Cancer* **34**, 383–387. Primary liver cancer and esophageal basal cell hyperplasia in rats caused by *Fusarium moniliforme*.

Melmed, R.N., Ishai-Michaeli, R. and Yagen, B. (1985) *Biochem. Pharmacol.* **32**, 2809–2812. Differential inhibition by T-2 toxin of total protein, DNA and isoprenoid synthesis by the cultured macrophage cell line J774.

Mirocha, C.J., Pathre, S.V., Schauerhamer, B. and Christensen, C.M. (1976) *Appl. Environ. Microbiol.* **32**, 553–556. Natural occurrence of *Fusarium* toxins in feedstuffs.

Patterson, D.S.P. (1983) In: *Trichothecenes – Chemical, Biological and Toxicological Aspects* (Ueno, Y. ed.). Developments in Food Science 4. Amsterdam: Elsevier Press, pp. 259–264. Trichothecenes: toxicoses and natural occurrence in Britain.

Purchase, I.F.H., Tustin, R.C. and van Rensburg, S.J. (1975) *Food Cosmet. Toxicol.* **13**, 639–647. Biological testing of food grown in the Transkei.

Robbana-Barnat, S., Loridon-Rosa, B., Cohen, H., La Farge-Frayssinet, C.,

Neish, G.A. and Frayssinet, C. (1987) *Food Addit. Contam.* 4, 49–55. Protein synthesis inhibition and cardiac lesions associated with deoxynivalenol ingestion in mice.

Robinson, T.S., Mirocha, C.J., Kurtz, H.J., Behrens, J.C., Chi, M.S., Weaver, G.A. and Nystrom, S.D. (1979) *J. Dairy Sci.* 62, 637–641. Transmission of T-2 toxin into bovine and porcine milk.

Rodricks, J.V., Hesseltine, C.W. and Mehlman, M.A. (1977) *Mycotoxins in Human and Animal Health*. Park Forest South, Illinois: Pathotox Publications.

Rogers, C.G. and Heroux-Metcalf, C. (1983) *Cancer Lett.* 20, 29–35. Cytotoxicity and absence of mutagenic activity of vomitoxin (4-deoxynivalenol) in a hepatocyte-mediated mutation assay with V79 Chinese hamster lung cells.

Russell, C. and Jones, J.H. (1972) *J. Med. Microbiol.* 6, 275–279. Effects of oral inoculation of *Candida albicans* in tetracycline-treated rats.

Sakamoto, T., Swanson, S.P., Yoshizawa, T. and Buck, W.B. (1986) *J. Agric. Food Chem.* 34, 698–701. Structures of new metabolites of diacetoxyscirpenol in the excreta of orally administered rats.

Schoental, R. and Joffe, A.Z. (1974) *J. Pathol.* 112, 37–42. Lesions induced in rodents by extracts from cultures of *Fusarium poae* and *F. sporotrichioides*.

Schoental, R., Joffe, A.Z. and Yagen, B. (1979) *Cancer Res.* 39, 2179–2189. Cardiovascular lesions and various tumors found in rats given T-2 toxin, a trichothecene metabolite of *Fusarium*.

Schoental, R. (1980) *Prev. Med.* 9, 159–161. A corner of history: Moses and mycotoxins.

Schoental, R. (1985) *Adv. Cancer Res.* 45, 217–290. Trichothecenes, zearalenone and other carcinogenic metabolites of *Fusarium* and related microfungi.

Schwenk, S., Altmayer, B. and Eichhorn, K.W. (1988) *J. Chromatogr.* 448, 424–427. Simultaneous detection of trichothecenes and rosenonolactone in grape juice and wine by capillary gas chromatography.

Seeley, T.D., Nowicke, J.W., Meselson, M., Guillemin, J. and Akratanakul, P. (1985) *Sci. Am.* 253, 122–131. Yellow rain.

Steyn, P.S., Vleggaar, R., Rabie, C.J., Kreik, N.P.J. and Harrington, J.S. (1978) *Phytochemistry* 17, 949–951. Trichothecene mycotoxins from *Fusarium sulphureum*.

Stoloff, L. (1982) In: *Carcinogens and Mutagens in the Environment* (Stich, H.F. ed.). Boca Raton: CRC Press, pp. 97–120. Mycotoxins as potential environmental carcinogens.

Stoner, G.D., Pettis, W., Haugen, A., Jackson, F. and Harris, C.C. (1981) *In Vitro* 17, 681–688. Explant culture of rat esophagus in a chemically defined medium.

Suneja, S.K., Ram, G.C. and Wagle, D.S. (1983) *Toxicol. Lett.* 18, 73–76. Effects of feeding T-2 toxin on RNA, DNA and protein contents of liver and intestinal mucosa of rats.

Swanson, S.P., Nicoletti, J., Rood, H.D., Buck, W.B. and Cote, L.M. (1987) *J. Chromatogr.* 414, 335–342. Metabolism of three trichothecene mycotoxins, T-2 toxin, diacetoxyscirpenol and deoxynivalenol by bovine rumen microorganisms.

Tanaka, T., Hasegawa, A., Matsuki, Y., Lee, U.S. and Ueno, Y. (1986) *Food Addit. Contam.* 3, 247–252. A limited survey of *Fusarium* mycotoxins nivalenol, deoxynivalenol and zearalenone in 1984 UK harvested wheat and barley.

Tuyns, A. (1979) In: IACR Internal Technical Report 70/003 (Serenko, A.F. and Romanski, A.A. eds.). Cancer morbidity and mortality data in USSR.

Ueno, Y., Ishikawa, Y., Amakai, K., Nakajima, M., Saito, M., Enomoto, M. and Ohtsubo, K. (1970) *Jpn. J. Exp. Med.* **40**, 33–38. Comparative study of skin necrotizing effect of scirpene metabolites of *Fusarium*.

Ueno, Y., Sato, N., Ishii, K., Sakai, H., Tsunoda, H. and Enomoto, M. (1973a) *Appl. Microbiol.* **25**, 699–704. Biological and chemical detection of trichothecene mycotoxins of *Fusarium* species.

Ueno, Y., Jakajima, M., Sakai, K., Ishu, K., Sato, N. and Shimada, N. (1973b) *J. Biochem.* **74**, 285–296. Comparative toxicology of trichothecene mycotoxins: inhibition of protein synthesis in animal cells.

Ueno, Y. and Matsumoto, H. (1975) *Chem. Pharmacol. Bull.* **23**, 2439–2442. Inactivation of some thiol-enzymes by trichothecene mycotoxins from *Fusarium* species.

Ueno, Y. (1977) In: *Mycotoxins in Human and Animal Health* (Rodricks, J.V., Hesseltine, C.W. and Mehlman, M.A., eds.). Park Forest South, Illinois: Pathotox Publications, pp. 189–207. Tricothecenes: overview address.

Ueno, Y., Kubota, K., Ito, T. and Nakamura, Y. (1978) *Cancer Res.* **38**, 536–542. Mutagenicity of carcinogenic mycotoxins in *Salmonella typhimurium*.

Ueno, Y. (1980) *Adv. Nutr. Res.* **3**, 301–354. Trichothecene mycotoxins, mycology, chemistry and toxicology.

Ueno, Y. (1983) *Trichothecenes – Chemical, Biological and Toxicological Aspects.* Development in Food Science No. 4. Amsterdam: Elsevier.

Ueno, Y. (1985) CRC Critical Reviews in Toxicology 14, Boca Raton: CRC Press, pp. 99–132. The toxicology of mycotoxins.

Wehner, F.C., Marasas, W.F.O. and Thiel, P.G. (1978) *Appl. Environ. Microbiol.* **35**, 659–662. Lack of mutagenicity to *Salmonella typhimurium* of some *Fusarium* mycotoxins.

Wiebe, L.A. and Bjeldanes, L.F. (1981) *J. Food Sci.* **46**, 1424–1426. Fusarin C, a mutagen from *Fusarium moniliforme* grown on corn.

Wilson, T.M., Nelson, P.E. and Krepp, C.R. (1985) *Carcinogenesis* **6**, 1155–1160. Hepatic neoplastic nodules, adenofibrosis, and cholangiocarcinomas in male Fischer 344 rats fed corn naturally contaminated with *Fusarium moniliforme*.

Wyllie, T.D. and Morehouse, L.G. (eds.). *Mycotoxic Fungi, Mycotoxins, Mycotoxicoses.* New York: Marcel Dekker. Vol. 1 (1977) Mycotoxic fungi and chemistry of mycotoxins; vol. 2 (1978) Mycotoxicoses of domestic and laboratory animals, poultry, and aquatic invertebrates and vertebrates; vol. 3 (1978) Mycotoxicoses of man and plants: mycotoxin control and regulatory practices.

Xia, Q.J. (1984) In: *Carcinoma of the Esophagus and Gastric Cardia* (Huang G.J. and K'ai, W.Y. eds.). Berlin: Springer, pp. 53–76. Carcinogenesis in the esophagus.

Yang, C.S. (1980) *Cancer Res.* **40**, 2633–2644. Research on esophageal cancer in China: a review.

Yoshizawa, T., Swanson, S.P. and Mirocha, C.J. (1980) *J. Appl. Environ. Microbiol.* **40**, 901–906. *In vitro* metabolism of T2 toxin in rats.

Yoshizawa, T., Mirocha, C.J., Behrens, J.C. and Swanson, S.P. (1981) *Food Cosmet. Toxicol.* **19**, 31–39. Metabolic fate of T-2 toxin in a lactating cow.

10

Dietary deficiencies: micronutrients, fresh plant food and protective factors

Introduction

The esophageal carcinogens which people frequently encounter, for example nitrosamines in food, drink and tobacco, are at sufficiently high levels of exposure to cause cancer only if the esophageal epithelium is predisposed by additional insults (van Rensburg 1981). Many authors have stressed the multifactorial nature of esophageal cancer, and the likelihood that the disease is the result of a site-specific carcinogen acting on nutritionally predisposed tissue. While alcohol and tobacco are the major secondary risk factors in the West, nutritional status is more important in less affluent communities, especially China, Iran and Africa. A large number of surveys have shown that low consumption of fresh fruit and vegetables is associated with cancers at various sites, including the esophagus. Both epidemiological studies and animal experiments have shown riboflavin deficiency and zinc deficiency to have especially adverse effects on the esophagus. Whether the protective action of fruit and vegetables is due entirely to their vitamin and mineral content, or whether other factors are also involved, has yet to be determined.

Esophageal cancer more than the majority of other cancers is a disease of poor rural areas with inefficient agriculture, or of groups of people elsewhere with the lowest socioeconomic status (Day et al. 1982). The cancer is not the result of one major nutritional deficiency, as with the typical deficiency diseases such as pellagra and scurvy, but is associated with general low nutrition.

Nutritional deficiencies are caused not only by a low intake of appropriate foods, but also by malabsorption from the alimentary tract, as occurs for example where unleavened bread made from lightly milled whole wheat forms the major item in the diet. Minerals become bound to the phytate, inositol hexaphosphate, which is present in high concentrations in cereals but is destroyed by leavening, and minerals are bound also to the complex carbohydrate fibers in the bread. They are therefore not biologically available. Another example of unavailability occurs with alcoholics. Not only is the consumption of other food reduced if more than about 900 calories per day are derived from alcohol, but ethanol also decreases the absorbability of riboflavin, zinc and other micronutrients (McCoy *et al.* 1980).

Other causes of malabsorption are disorders of the small intestine. Celiac disease is a familial condition, with about 10% of first degree relatives being affected, and zinc deficiency has been observed in patients who did not respond to gluten-free diets (Love *et al.* 1978). The disease has been associated with lymphoma and carcinomas of the tongue, stomach, colon, rectum and anus, but especially of the esophagus (Harris *et al.* 1967). The patients had a long history of celiac disease, the most frequent location of the tumor in the esophagus being in the middle or lower third. In general, similar malignancies were found also by Holmes *et al.* (1976).

Evidence for the role of nutrient deficiencies in the etiology of esophageal cancer is discussed from the aspect of epidemiological surveys which study the association with consumption of fruit, vegetables, cereals and other food items, and also from the aspect of specific vitamins and minerals.

Many case–control studies and population surveys have studied the nature of the food items consumed. This is of special interest where the diet is restricted to a staple food, for example maize, sorghum or rice. Other studies have concentrated on certain micronutrients and measured, for example, zinc status by hair and blood analyses, and riboflavin status by studying intake and blood levels. The work has been carried out mainly in regions with a high incidence of esophageal cancer, as in Southern Africa, Iran, China, France and in certain populations in the USA. As the surveys have considered the nature of the diet and the levels of consumption of several micronutrients simultaneously, the epidemiological work will be described after a brief discussion of the micronutrients which are most likely to be relevant.

Specific micronutrients
Zinc
Although it has been known for many years that zinc is an essential trace element for man, the ubiquity of the mineral in food made it seem unlikely that the low requirement would not be met. Symptoms of zinc deficiency, however, were first reported around 1961 in certain regions of Egypt and Iran (Prasad 1983). The rate of esophageal cancer is exceptionally high in the regions of Iran where zinc deficiency was

observed, while it is not especially high in Egypt. Zinc deficiency *per se* therefore does not appear to be a sufficient cause of esophageal cancer.

The highest levels of zinc exist in the more expensive foods, for example in meat, fish and green leafy vegetables, and deficiencies in intake are therefore more likely to occur in families with a low socioeconomic status. In addition, there may be a low bioavailability of zinc, usually as a result of a high consumption of unleavened wholegrain bread in which, as previously explained, the fibre and phytate reduced absorption of zinc from the intestine.

In the USA, the diets of certain hospitals, and of teenagers consuming unbalanced diets with a high proportion of soft drinks, are also low in zinc (Osis *et al.* 1972). Excessive intake of alcohol is another cause of zinc deficiency (Prasad 1979; and see Chapter 6). Deficiency in the USA occurs also in poor families, especially in children, pregnant and lactating women, in the elderly, and where there is an increased urinary excretion of zinc, as in patients on drugs which are chelating agents (Prasad 1983).

The optimum dietary zinc intake is not known. While there is no recommended daily allowance in the UK, the US Food and Drug Administration have recommended a daily intake of 15 mg. This is not a daily requirement, but an estimate believed to exceed the requirements of most people. On this basis, the diets of people in the west of Scotland, the region with the highest rate of esophageal cancer for women in Europe, were found by analysis of typical cooked meals to provide insufficient zinc. It is possible that subclinical zinc deficiency is widespread. The level of deficiency for women (49 %) was higher than for men (33 %) (Lyon *et al.* 1979).

Zinc status is difficult to assess from determination of zinc intake in food combined with estimates of the zinc contents of foods. This is partly on account of the variable bioavailability, and also because of the variations in the levels of zinc content of the same food item in different regions. Thus the zinc content of most grains, leaves and legumes was increased when superphosphate was used as a fertilizer.

A more accurate assessment of zinc status might therefore be expected to come from estimates of zinc in hair or in plasma. If the hair has been growing normally, the zinc content is a useful index of chronic zinc status (Prasad 1979). When there is a severe zinc deficiency, however, the growth of hair is retarded, and the longer residence time of the growing hair in the follicle allows it to pick up more zinc, so that the concentration may not be reduced (Sandstead *et al.* 1982). Severe protein-calorie malnutrition also reduces the length and diameter of the hair which is produced; in kwashiorkor the fiber production falls to 10 % of normal, and zinc content may or may not be reduced. In addition, sex hormones and contraceptives affect not only pubic and axillary hair but also head hair, and the dietary intake of other minerals and of vitamins is another factor which affects the zinc in hair (Bland 1983). Plasma zinc is often studied in addition to hair zinc, but even normal plasma levels do not rule out zinc deficiency (Sandstead *et al.* 1982).

In spite of these difficulties, a variety of methods has been used to assess the zinc status of patients with esophageal cancer, and of people in high-risk areas. It was found that the levels of zinc in hair in the high cancer region of Iran was low compared with that of populations in Tehran, where the levels were similar to those in Baltimore, USA (Mobarhan *et al.* 1980). The low levels were thought to be due to the high fibre/phytate content of the diet. Plasma zinc was found to be below normal in esophageal cancer patients in Washington, DC, and here the cause was probably alcohol consumption (Mellow *et al.* 1983). Similar data on patients from other regions of the USA have been reported, with a marginal zinc deficiency in many middle-income families (Rose 1983). In spite of a low concentration of zinc in plasma of cancer patients, however, biopsies of esophageal cancer tissue contained similar levels to control samples (Lipman *et al.* 1987).

Animal experiments relating zinc deficiency to esophageal cancer
The esophagus was found to be the organ most severely affected by zinc deficiency in the rat (Follis *et al.* 1941). The buccal cavity and skin showed similar but less pronounced changes. In the esophagus, the basal cells were more numerous and closely packed, the numbers of overlying cells were increased, and the outermost cells did not lose their nuclei in the normal way, so that a thick layer of partially keratinized cells developed. Overall the changes could have resulted from delayed keratinization, or from an increase in proliferation of the basal cells. The pathology was similar to that of certain skin lesions in man, such as psoriasis. The changes were found to be rapidly reversible, as intraperitoneal injection of zinc resulted in recovery of all cell layers in about 2 days, with disappearance of the abnormal cells (Barney *et al.* 1968). Recovery in the testis, however, did not occur, and after 16 days the spermatogenesis time was still prolonged. Zinc deficiency produced lesions, including hyperplasia, in the esophagus of the fetal rat, at levels of deficiency which had no effect on the mother (Diamond *et al.* 1970, 1971). The symptoms of zinc deficiency were so characteristic and pronounced that the suggestion was made that they should be used as an indicator of the deficiency state. The esophagus was stunted to between two thirds and one half the size of the organ in normal

full-term fetuses, but in spite of this there was an increase in the number of cells per unit length in the basal layer. This was assumed by the authors to result from hyperplasia rather than from inhibition of differentiation. The paradox of hyperplasia with overall stunting was not explained.

An increase in the mitotic index of the esophageal and buccal mucosa was reported by Fell *et al.* (1973). Thus, while there is atrophy and a decrease in rate of cell proliferation in other organs studied, including the small intestine (Suthon *et al.* 1985), an opposite effect occurred in the mucosa of the esophagus and oral cavity. The possibility that the upper digestive tract might be protected by sequestering zinc was studied by Gerson *et al.* (1985), but the zinc content of oral epithelium was reduced by half during a period of zinc deficiency.

The effect of zinc deficiency on the zinc content of various tissues in the rat showed zinc levels to decrease in several organs, including esophagus, kidneys, muscles, testes and bone (Prasad *et al.* 1967). The activities of the zinc-dependent enzymes also decreased, the nature of the enzyme concerned varying with the organ. In the esophagus a decrease was measured in malic dehydrogenase, alcohol dehydrogenase, and NADH diaphorase. The activities increased rapidly after repletion of the diet with zinc. The reasonable suggestion was made that the manifestations of zinc deficiency are caused by lack of zinc-dependent enzymes. Where studied, similar enzyme deficiencies were detected in man (Prasad 1979). The problem of why zinc deficiency should increase the rate of cell replication in the esophagus and buccal mucosa while inhibiting replication in other organs does not, therefore, appear to be explained by the resulting changes in organ levels of zinc-dependent enzymes.

A way in which zinc deficiency could increase the incidence of esophageal cancer is by enhancing the action of chemical carcinogens. Thus zinc deficiency was shown to increase the esophageal carcinogenicity of *N*-nitroso-methylbenzylamine (NMBzA) (Fong *et al.* 1978) and of precursors of the nitrosamine (Fong *et al.* 1974). Glutathione transferases offer protection against a range of electrophilic carcinogens through conjugation with glutathione, and it was found that the activity of glutathione transferase in the esophagus of zinc-deficient rats was decreased (Lee *et al.* 1986). Possibly as a result of this, there was an increase in the level of acid-soluble sulfhydyl groups. An alternative, or possibly an additional, mechanism of action, however, is the enhanced microsomal metabolism of NMBzA (Barch *et al.* 1984).

Mediation of zinc deficiency in esophageal carcinogenesis
While it is possible that changes in the metabolism of carcinogens are involved in the link between zinc deficiency and esophageal cancer, it is probable that also involved is the dramatic proliferative effect on the esophagus, which contrasts with its inhibitory action on almost all other organs. Since the discovery in 1940 that zinc was essential to the activity of carbonic anhydrase, more than 200 zinc metalloenzymes have been recorded (Prasad 1984). The metal is located at the active site of the enzyme and participates in the catalytic process. Among the enzymes which are zinc dependent are DNA and RNA polymerases. It is therefore surprising that an increase in cell replication in the esophagus could occur under conditions of zinc deficiency.

It has often been suggested that zinc deficiency has a direct fundamental effect on gene expression, and that this differs in esophagus from that in most other organs. The effect of zinc on cell replication and nuclear composition in the protozoan *Euglena gracilis* has been studied for many years, and changes in the amounts and types of histones and non-histone proteins have been recorded. Alterations in nuclear proteins could be responsible for changes in gene expression, with repression being the main result, but with some genes being selectively activated (Czupryn *et al.* 1987). Similar studies in the esophagus and in contrasting tissues would be of much interest.

There are several additional ways in which zinc can have a fundamental effect on the cell, of which its role in the functioning of the plasma membrane and in vitamin A metabolism (Smith *et al.* 1973) are but two. At present it can only be concluded that the contrasting effect of zinc deficiency in the esophagus compared with other organs, and its mediation in esophageal cancer, cannot be explained. Deplorably, little is apparently being done to elucidate the effects of deficiency on gene functioning or on enzyme activities in the esophagus. These will need to be understood before the mechanisms involved in its association with esophageal cancer can be elucidated.

Riboflavin
Deficiency of riboflavin commonly occurs in regions with a high rate of esophageal cancer, but it is associated with deficiencies of other micronutrients, including zinc, magnesium, molybdenum, vitamin A and nicotinamide. This is on account of the fact that minerals and vitamins occur at the highest levels in similar foods, for example milk, eggs, meat, fish and green leafy vegetables. The deficiencies therefore occur together in

populations in which cereals form the staple diet. Because the micro-nutrients are at their highest levels mainly in the more expensive foods, deficiencies occur in poor rural communities, and in groups of people with the lowest socioeconomic status. As in the case of zinc, the human body has no means of storing riboflavin, so that deficiency develops very rapidly when the supply is inadequate. This is important in view of the intermittent nature of the inadequate supply – for example in winter but not in summer in remote cold regions. However, as with zinc, prolonged deficiency can exist in a country, for example in The Gambia, which does not have a high rate of esophageal cancer. The very probable explanation is that riboflavin deficiency can increase the vulnerability of the esophagus to environmental carcinogens, and the extent of exposure to the initiating carcinogens varies in different locations.

Some of the first evidence linking deficiency of riboflavin and iron with esophageal cancer came from studies of the Plummer–Vinson syndrome, as discussed in Chapter 3. In regions where people suffered from intermittent periods of deficiency, as in remote regions in Sweden, Norway, Scotland and Wales during winter, women presented first with anemia, and often later with esophageal cancer (Wynder *et al.* 1978; Schottenfeld *et al.* 1982; Byers *et al.* 1984). Improvements in the diet, including the addition of riboflavin to bread, reduced the incidence of the disease in Sweden, so that Scotland is now the European country with the highest incidence of esophageal cancer in women (Day *et al.* 1982). The explanation of the importance of intermittent periods of deficiency could be that the basal cells become initiated for malignancy by environmental carcinogens during the period of riboflavin deficiency, but cancer growth is held in check by poor nutrition. In summer, when micronutrient intake is adequate, the growth of the 'sleeping' cancer cells is stimulated.

Other epidemiological evidence for an association of riboflavin deficiency with esophageal cancer is discussed with the other micro-nutrient deficiencies in a later section.

Animal experiments

Good evidence that riboflavin deficiency can promote esophageal cancer is given by the effect of deficiency on the esophagus of experimental animals. It was soon discovered that riboflavin deficiency had a dramatic effect on the esophagus, as conspicuous among the profusion of congenital malformations resulting from maternal deficiency was the complete absence of an esophagus (Kalter 1959). The pharynx ended in a thread derived from the peripheral muscle layers of the esophagus, and this soon disappeared. The space in the thorax normally occupied by the esophagus was taken up by connective tissue, the esophagus sometimes reappearing in the abdomen, but often not reappearing at all.

The effect of riboflavin deficiency in mice was described by Wynder *et al.* (1965). The pathology included atrophy and hyperkeratization of the skin, tongue, esophagus and forestomach. The first microscopic changes to be detected were in the squamous epithelium of the esophagus and forestomach, with atrophy, irregular thinning, and hyperkeratosis which was so marked that it led to almost complete obstruction of the lumen of the esophagus. In the skin atrophy was followed by hyperplasia (Wynder *et al.* 1970). As this unexpected response did not occur during starvation, it was suggested to be a result specific to riboflavin deficiency. The facts that similar changes are associated with riboflavin and iron deficiencies in the Plummer–Vinson syndrome, and that respiratory enzymes require riboflavin and iron to function, led Wynder *et al.* to suggest that respiratory enzymes were involved in neoplasia, as had been previously suggested by Warburg (1956). The swelling and damage to liver mitochondria which occur in riboflavin-deficient rats supported this view. This type of deficiency state could act as a stimulus to convert dormant tumor cells into cancer cells (Wynder *et al.* 1965).

The concept was strongly supported by subsequent experiments which showed that the skin of riboflavin-deficient mice was more susceptible to the effect of 7,12-dimethylbenz[*a*]anthracene (DMBA) promoted by croton oil than was normal skin (Wynder *et al.* 1975). In addition, one of the respiratory enzymes, aryl hydrocarbon hydroxylase, thought to be involved in the carcinogenic activity of DMBA, was induced in liver by riboflavin deficiency (Wynder *et al.* 1975). It was pointed out that similar studies in epithelial cells, although more difficult, are needed.

As the baboon is an animal with many morphological and physiological similarities to humans, it is significant that the esophagus of these animals responded to riboflavin deficiency in a similar way to that of rats and mice. Complete riboflavin deficiency in the baboon resulted in atrophy, ulcers and, interestingly, some hyperplastic esophageal lesions which were thought to be precancerous (Foy *et al.* 1977). In a more detailed study, Foy *et al.* (1984) described numerous mitotic figures in the esophageal epithelium, not only in the basal cells but also in overlying cells, these regions of esophagus being distinguishable from carcinoma only by the absence of invasion of the muscle layers. It was suggested that these lesions predispose the esophagus to carcinogens. As it is unlikely that man often suffers from a complete absence of riboflavin, it would be of much interest to study the effect of lower levels of deficiency on the carcinogenicity of the well-studied NMBzA.

Possible mechanisms operative in the association of riboflavin deficiency with esophageal cancer
The fact that the enzymes formed from riboflavin – flavine adenine dinucleotide (FAD) and flavomononucleotide (FMN) – are essential for the activity of many oxidases and dehydrogenases, probably explains why riboflavin is essential for maintaining the integrity of epithelial cells, including those of the esophagus. The breakdown of normal structure resulting from deficiency could predispose the epithelium to carcinogens. Alternatively, as flavo enzymes are an essential part of the mixed-function oxidase system which is responsible for the detoxication or activation of many carcinogens (Yang 1974), increased vulnerability could be the result of altered metabolism of the carcinogen.

An additional way in which riboflavin deficiency may act is by its effect on metabolism of iron. Both riboflavin deficiency and iron deficiency occur extensively in poor rural areas which have high rates of esophageal cancer, and human studies and animal experiments have shown an association between riboflavin status and iron metabolism. Deficiency of riboflavin decreases the absorption of iron from the intestine (Adelekan *et al.* 1986*a*). The decreased activity of NADH–FMN oxidoreductase (ferrireductase) results in an accumulation of iron in the duodenum, with the subsequent loss of iron when the cells are exfoliated. Another result of decreased activity of the oxidoreductase is the decreased mobilization of iron from storage compartments (Adelekan *et al.* 1986*b*). One effect is the decreased synthesis of hemoglobin, which leads to anemia, and is associated with a high rate of esophageal cancer, as in the Plummer–Vinson syndrome already mentioned. The change in iron status, in addition to the riboflavin deficiency itself, is detrimental to normal functioning of respiratory enzymes. Only further work on populations with a high incidence of esophageal cancer can determine which mechanisms are involved in the tragic human situations.

Vitamin A
This vitamin is essential for maintenance of the normal state of replication and differentiation of epithelial tissues, and there has been much discussion of the importance of retinoids in the prevention and treatment of epithelial tumors. The main symptoms of vitamin A deficiency are blindness in children or, if the deficiency is less severe, defective vision in dim light, and skin lesions. A definite association with esophageal cancer has not yet been demonstrated. Experimental work is very limited and contradictory. Thus it was shown that treatment of rats with 13-*cis*-

retinoic acid after injection of N-nitroso-methylbutylamine (NMBA) slightly reduced the esophageal tumor-related mortality rate (Moon et al. 1982). On the other hand, vitamin A deficient rats failed to develop esophageal tumors following NMBzA treatment (van Rensburg et al. 1981). The explanation put forward was that vitamin A may protect against some cancers by preventing the conversion of secretory epithelia to squamous epithelia, but worsen cancer of the esophagus, an organ in which the epithelium is normally squamous.

Vitamin A deficiency alone caused changes in the esophagus which suggested a disorder of epithelial differentiation, including thinning of the epithelium and abnormalities of the basal cells, but deficiency was not found to have an effect on basal cell replication (Mak et al. 1987). By contrast, vitamin A deficiency increased the activity of ornithine decarboxylase, an enzyme implicated in the initial stages of cellular proliferation (Daliam et al. 1988). Obviously more work along these lines would be very valuable. The epidemiological evidence for an adverse effect of vitamin A consumed in animal fat and of the protective action of β-carotene in fruit and vegetables is discussed later.

Nicotinamide

The introduction of maize (or corn, Zea mays) from the New World into Europe and Africa coincided with the appearance of pellagra in communities where the cereal became the staple or at least a major part of the diet. Nicotinamide in maize occurs in a form which is not absorbed from the alimentary tract, and maize is defective also in the amino acid tryptophan, the metabolism of which leads to the formation of a limited amount of nicotinamide. As dermatitis is a major symptom of pellagra, it seemed likely that other epithelial organs, including the esophagus, might be injured by nicotinamide deficiency. Studies of patients with pellagra showed esophagitis ranging from mild to severe in all patients examined, a proportion of the cases improving when treated with nicotinamide (Segal et al. 1990). It is probable that the symptoms were alleviated in only a proportion of the patients because the esophagitis, as well as pellagra, was caused by a combination of deficiencies of several micronutrients. While pellagra is due to a gross deficiency of, mainly, nicotinamide, more prolonged deficiency is likely to cause chronic esophagitis, and so predispose the esophagus to carcinogens.

Studies in Africa very strongly suggested that esophageal cancer did not follow the consumption of maize per se, but of maize infected with the mold Fusarium (see Chapter 9). Northern Italy is another region with a high incidence of esophageal cancer, and is also one of the few examples of a highly developed area where maize has been the most widely grown cereal. Here a highly significant association was detected between frequent intake of maize and oral, pharyngeal and esophageal cancer (Franceschi *et al.* 1990). The association, however, was evident only in those individuals who also reported heavy drinking. It is possible that a high maize consumption alone tends to cause deficiencies and so enhance esophageal cancer, but further insults from either alcohol consumption or mycotoxins are necessary to cause the symptomatic disease.

Vitamin C

With reference to vitamin C, there is considerable epidemiological evidence for an association of deficiency of the vitamin with esophageal cancer, and some theoretical basis for the association. Thus vitamin C inhibits the formation of nitrosamines in the stomach (see Chapter 5) and, as it is an antioxidant, it could protect cell membranes from oxidative damage. But there appears to be no direct experimental evidence for an adverse effect of vitamin C deficiency on esophageal cancer.

Molybdenum

Another factor the deficiency of which is often mentioned in epidemiological surveys is molybdenum. It is said that not long ago the grass grew knee-high over the whole of the Transkei, and the incidence of esophageal cancer was low. Gradually certain areas became less fertile and lost their knee-high grass, and at the same time, from around 1943, there was an increase in esophageal cancer. Plants in the gardens in the regions of the Transkei in which there was a high incidence of esophageal cancer showed signs of molybdenum deficiency, and treatment with molybdenum reduced the extent of withering (Burrell *et al.* 1966). The gardens were deficient also in iron, copper, zinc and other trace elements, these micronutrient deficiencies causing the plants to become more prone to infection by molds. In addition, with the reduced fertility of the soil, the women were compelled to make use not only of the staple foods, maize, pumpkin, beans and potatoes, but of many weeds, such as milky thistle and black nightshade, which may contain carcinogens. The association of molybdenum deficiency with molybdenum as a fertilizer increased the molybdenum content and decreased the nitrate and nitrite in plants.

An additional mechanism by which molybdenum deficiency could affect esophageal cancer is by enhancing the action of carcinogens. Thus it was found that addition of molybdenum to the drinking water reduced the esophageal carcinogenesis induced by N-nitrososarcosine ethyl ester in rats (Luo *et al.* 1983). A high-molybdenum diet also decreased the incidence of tumors in rats treated with NMBzA (Komada *et al.* 1990). Stimulation of the molybdenum-dependent flavo enzyme xanthene oxidase, possibly the rate-limiting factor in purine catabolism, was thought to be involved. But there appears to be no experimental evidence that deficiency of molybdenum below normal values causes an increase in the incidence of esophageal cancer.

Dietary deficiencies and epidemiology

While cancer of the breast and colon are related to affluence, esophageal cancer is a disease of poverty, a poor diet often largely restricted to one staple food item, and a lack of micronutrients, fresh fruit and vegetables. This situation exists in South Africa, Iran, China, Puerto Rico, and among groups of people with a low socioeconomic status in New York and Washington, DC. Possibly the only affluent region of the world with a high rate of esophageal cancer is in northern France, where the protective factors in good food cannot compete with the high consumption of spirits.

The subject of esophageal cancer and diet has been discussed in several reviews (Byers 1984; Tuyns 1985; Cook 1985; Howe 1986; Day *et al.* 1982*a, b*; Dowlatshaki *et al.* 1984). These surveys have repeatedly stressed the link with a low intake of fresh fruit and vegetables. Plant foods supply not only the fine balance which is needed between minerals, vitamins and antioxidants, but probably also provide various protective factors. People habitually taking vitamin supplements do not have a lower risk for cancer (Van Rensburg 1982). In an extensive survey in northern Italy, it was shown that for vegetables there was a consistent pattern of protection for all epithelial cancers, with relative risks in the upper tertile ranging from 0.2 for esophagus, liver and larynx, to 0.7 for breast. All the trends of risk were in the same direction, and were significant for all carcinomas except that of gallbladder. Similarly, for fruit, the relative risks were 0.2–0.3 for oral cavity, pharynx, esophagus and larynx (Negri *et al.* 1991). Certain chemicals which occur in commonly consumed plant foods have been shown to inhibit nitrosamine-induced esophageal cancer in animals (see Chapter 5). These include various phenols, for example ellagic acid, cinnamic acid, coumarins, indoles, isothiocyanates, and diallyl sulfide. The possible use of these chemicals for cancer prevention merits urgent investigation.

Southern Africa

The situation in Southern Africa is possibly unique in that there is an abrupt change in incidence of esophageal cancer at a political border

(Haas *et al.* 1978). At the turn of the century the use of maize as a food crop increased and began to replace sorghum in certain regions of Africa, and with the spread of maize there was an increase in the rate of esophageal cancer. In 1930 the Uganda government discouraged the cultivation of maize, and bananas, sorghum, yams, cassava, rice and millet remained the staple foods. In Kenya on the other hand the spread of maize was encouraged, and an abrupt drop in the cancer rate developed on the Ugandan side of the border. This did not appear to be explained by geological or cultural changes, and the possibility arose that a diet composed mainly of maize was defective in certain micronutrients. Maize is widely consumed also in the USA, where in general the cancer rate is low, but here the very varied nature of the diet would supply adequate nutrients.

In South Africa it was shown that people living in the high-risk areas had a long-standing deficiency of certain micronutrients, notably riboflavin, nicotinamide, zinc and magnesium (van Rensburg 1981). The staple foods in the high-risk areas were maize and wheat, while in the low-risk areas they were sorghum, millet, cassava and yams. The deficiency in magnesium was shown to correlate best with the incidence of esophageal cancer world-wide (van Rensburg 1983).

The differences in cancer rates among the different populations were very striking. In human populations surviving mainly on millet the esophageal cancer incidence was around 0.4 cases per 100000 males, while in those eating mainly maize or wheat it was 50.5 per 100000 males (van Rensburg *et al.* 1985). The results of animal experiments gave strong support to these concepts (van Rensburg *et al.* 1985, 1986). Rats were fed various diets either before, during and after, or only after, treatment with the esophageal carcinogen NMBzA. A similar incidence of tumors developed in animals fed maize, wheat, commercial bird-resistant sorghum, bananas, or polished rice, but the rate was strikingly lower in rats fed millet, red sorghum, brown rice, or potatoes. The addition of certain micronutrients to the group known to be deficient eliminated the difference. The group of micronutrients involved was riboflavin, nicotinamide, zinc and magnesium, but the response was not consistently related to any one particular item. Protection occurred when the supplements were not given until after tumor initiation with NMBzA, a result strongly suggesting that the defective diets acted by stimulating growth of the lesions rather than by exerting a specific effect on nitrosamine metabolism. As previously discussed, however, there is evidence that zinc deficiency does alter the metabolism of NMBzA.

An alternative explanation of the association of esophageal cancer with a staple diet of maize is that the link is not with maize *per se* but with maize

260 *Dietary deficiencies*

contaminated by the mold *Fusarium*. Very probably both micronutrient deficiency and the action of mycotoxins are involved (Chapter 9).

In addition to deficiencies in the diet in high-risk cancer regions in the Transkei, it is possible that toxic or carcinogenic plants are consumed. In order to test this possibility, groups of rats were fed either a diet of maize and beans, or a full Transkei diet including imifino (*Solanum nigrum*), the fruit used to curdle milk (Purchase *et al.* 1975). Animals receiving the latter diet developed liver lesions and epithelial cell dysplasia in the esophagus. Dietary deficiencies and consumption of toxic plants would combine to increase the vulnerability of the esophagus to carcinogens.

Iran and Central Asia

The high incidence 'cancer belt' extends from Iran through Soviet Central Asia, Afghanistan, Siberia and Mongolia to north-west China. While esophageal cancer has been known to be an exceptional hazard in China since antiquity, it was not until the end of the 1960s that it became widely known that Iran was also an especially high-risk area. The high incidence was probably not of recent origin, however, as it had been described in Persian manuscripts 800 years previously (quoted in Ghadirian 1987). Initial studies were carried out by Kmet *et al.* (1972). The high rate areas were in the north-east of Iran, with a sharp decrease in incidence on moving west along the southern littoral of the Caspian Sea. Among the especially high-risk areas of the eastern littoral are the Gonbad district, settled by Turkomans, and Azerbaijan. This region has a low rainfall, and is comprised of low-lying steppe, semi-desert or desert. The people are nomads or semi-nomads, rearing sheep and goats, so that their diet includes the milk and yoghurt provided by these animals. But the staple diet is unleavened bread prepared from wheat or barley, and tea. While the supply of calories is generally adequate, the diet is deficient in vitamins and trace minerals. This has a greater impact on the women, who are more-or-less permanently pregnant, and who breast feed their children for 18 months to 2 years (Kmet *et al.* 1980). This may explain why the rate of esophageal cancer in the Gonbad region is higher for women than for men. As the long period of breast-feeding delays the introduction of supplementary food for the children, it could explain why pre-school children are not only deficient in micronutrients, but also suffer from protein-calorie malnutrition.

The west of the littoral Caspian, on the other hand, is located under the slopes of the mountains, and enjoys a high rainfall, hot summers, and milder winters than the adjacent areas. There is a flourishing cultivation of fruit, vegetables and rice, a cereal which does not reduce the bioavailability of minerals as does the unleavened bread of the high-risk regions. Tea is consumed in the low-risk as well as in the high-risk areas, and dietary deficiencies rather than hot tea appear to be the major hazard. The period of breast-feeding babies is shorter than in the high cancer incidence area.

A more extensive investigation was carried out by the Joint Iran–IARC Study Group (1977). A series of epidemiological surveys attempted to identify the major risk factors, and the nature of the population, local agriculture, climate, vegetation and geology in 15 regions were studied. The dry, saline, alkaline soil in the high-risk areas resulted in a bare steppe environment, with virtually no cultivation of fruit or vegetables. The diet was tested for carcinogens, including polycyclic hydrocarbons, aflatoxin and nitrosamines, but the levels were low in all areas studied. The results of the investigations confirmed the previous implication of dietary deficiencies being the major hazard.

Similar surveys by Hormozdiari *et al.* (1975) revealed that bread, tea and sugar were the sole items of diet in the high-incidence villages examined during the period studied. There was a consequent low intake of vitamins A and C, riboflavin, and animal protein. Case–control studies strongly associated the risk of esophageal cancer with a low intake of fresh fruit and vegetables (Cook-Mozaffari *et al.* 1979). The consumption of sheep's milk and yoghurt was not thought to be relevant.

The dietary deficiencies were reflected in incidence rates for other cancers, but the effect on esophageal cancer was the most marked (Cook-Mozaffari *et al.* 1979). It is surprising that given the striking variations in climate and landscape in different regions of the Caspian littoral, the geographic distribution of other cancers is not more dramatic. Preliminary studies of cancer of the stomach, however, have suggested that it may mirror that of the esophagus (Nadim *et al.* 1986).

A more recent survey showed that dietary deficiencies are still a major hazard in high-risk areas. Thus only 5% of the Turkoman families purchased vegetables from visits to markets in neighbouring towns, the remaining 95% simply not eating vegetables at all. Several additional possible hazards were detected (Ghadirian 1987). These included the special diet of a mixture of crushed sour pomegranate seeds and black pepper which is given to pregnant women. This could well irritate the esophagus and so increase the vulnerability to carcinogens. Also, although tea is widely consumed, the inhabitants of the high-risk areas drank more tea and at a higher temperature. One pot of tea, about 1 litre, is normally prepared per person. Interestingly food was found to be consumed three to four times faster in the high-risk areas. Eating more quickly could result in food being swallowed without sufficient chewing, another factor which could cause irritation to the esophagus.

The high rate of esophageal cancer in the east of the Caspian littoral does not stop at the political border, but extends into the Central Asian republics of the Soviet Union. An enterprising survey of the Uzbek area was carried out by Zaridze *et al.* (1985). All male residents 55–69 years of age in a local authority were invited to attend a medical examination and to answer questions relating to diet and other factors. Of the 1506 men who presented themselves, blood analyses showed 86 % to have low riboflavin levels, 79 % low carotinoids, and 14 % low vitamin A. Chronic esophagitis, a condition through to be a precursor of esophageal cancer, was diagnosed in 60 % of the people examined. The frequency of esophagitis was not affected by the use of nass, a type of chewing tobacco made with local tobacco, ash, cotton oil or sesame seed oil, and, in the Uzbek area, high levels of lime. The survey therefore supported other studies in suggesting that certain nutritional deficiencies could be responsible for the condition.

China

As in Iran, the diet consumed in the high cancer incidence areas in China is very restricted, often being limited to millet gruel, pickled vegetables and tea. In addition to the hazards presented by the presence of molds in the pickles, of nitrosamines and their precursors in the food and in the poor water supply, and of contamination of the cereals by needles of silica, it is obvious that nutritional deficiencies could well be involved. While the calorie intake in the notorious Linxian district was adequate, there was a low intake of vitamins A and C, riboflavin, animal protein, fat, fresh vegetables and fruit (Li *et al.* 1980, 1984, 1989). Symptoms of riboflavin deficiency, i.e. cheilosis, glossitis and burning of the tongue, were common. The levels of certain trace elements, including zinc, molybdenum and magnesium, were low in the drinking water. Biochemical analyses of hair, plasma and urine of cancer patients confirmed these deficiencies. Later studies measured blood levels of riboflavin, vitamin A, β-carotene and zinc in the high-incidence Linxian district and the lower-incidence Jiaoxian district (Thurnham *et al.* 1985). Riboflavin deficiency in Linxian was as severe as anywhere in the world, and only riboflavin status correlated with esophageal cancer. By the time this survey was carried out, more wheat and maize, and less millet, sorghum and rice were being consumed, but cereals and potato still provided 90 % of the protein intake. The better riboflavin status reported by Yang *et al.* (1982) was probably due to the fact that their surveys were carried out in September, at the end of summer, when some seasonal vegetables had been available, while those of Thurnham *et al.* were carried out in May.

The importance of consumption of fresh fruit was illustrated again in the widespread survey of Guo *et al.* (1990).

A double-blind intervention study at first gave disappointing results. Supplementation of the diet in the Linxian area with riboflavin, retinol and zinc for 13.5 months did not influence the prevalence of precancerous lesions, i.e. esophagitis with or without atrophy or dysplasia (Munoz *et al.* 1985). It is possible that, as with chronic atrophic gastritis, a precursor lesion of gastric cancer, the changes in the esophagus are irreversible.

Although no difference had been detected between the treated and the placebo groups in the occurrence of histologically detectable precancerous lesions, there was the possibility that an effect could be detected if an earlier end point was used. Smears of exfoliated cells from the esophagus were obtained during endoscopy after treatment, and a statistically significant reduction was observed in the prevalence of micronuclei in the treated group (Munoz *et al.* 1987). Although the relevance of micronuclei in carcinogenesis is unknown, it is very probable that these lesions provide a measure of genetic damage.

A complicating factor in the intervention study was the increase in blood retinol which occurred in the placebo as well as in the treated group. When the data were re-examined by logistic regression analysis, it was found that an improvement in blood retinol, irrespective of treatment, associated with a lower incidence of precancerous lesions (Wahrendorf *et al.* 1988). The increase in the placebo group was probably due to the difference in time of year of the initial and final observations. The first measurements were made during September but, as the subjects were busy harvesting the crops in September, the final studies were made in October/November of the following year. A better supply of vegetables would have been available after harvest, and the intake of β-carotene and hence the blood levels of retinol would have increased. Detailed biochemical studies of plasma samples obtained in the trial confirmed this conclusion (Thurnham *et al.* 1988). The suggestion from this study is therefore that an improvement in retinol status is associated with a decrease in precancerous lesions. As riboflavin status improved only during the first 2 months, and then remained constant, it is probable that an increase in riboflavin levels would also produce a beneficial effect on the esophagus.

Europe
Nutritional deficiency is associated with esophageal cancer mainly in areas with infertile soil and underdeveloped agriculture, where poor

rural communities are limited in their staple diet. However, cancer occurs also in poor groups of people in the more affluent West, where high alcohol consumption reduces the intake of micronutrients, and in remote areas where the supply of fresh food is limited, especially in winter. Thus until recently the highest rate of esophageal cancer for women in Europe occurred in isolated regions in Sweden, but after improvements had been made to the national diet the rate of cancer decreased, so that now Scottish women have the highest rate for women in Europe. Although case–control studies have not been carried out, it has been pointed out that the supply of fresh food in remote regions in Scotland is limited. The mountainous terrain and the inclement climate make the cultivation and transport of food difficult (Kemp *et al.* 1985).

As might have been expected, studies of diet in the affluent north of France, with its reputation for good food, revealed no dramatic dietary deficiencies (Tuyns *et al.* 1985; Tuyns 1987). However, case–control studies even here showed that a higher intake of animal protein, polyunsaturated fats, β-carotene and zinc decreased the cancer risk, while vitamin A, as consumed in butter, was associated with a higher risk.

Very similar results were obtained in a case–control study in the high cancer rate region of north-east Italy (Decarli *et al.* 1987). As in France, meat, fish, fresh green vegetables and fruit, and β-carotene were protective, while retinol intake was associated with an increased risk. As discussed previously, it is possible that a high consumption of maize in this area results in a deficiency of nicotinamide (Franceschi *et al.* 1990).

USA and Japan

In the USA also, groups of the population in regions with higher than average rates of esophageal cancer were found to have a lower consumption of certain foods. Thus case–control studies showed that cancer patients in New York (Wynder 1961) and in Roswell Park (Mettlin 1981) consumed slightly reduced quantities of green and yellow vegetables, eggs, and milk than did the controls.

Detailed studies of alcohol and tobacco consumption and of diet were carried out among black men in Washington, DC (Pottern *et al.* 1981; Ziegler *et al.* 1981). Although the main association of esophageal cancer was with alcohol consumption, a twofold difference existed between cases and controls in levels of consumption of fresh or frozen meat, fish, fruit, vegetables and dairy produce. No significant differences were revealed in the consumption of coffee, tea (even when this was drunk 'burning hot'), or hot spices and peppers. Apparently deficiencies were not related to any specific micronutrient, but lower intakes of vitamin A, β-carotene, vitamin C, thiamine and riboflavin were associated with cancer. The methods used to cook the food were related to risk, those who baked or grilled being at lower risk than those who fried. The exact reason for this was not understood.

Similar data were found yet again in case–control studies in Los Angeles, California (Yu *et al.* 1988). Even where alcohol and tobacco were the main hazards, low consumption of fruit, vegetables and whole grain bread increased the risk. Case–control studies in three counties in western New York replicated earlier findings that ingestion of vitamin A as retinol in dairy produce associated with increased risk, while β-carotene in fruit and vegetables was protective (Graham *et al.* 1990).

The situation in Japan is similar to that found in the USA and Europe. After allowing for the main risk factors for esophageal cancer, i.e. consumption of alcohol (especially spirits), tobacco and, in the case of Japan, of bracken, risk was associated with a low intake of meat and fruit (Hirayama 1979). A more detailed study showed that salty food and excessive rice consumption increased the risk, while fruit, raw vegetables, seaweed and meat were protective (Nakachi *et al.* 1988). The effect of meat was probably complex, being due in part to its content of riboflavin, nicotinic acid and zinc. Seaweed, widely consumed in Japan after frying and also in biscuits, is a good source of riboflavin and zinc.

In summary, the conclusion from studies in high-incidence areas in South Africa and the Iran/China cancer belt, and the moderate cancer regions of Europe, USA and Japan, is unambiguous. Fresh fruit and vegetables are protective, partly but not necessarily entirely as a result of their vitamin and mineral content. This undisputed fact should be proclaimed to the general public as the most certain and easy to follow dietary guideline.

References

Adelekan, D.A. and Thurnham, D.I. (1986*a*) *Br. J. Nutr.* **56**, 171–179. Influence of riboflavin deficiency on absorption and liver storage of iron in the growing rat.

Adelekan, D.A. and Thurnham, D.I. (1986*b*) *J. Nutr.* **116**, 1257–1265. Effects of combined riboflavin and iron deficiency on the haematological status and tissue iron concentrations in the rat.

Armstrong, B.K., McMichael, A.J. and MacLennan, R. (1982) In: *Cancer Epidemiology and Prevention* (Schottenfeld, D. and Fraumeni, J.F. eds.). Philadelphia: Saunders, pp. 419–433. Diet.

Barch, D.H., Keummerle, S.C., Hollenberg, P.F. and Iannaccone, M. (1984) *Cancer Res.* **44**, 5629–5633. Esophageal microsomal metabolism of *N*-nitroso-methylbenzylamine in zinc deficient rats.

Barney, G.H., Orgebin-Crist, M.C. and Macapinlap, M.P. (1968) *J. Nutr.* **95**, 520–534. Genesis of esophageal parakeratosis and histologic changes in the testes of the zinc deficient rat and their reversal by zinc repletion.

Basu, T.K., Chan, U. and Fields, A. (1984) In: *Vitamins, Nutrition and Cancer* (Prasad, A.S. ed.). Basel: Karger, pp. 33–45. Vitamin A (retinol) and epithelial cancer in man.

Bland, J. (1983) *Hair Tissue Mineral Analysis.* Wellingborough: Thorsons.

Burrell, R.J., Roach, W.A. and Shadwell, A. (1966) *J. Natl. Cancer Inst.* **36**, 201–214. Esophageal cancer in the Bantu of Transkei associated with mineral deficiency in garden plants.

Byers, T. and Graham, S. (1984) *Adv. Cancer Res.* **41**, 1–69. Epidemiology of diet and cancer.

Cook-Mozaffari, P.J., Azordegan, F., Day, N.E., Ressicaud, A., Sabai, D. and Aramesh, B. (1979) *Br. J. Cancer* **39**, 293–309. Esophageal cancer studies in the Caspian littoral of Iran: results of a case–control study.

Cook-Mozaffari, P.J.. (1985) In: *Cancer Risks and Prevention* (Vessey, M.P. and Gray, M. eds.). Oxford: Oxford University Press, pp. 15–43. The geography of cancer.

Cooperman, J.M. and Lopez, R. (1984) In: *Handbook of Vitamins* (Machleni, L.J. ed.). New York: Marcel Dekker, pp. 299–327. Riboflavin.

Czupryn, M., Falchuk, K.H. and Vallee, B.L. (1987) *Biochemistry* **26**, 8263–8269. Zinc deficiency and metabolism of histones and non-histone proteins in *Euglena gracilis.*

Daliam, A., Savoure, N., Ramee, M.P., Desrues, B., Dazard, L. and Nicol, M. (1988) *Carcinogenesis* **9**, 2161–2164. Ornithine decarboxylase basal activation in liver, esophagus and lung of vitamin A deficient rats, and the effect of retinoic acid.

Day, N.E. and Munoz, N. (1982*a*) In: *Cancer Epidemiology and Prevention* (Schottenfeld, D. and Fraumeni, J.F. eds.). Philadelphia: Saunders, pp. 596–623. Esophagus.

Day, N.E., Munoz, N. and Ghadirian, P. (1982*b*) In: *Epidemiology of Cancer of the Digestive Tract* (Correa, P. and Haenszel, W. eds.). Amsterdam: Martinus Nijhoff, pp. 21–57. Epidemiology of esophageal cancer: a review.

Decarli, A., Lianti, P., Negri, E., Franceschi, S. and La Vecchia, C. (1987) *Nutr. Cancer* **10**, 29–37. Vitamin A and other dietary factors in the etiology of esophageal cancer.

Diamond, I. and Hurley, L.S. (1970) *J. Nutr.* **100**, 325–329. Histopathology of zinc-deficient fetal rats.

Diamond, I., Swenerton, H. and Hurley, L.S. (1971) *J. Nutr.* **101**, 77–84. Testicular and esophageal lesions in zinc-deficient rats and their reversibility.

Dowlatshahi, K. and Mobarhan, S. (1984) In: *Frontiers in Gastrointestinal Cancer* (Levin, B. and Riddel, R.H. eds.). Amsterdam: Elsevier, pp. 1–17. Diet and environment in the etiology of esophageal carcinoma.

Fell, B.F., Leigh, L.C. and Williams, R.B. (1973) *Res. Vet. Sci.* **14**, 317–325. The cytology of various organs in zinc-deficient rats with particular reference to the frequency of cell division.

Follis, R.H., Day, H.G. and McCollum, E.V. (1941) *J. Nutr.* **22**, 223–237. Histologic studies of the tissues of rats fed a diet extremely low in zinc.

Follis, R.H. (1966) In: *Zinc Metabolism* (Prassad, A.S. ed.). Northridge, C.A.: Springfield Publishing, pp. 129–141. Pathology of zinc deficiency.

Fong, L.Y.Y. and Newberne, P.M. (1978) *J. Natl. Cancer Inst.* **61**, 145–150. Zinc deficiency and methylbenzylnitrosamine-induced esophageal cancer in rats.

Fong, L.Y.Y., Lee, J.S.K., Chan, W.C. and Newberne, P.M. (1984) *J. Natl. Cancer Inst.* **72**, 419–425. Zinc deficiency and the development of esophageal and forestomach tumors in Sprague–Dawley rats fed precursors of *N*-nitroso-benzylmethylamine.

Foy, A. and Mbaya, V. (1977) *Progr. Food Nutr. Sci.* **2**, 357–394. Riboflavin.

Foy, H. and Kondi, A. (1984) *J. Natl. Cancer Inst.* **72**, 941–948. The vulnerable esophagus: riboflavin deficiency and squamous cell dysplasia of the skin and the esophagus.

Franceschi, S., Bidoli, E., Baron, E.A. and La Vecchia, C. (1990) *J. Natl. Cancer Inst.* **82**, 1407–1411. Maize and risk of cancers of the oral cavity, pharynx and esophagus in north-eastern Italy.

Gerson, S.J., Meyer, J. and Gandor, D. (1985) *J. Nutr.* **115**, 820–823. Decreased zinc concentration does not lead to atrophy of rat oral epithelium.

Ghadirian, P. (1987) *Nutr. Cancer* **9**, 147–157. Food habits of the people of the Caspian littoral of Iran in relation to esophageal cancer.

Graham, S., Marshall, J., Haughey, B., Brasure, J., Freudenheim, J., Zielezny, M., Wilkinson, G. and Nolan, J. (1990) *Am. J. Epidemiol.* **131**, 454–467. Nutritional epidemiology of cancer of the esophagus.

Groenewald, G., Langenhoven, M.L., Beyers, M.J.C., du Plessis, J.P., Ferreira, J.J. and van Rensburg, S.J. (1981) *S. Afr. Med. J.* **60**, 964–967. Nutrient intakes among rural Transkeians at risk for esophageal cancer.

Guo, W., Li, J.Y., Blot, W.J., Hsing, A.W., Chen, J. and Fraumeni, J.F. (1990) *Nutr. Cancer* **13**, 121–127. Correlations of dietary intake and blood nutrient levels with esophageal cancer mortality in China.

Haas, J.F. and Schottenfeld, D. (1978) In: *Gastrointestinal Tract Cancer* (Lipkin, M. & Good, R.A. eds.). New York: Plenum Press, pp. 145–172. Epidemiology of esophageal cancer.

Harris, O.D., Cooke, W.T., Thompson, H. and Waterhouse, J.A.H. (1967) *Am. J. Med.* **42**, 899–911. Malignancy in adult coeliac disease and idiopathic steatorrhoea.

Hirayama, T. (1979) *Nutr. Cancer* **1**, 67–81. Diet and cancer.

Holmes, G.K., Stokes, P.L., Sorahan, T.M., Prior, P., Waterhouse, J.A.H. and Cooke, W.T. (1976) *Gut* **17**, 612–619. Coelic disease, gluten-free diet, and malignancy.

Hormozdiari, H., Day, N.E., Aramesh, B. and Mahboubi, E. (1975) *Cancer Res.* **35**, 3493–3498. Dietary factors and esophageal cancer in the Caspian littoral of Iran.

Howe, G.M. (1986) *Global Cancerology*. Edinburgh: Churchill Livingstone.

Jaskiewicz, K. and Marasas, W.F.O. (1988) *Anticancer Res.* **8**, 711–716. Association of esophageal cytological abnormalities with vitamin and lipotope deficiencies in populations at risk for esophageal cancer.

Joint Iran-IARC Study Group (1977) *J. Natl. Cancer Inst.* **59**, 1127–1138. Esophageal cancer studies in the Caspian littoral of Iran: results of population studies. A prodrome.

268   Dietary deficiencies

Kalter, H. (1959) *Pediatrics* **23**, 222–230. Congenital malformations induced by riboflavin efficiency in strains of inbred mice.

Kemp, I., Boyle, P., Smans, M. and Muir, C. (1985) *Atlas of Cancer in Scotland*. IARC Scientific Publication No. 72. Lyon: IARC.

Kmet, J. and Mahboubi, E. (1972) *Science* **175**, 846–853. Esophageal cancer in the Caspian littoral of Iran: initial studies.

Kmet, J., McLaren, D.S. and Siassi, F. (1980) *Adv. Mod. Hum. Nutr.* **1**, 343–365. Epidemiology of esophageal cancer with special reference to nutritional studies among the Turkoman of Iran.

Komada, H., Kise, Y., Nakagawa, M., Yamamura, M., Hioki, K. and Yamanoto, M. (1990) *Cancer Res.* **50**, 2418–2422. Effect of dietary molybdenum on esophageal carcinogenesis in rats induced by N-methyl-N-benzylnitrosamine.

Lee, J.S.K. and Fong, L.Y.Y. (1986) *Carcinogenesis* **7**, 1111–1113. Decreased glutathione transferase activities in zinc-deficient rats.

Li, M.X. and Cheng, S.J. (1984) In: *Carcinoma of the Esophagus and Gastric Cardia* (Huang, G.J. and K'ai, W.Y. eds.). Berlin: Springer, pp. 25–51. Etiology of carcinoma of the esophagus.

Li, M., Li, P. and Li, B. (1980) *Adv. Cancer Res.* **33**, 173–249. Recent progress in research on esophageal cancer in China.

Li, J.Y., Ershow, A.G., Chen, Z.J., Wacholder, S., Li, G.Y., Guo W., Li, B. and Blot, W.J. (1989) *Int. J. Cancer* **43**, 755–761. A case–control study of cancer of the esophagus and gastric cardia in Linxian.

Lipman, T.O., Diamond, A., Mellow, M.H. and Patterson, K.Y. (1987) *J. Am. Coll. Nutr.* **6**, 41–46. Esophageal zinc content in human squamous esophageal cancer.

Love, A.H.G., Elmes, M., Golden, M.K. and McMaster, D. (1978) In: *Perspectives in Coeliac Disease* (McNicholl, B., McCarthy, C.F. and Fottrell, P.F. eds.). Lancaster: MTP Press, pp. 335–342. Zinc deficiency and coeliac disease.

Luo, X.M., Wei, H.J. and Yang, S.P. (1983) *J. Natl. Cancer Inst.* **71**, 75–80. Inhibitory effects of molybdenum on esophageal and forestomach carcinogenesis in rats.

Lyon, T.D.B., Smith, H. and Smith, L.B. (1979) *Br. J. Nutr.* **42**, 413–416. Is there a zinc deficiency in the west of Scotland?

Mak, K.M., Leo, M.A. and Lieber, C.S. (1987) *Gastroenterology* **93**, 362–370. Effect of ethanol and vitamin A deficiency on epithelial cell proliferation and structure in the rat esophagus.

McCoy, G.D., Hecht, S.S. and Wynder, E.L. (1980) *Prev. Med.* **9**, 622–629. The roles of tobacco, alcohol and diet in the etiology of upper alimentary and respiratory tract cancers.

Mellow, M.H., Layne, E.A. and Lipman, T., Krushik, M., Hostetler, C. and Smith, J.C. (1983) *Cancer* **51**, 1615–1620. Plasma zinc and vitamin A in human squamous carcinoma of the esophagus.

Mettlin, C., Graham, S., Priore, R., Marshall, J. and Swanson, M. (1981) *Nutr. Cancer* **2**, 143–147. Diet and cancer of the esophagus.

Mobarhan, S., Dowlatshahi, K. and Diba, Y.Y. (1980) *Am. J. Clin. Nutr.* **33**, 940. Hair zinc levels from a normal population in North-East Iran with a high incidence of esophageal carcinoma.

Moon, R.C. and McCormick, D.L. (1982) *J. Am. Acad. Dermatol.* **6**, 809–814. Inhibition of chemical carcinogenesis by retinoids.

Munoz, N., Wahrendorf, J., Bang, L.J., Crespi, M., Thurnham, D.I., Day, N.E., Ji, Z.H., Grassi, A., Yan, L.W., Lin, L.G., Quan, L.Y., Lang, Y.Q., Yun, Z.C., Fang, Z.S., Yao, L.J., Correa, P., O'Connor, G.T. and Bosch, X. (1985) *Lancet* **ii**, 111–114. No effect of riboflavine, retinol, and zinc on prevalence of precancerous lesions of esophagus.

Munoz, N., Hiyashi, M., Bang, L.J., Wahrendorf, J., Crespi, M. and Bosch, F.X. (1987) *J. Natl. Cancer Inst.* **79**, 687–691. Effect of riboflavin, retinol and zinc on micronuclei of buccal mucosa and of esophagus: a randomized double-blind interventional study in China.

Nakachi, K., Imai, K., Hoshiyama, Y. and Sasaba, T. (1988) *J. Epidemiol. Comm. Health* **42**, 355–364. The joint effects of two factors in the etiology of esophageal cancer in Japan.

Negri, E., La Vecchia, C., Franceschi, S., D'Avanzo, B. and Parazzini, F. (1991) *Int. J. Cancer* **48**, 350–354. Vegetable and fruit consumption and cancer risk.

Osis, D., Kramer, L., Waitrowski, E. and Spencer, H. (1972) *Am. J. Clin. Nutr.* **25**, 582–588. Dietary zinc intake in man.

Pottern, L.M., Morris, L.E., Blot, W.J., Ziegler, R.G. and Fraumeni, J.F. (1981) *J. Natl. Cancer Inst.* **67**, 777–783. Esophageal cancer among black men in Washington, DC. I. Alcohol, tobacco, and other risk factors.

Prasad, A.S., Oberleas, D., Wolf, P. and Horwitz, P. (1967) *J. Clin. Invest.* **46**, 549–557. Studies on zinc deficiency: changes in trace elements and enzyme activities in tissues of zinc-deficient rats.

Prasad, A.S. (1979) *Zinc in Human Nutrition.* Boca Raton: CRC Press.

Prasad, A.S. (1983) *Nutr. Rev.* **41**, 197–208. Clinical, biochemical and nutritional spectrum of zinc deficiency in human subjects.

Prasad, A.S. (1984) *Fed. Proc.* **43**, 2829–2834. Discovery and importance of zinc in human nutrition.

Purchase, I.F.H., Tustin, R.C. and van Rensburg, S.J. (1975) *Food Cosmet. Toxicol.* **13**, 639–647. Biological testing of food grown in the Transkei.

Rodgers, A.E., Sanchez, C., Feinsted, F.M. and Newberne, P.M. (1974) *Cancer Res.* **34**, 96–99. Dietary enhancement of nitrosamine carcinogenesis.

Rose, D.P. (1983) In: *Environmental Aspects of Cancer: The Role of Macro and Micro Components of Foods* (Wynder, E.L., Leveille, G.A., Weisberger, J.H. and Livingstone, G.E. eds.). New Jersey and London: Food and Nutrition Press, pp. 127–156. Micronutrients in carcinogenesis.

Sandstead, H.H., Henricksen, L.K., Greger, J.L., Prasad, A.S. and Good, R.A. (1982) *Am. J. Clin. Nutr.* **36**, 1046–1059. Zinc nutriture in the elderly in the relation to taste acuity, immune response, and wound healing.

Segal, I., Hale, M., Demetriou, A. and Mohamed, A.E. (1990) *Nutr. Cancer* **14**, 233–238. Pathological effects of pellagra on the esophagus.

Smith, J.C., McDaniel, E.G., Fann, F.F. and Halstead, J.A. (1973) *Science* **181**, 954–955. Zinc: a trace element essential in vitamin A metabolism.

Southon, S., Livesey, G., Gee, J.M. and Johnson, I.T. (1985) *Br. J. Nutr.* **53**, 595–603. Intestinal cellular proliferation and protein synthesis in zinc-deficient rats.

270   *Dietary deficiencies*

Sporn, M.B. and Newton, D.L. (1981) In: *Inhibition of Tumor Induction and Development*. (Zadek, M.S. and Lipkin, M. eds.). New York: Plenum Press, pp. 71–100. Retinoids and chemoprevention of cancer.

Thurnham, D.I., Zheng, S.F., Munoz, N., Crespi, M., Grassi, A., Hambridge, K.M. and Chai, T.F. (1985) *Nutr. Cancer* 7, 131–143. Comparison of riboflavin, vitamin A and zinc status of Chinese populations at high and low risk for esophageal cancer.

Thurnham, D.I., Munoz, N., Lu, J.B., Wahrendorf, J., Zheng, S.F., Hambidge, K.M. and Crespi, M. (1988) *Eur. J. Clin. Nutr.* 42, 647–660. Nutritional and haematological status of Chinese farmers: the influence of 13.5 months treatment with riboflavin, retinol and zinc.

Tuyns, A.J., Riboli, E. and Doornbos, G. (1985) In: *Diet and Human Carcinogenesis* (Joossens J.V., Hill, M.J. and Geboers, J. eds.). Amsterdam: Excerpta Medica, pp. 71–79. Nutrition and cancer of the esophagus.

Tuyns, A.J., Riboli, E., Doornbos, G. and Pequignot, G. (1987) *Nutr. Cancer* 9, 81–92. Diet and esophageal cancer in Calvados, France.

van Helden, P.D., Beyers, A.D., Bester, A.J. and Jaskiewicz, K. (1987) *Nutr. Cancer* 10, 247–255. Esophageal cancer: vitamin and lipotrope deficiencies in an at-risk South African population.

van Rensburg, S.J. (1981/1) *J. Natl. Cancer Inst.* 67, 243–251. Epidemiologic and dietary evidence for a specific nutritional predisposition to esophageal cancer.

van Rensburg, S.J., Kruger, E.F., Louw, M.E.J. and du Plessis, J.P. (1981/2) *Nutr. Rep. Int.* 24, 1123–1131. Vitamin A status and cancer risk: epidemiological and experimental evidence for a positive association.

van Rensburg, S.J., Benade, A.S., Rose, E.F. and du Plessis, J.P. (1983) *Nutr. Cancer* 4, 206–216. Nutritional status of African populations predisposed to esophageal cancer.

van Rensburg, S.J., Hall, J.M. and du Bruyn, D.B. (1985) *J. Natl. Cancer Inst.* 75, 561–566. Effect of various dietary staples on esophageal carcinogenesis induced in rats by simultaneously administered N-nitrosomethylbenzylamine.

van Rensburg, S.J., Hall, J.M. and Gathercole, P.S. (1986) *Nutr. Cancer* 8, 163–170. Inhibition of esophageal carcinogenesis in corn-fed rats by riboflavin, nicotinic acid, selenium, molybdenum, zinc and magnesium.

Wahrendorf, J., Munoz, N., Jian-Bang, L., Thurnham, D.I., Crespi, M. and Bosch, F.X. (1988) *Cancer Res.* 48, 2280–2283. Blood retinol, zinc and riboflavin status in relation to precancerous lesions of the esophagus: findings from a vitamin intervention trial in the People's Republic of China.

Warburg, O. (1956) *Science* 123, 309–314. On the origin of cancer cells.

Warwick, G.P. (1973) *Adv. Cancer Res.* 17, 81–229. Some aspects of the epidemiology and etiology of esophageal cancer with particular emphasis on the Transkei, South Africa.

Wynder, E.L. and Bross, I.J. (1961) *Cancer* 14, 389–413. A study of etiological factors in cancer of the esophagus.

Wynder, E.L. and Klin, U.E. (1965) *Cancer* 18, 167–180. The possible role of riboflavin deficiency in epithelial neoplasia. I. Epithelial changes of mice in simple deficiency.

Wynder, E.L. and Chan, P.C. (1970) *Cancer* 26, 1221–1224. The possible role of riboflavin deficiency in epithelial neoplasia. II. Effect on skin tumor development.

Wynder, E.L., Hoffmann, D., Chan, P. and Reddy, B. (1975) In: *Persons at High Risk of Cancer – An Approach to Cancer Etiology and Control* (Fraumeni, J.F. ed.). New York: Academic Press, pp. 485–501. Interdisciplinary and experimental approaches: metabolic etiology.

Wynder, E.L., Hoffmann, D., McCoy, G.D., Cohen, L.A. and Reddy, B.S. (1978) In: *Carcinogenesis*, vol. 2. *Mechanism of Tumor Promotion and Co-carcinogenesis* (Slaga, T.J., Sivak, A. and Boutwell, R.K. eds.). New York: Raven Press, pp. 59–77. Tumour promotion and co-carcinogenesis as related to man and his environment.

Yang, C.S. (1974) *Arch. Biochem. Biophys.* **160**, 623–630. Alterations of the aryl hydrocarbon hydroxylase system during riboflavin depletion and repletion.

Yang, C.S. (1980) *Cancer Res.* **40**, 2633–2644. Research on esophageal cancer in China: a review.

Yang, C.S., Miao, J., Yang, W., Huang, M., Wang, T., Xue, H., You, S., Lu, J. and Wu, J. (1982) *Nutr. Cancer* **4**, 154–164. Diet and vitamin nutrition of the high esophageal cancer risk population in Linxian, China.

Yang, C.S., Sun, Y., Yang, Q., Miller, K.W., Li, G., Zheng, S-F., Ershow, A.G., Blot, W.J. and Li, J. (1984) *J. Natl. Cancer Inst.* **73**, 1449–1453. Vitamin A and other deficiencies in Linxian, a high esophageal cancer incidence area in northern China.

Yu, M.C., Garabrant, D.H., Peters, J.M. and Mack, T.M. (1988) *Cancer Res.* **48**, 3843–3848. Tobacco, alcohol, diet, occupation and cancer of the esophagus.

Zaridze, D.G., Blettner, M., Trapeznikov, N.N., Kuvshinov, J.P., Matiakin, E.G., Poljakov, B.P., Poddubni, B.K., Parshikova, S.M., Rottenberg, V.I., Chamrakulov, F.S., Chodjaeva, M.C., Stich, H.F., Rosin, M.P., Thurnham, D.I., Hoffmann, D. and Brunnemann, K.D. (1985) *Int. J. Cancer* **36**, 153–158. Survey of a population with a high incidence of oral and oesophageal cancer.

Ziegler, R., Morris, L., Blot, W., Pottern, L.M., Hoover, R. and Fraumeni, J.F. (1981) *J. Natl. Cancer Inst.* **67**, 1199–1206. Esophageal cancer among black men in Washington DC. II. Role of nutrition.

11

Possible mechanisms involved in carcinogenesis

Molecular mechanisms

In the majority of human and experimental cancers, genetic damage is believed to be the initial cause of the disease. Of all the huge number of chemicals which have been tested for carcinogenesis, only N-nitroso compounds have been found to be potent carcinogens for the esophagus. As far as they have been studied, all the nitrosamines which affect the esophagus are metabolized by the target organ, and alkylate DNA at the O^6-position of guanine. The mutagenic base which is formed is removed rapidly from liver and several other organs, but not from esophagus (see Chapter 5). As human exposure to nitrosamines from a variety of sources, or formation of the compounds in the stomach, is probably universal, at present these compounds are the main contenders as initiators of esophageal cancer.

In general, very low levels of exposure to carcinogens result in malignancy only if the effects are promoted by a second insult. In animal experiments this can be a high dose of the carcinogen *per se*, so that it causes cellular damage and restorative hyperplasia. It could well be this increase in replication which is responsible for the promoting effect. In man, consumption of alcoholic beverages is the main cause of esophageal cancer in the West, and intubation of ethanol, especially of ethanol containing the fusel alcohols which are present in many spirits, causes an increase in basal cell replication without initial histological signs of damage (see Chapter 6). In other high-incidence areas, as in the Iran to China 'cancer belt', and in regions of Africa, the secondary hazard is not always alcohol but may be dietary factors, and many of these have also been shown to cause an increase in cell replication in the esophagus.

There are several ways in which an increase in basal cell replication could promote carcinogenesis. A round of DNA replication may be essential in order to convert the lesion into a change in base sequence, and this would have to occur before repair enzymes had removed the alkyl adduct from the DNA. Alternatively, or in addition, an increase in the number of initiated cells might be necessary in order to allow them to reach a 'critical mass', which has been postulated to be necessary before independent uncontrolled replication can take place. Another possibility is that an increase in the mitotic rate is essential to increase the opportunities for further mutations to occur. Several additional mutations after the initiating event have been shown to be necessary to produce the biochemical changes which result in uncontrolled growth (see next section).

The changes in biochemical mechanisms which accompany carcinogenesis have been studied largely with the aim of finding a marker for use as a means of detecting cancer at the early stages, when prevention of further development may be possible. The initial work on γ-glutamyl transferase, and studies on microfilaments, are described in Chapter 2. Many biochemical responses to carcinogens, for example the increase in ornithine decarboxylase which occurs in Barrett's esophagus, usually occur with any increase in replication, and are not specifically associated with disease. More significant is the appearance of keratin species not seen in normal esophageal cells (see Chapter 2) (Scaramuzzino *et al.* 1986; Banks-Schlegel *et al.* 1984, 1986*a*) and of various ectopic tumor-associated antigens, including human chorionic gonadotropin, human placental lactogen, α-fetoprotein, carcinoembryonic antigen, and non-specific cross-reacting antigen (Burg-Kurland *et al.* 1986). The significance of these changes has been discussed by Lipkin (1988).

A more relevant change which might be expected to account for the increased rate of cell replication is the increase in the number of epidermal growth factor (EGF) receptors found in various squamous cell carcinomas. Surprisingly, it was found that esophageal carcinomas contained lower quantities of EGF receptors than did normal esophageal epithelial cells, but that their affinity was increased (Banks-Schlegel *et al.* 1986*b*). There was no simple relationship between number, affinity, or growth-stimulatory response to EGF. Changes which alter the rate of tissue growth are obviously an important factor at the progression stage.

By some means the changes in the biochemistry of the cell lead to the succession of changes in structure described in Chapter 3, and the final result is autonomous uncontrolled growth, with immortalization of the malignant cells, but in many cases suffering and death of the patient.

Genetic changes

Studies of the nature of oncogene involvement and other genetic disturbances which occur in carcinogenesis could give insight into the etiology of the disease. Of the proto-oncogenes which have been shown to acquire transforming activity the *ras* gene, first identified in a virus which causes rat sarcomas, has been most often studied.

Activation has been detected in several human malignancies. With reference to the upper respiratory–intestinal tract, a low incidence of *ras* oncogene activation was detected in certain human squamous cell carcinomas, including those of the larynx (Rumsby *et al.* 1990). Disappointingly, however, examination of human esophageal squamous cell tumors from especially high-risk areas, i.e. from Normandy in France (Hollstein *et al.* 1988), and from South Africa (Victor *et al.* 1990), showed no evidence for the activation of K-*ras* or N-*ras*.

Mutagenic activation of the *ras* genes results from base substitutions in codons 12, 13 and 61. The DNA adduct, O^6-methylguanine, which is formed after nitrosamine exposure and metabolism, is known to induce guanine to adenine transition mutations which can activate the C-*ras* genes (Bartsch *et al.* 1984). In keeping with this, activation of Ha-*ras* was detected in rat esophageal papilloma induced by *N*-nitroso-*N*-methyl-benzylamine (NMBzA) (Wang *et al.* 1990; Barch *et al.* 1991). The occurrence in papillomas suggested that activation is an early event in carcinogenesis. As described in Chapter 5, suggestive evidence that nitrosamines are involved in human cancer was given by the elevated levels of O^6-methylguanine detected in samples of esophageal cancers from Linxian county in China (Umbenhauer *et al.* 1985). The failure to detect activation of *ras* until now in the human samples studied has not been explained, but it does not necessarily imply that this gene is not involved. As stressed by Hollstein *et al.* (1988), variations from one study to another of mutations in *ras* could be due to differences in sensitivity of the detection methods used, or to variations in the pathology of the specimens studied.

In addition to activation of cellular oncogenes which tend to induce the changes characteristic of cancer cells, loss of the genes which suppress these changes is also essential for the development of malignancy. The total number of suppressor genes active in any organ is unknown. Their loss or deletion, however, necessitates at least two mutations, as the suppressor genes occur in pairs, and both must be inactivated for their function to be lost entirely. Loss or deletion of specific segments of chromosomes has been detected mainly on numbers 5, 18 and 17, and in the case of esophageal squamous cell carcinomas deletion has been detected with high frequency in chromosome 17 (Wagata *et al.* 1991). The gene which is deleted, designated p53, codes for a nuclear phosphoprotein of molecular weight 53 000 that is involved in the control of cell proliferation and may have tumor-suppressing activity. Mutations in the p53 gene have been detected also in Barrett's esophagus (Casson *et al*. 1991), but it was pointed out that the frequency may reflect the susceptibility of proliferating esophageal epithelium to mutational events.

Amplification of transforming genes is another event which has been detected in human carcinogenesis. In the case of the esophagus, amplification of several genes has been detected, including the *erb* gene (Hollstein *et al*. 1988; Houldsworth *et al*. 1990). It was found that the epidermal growth factor receptor is homologous to the product of the avian erythroblastosis virus oncogene v-*erb*. Gene amplification is usually accompanied by enhanced gene expression, and data strongly suggest that an increase in epidermal growth factor receptor levels is associated with the development of human squamous cell cancers of the esophagus and lung (Ozawa *et al*. 1988; Hollstein *et al*. 1988; Houldsworth *et al*. 1990; Chen *et al*. 1991).

Amplification has also been detected of the *hst* gene in esophageal cancers, this time in a Japanese population (Tsuda *et al*. 1988, 1989). This transforming gene was first isolated from a human gastric cancer, and has frequently been detected in human malignancies. It codes for a protein related to fibroblast growth factor. In esophagus, the amplification may occur at a late stage in carcinogenesis, possibly when metastases begin to develop.

Another type of genetic change detected in malignancy is the non-random chromosome rearrangements which occur in gastric and esophageal adenocarcinomas (Rodriguez *et al*. 1990). Such changes could cause the abnormalities of differentiation which have been detected. An important feature in terminal cell differentiation in normal esophagus, the development of cross-linked envelopes, was reduced in carcinoma cells – a change suggesting a shift from a state of differentiation to one of proliferation (Banks-Schlegel *et al*. 1984, 1986).

As mentioned previously (Chapter 8), papilloma virus infection in conjunction with a possible esophageal carcinogen was implicated in esophageal cancer in cattle, and there is very limited evidence for a role in human esophageal cancer (Hansen *et al*. 1987). This heterogeneous group of DNA viruses has been implicated in several human squamous cell carcinomas, although absence of the viral DNA or viral antigens in experimental tumors of the alimentary tract shows that the viral genome is not essential for the development of malignancy. Studies of biopsies from patients in the Linxian region of China showed that human papilloma virus

DNA was frequently associated with hyperplastic or dysplastic cells adjacent to the carcinomas (Chang *et al.* 1990). Whether the viral infection is a cause or a result of the disease remains to be established.

Obviously an understanding of the changes in the functioning of the genetic material is at a very preliminary stage. At present, however, the advances in this area of cancer research are exceptionally rapid.

Future prospects

As environmental factors are responsible for causing almost all esophageal cancers, the prospects for taking preventive measures might be expected to be good. Disappointingly, even where the cause is certain, it has not yet been possible to make very great reductions in cancer incidence. A few causes have been established with certainty, as with the consumption of alcoholic beverages, especially when accompanied by smoking tobacco, and also chewing betel quids. Other factors have been established almost beyond reasonable doubt. Examples are the deficiency of certain micro-nutrients, especially of riboflavin and zinc, consumption of food or drink contaminated by *Fusarium* mycotoxins, and consumption of nitrosamines, the only chemical initiators so far characterized and present in food. Other factors associated with esophageal cancer merit urgent study. A neglected factor which is incriminated by a great deal of evidence but not yet by scientific surveys is the hazard presented by drinking hot black (i.e. fermented) tea without sufficient milk to precipitate the tannins. Consumption of bracken fronds is another very likely but not yet proven cause of esophageal cancer.

It is obvious that even when the causes are known with certainty or with a high degree of probability, it is difficult to take preventive measures. The complete banning of alcoholic beverages is unthinkable, and 'safe' doses are dependent on complex factors such as tobacco use and type of beverage consumed. Also it is obvious that dietary deficiencies around the world will take many years to remedy.

On the other hand, it should be possible to lower the incidence of esophageal cancer if research into the mechanisms involved in carcinogenesis is continued. For example, where spirits are the most hazardous type of drink, and if this is due to the high levels of fusel alcohols present in many spirits, it should be possible to reduce the concentrations of these complex alcohols without adversely affecting the organoleptic properties of the drinks. There are several other instances where safer products could be produced. For example, if the formation of nitrosamines is proved to be the cause of the risk presented by chewing betal quids or consuming food preserved by smoking, the addition of vitamin C to the quids, or a change in the composition of the smoke used, should reduce nitrosamine formation. If the way in which riboflavin or zinc deficiencies cause esophageal cancer was understood, it may then be possible to supplement diets of the populations at risk by supplying easily transported tablets instead of bulky perishable foods.

An important factor which has not received sufficient attention is the protective effect of a high consumption of fresh fruit and vegetables in the diet. A great many surveys, mentioned in Chapters 6, 10 and elsewhere, have illustrated this protective action. Although diet cannot negate the hazard of alcohol and tobacco, it can bring about a reduction in cancer incidence of the people at risk from these hazards. A recent study of the relationship between fruit and vegetable consumption and cancer risk for a number of sites was carried out in northern Italy (Negri *et al.* 1991). For both fruit and vegetables, there was consistent protection for all epithelial tumors, although not for non-epithelial lymphoid neoplasms.

The mechanisms underlying the protective action are not understood, but are very probably not due only to the micronutrient content of these foods. A variety of chemicals present in these foods have been shown to inhibit the metabolic activation of carcinogenic nitrosamines to scavenge electrophilic metabolites, and to remove free radicals which can damage the genetic material. When the details of these actions are understood, it may be possible to supplement diets with tablets of purified chemicals. But until questions of dose, time of administration, and possible unexpected harmful effects have been answered, the only safe procedure is to supply the fruit and vegetables themselves.

It was in 1982 that van Rensburg stated that we were on the brink of an era of cancer prevention (van Rensburg 1982). Now, 10 years later, we are very much nearer to this change in emphasis from cure to prevention.

References

Banks-Schlegel, S.P. and Harris, C.C. (1984) *Cancer Res.* **44**, 1153–1157. Aberrant expression of keratin proteins and cross-linked envelopes in human esophageal carcinomas.

Banks-Schlegel, S.P. and Quintero, J. (1986*a*) *Cancer Res.* **46**, 250–258. Growth and differentiation of human esophageal carcinoma cell lines.

Banks-Schlegel, S.P. and Quintero, J. (1986*b*) *J. Biol. Chem.* **261**, 4359–4362. Human esophageal carcinoma cells have fewer, but higher affinity epidermal growth factor receptors.

Barch, D.H., Jacoby, R.F., Brasitus, T.A., Radosevich, J.A., Carney, W.P. and Iannaccone, P.M. (1991) *Carcinogenesis* **12**, 2373–2377. Incidence of Harvey *ras* oncogene point mutations and their expression in methylbenzylnitrosamine-induced esophageal tumorigenesis.

Bartsch, H. and Montesano, R. (1984) *Carcinogenesis* **5**, 1381–1393. Relevance of nitrosamines to human cancer.

Burg-Kurland, C.L., Purnell, D.M., Combs, J.W., Hillman, E.A., Harris, C.C. and Trump, B.F. (1986) *Cancer Res.* **46**, 2936–2943. Immunocytochemical evaluation of human esophageal neoplasms and preneoplastic lesions for β-chorionic gonadotropin, placental lactogen, α-fetoprotein, carcinoembryonic antigen, and nonspecific cross-reacting antigen.

Casson, A.G., Mukhopadhyay, T., Cleary, K.R., Ro, J.Y., Levin, B. and Roth, J.A. (1991) *Cancer Res.* **51**, 4495–4499. p53 gene mutations in Barrett's epithelium and esophageal cancer.

Chang, F., Syrjanens, S., Shen, Q., Ji, H. and Syrayana, K. (1990) *Int. J. Cancer* **45**, 21–25. Human papillomavirus (HPV) DNA in esophageal precancer lesions and squamous cell carcinomas from China.

Chen, S., Chou, C., Wong, F., Chang, C. and Hu, C. (1991) *Cancer Res.* **51**, 1898–1903. Overexpression of epidermal growth factor and insulin-like growth factor-I receptors and autocrine stimulation in human esophageal carcinoma cells.

Hausen, zur H. and de Villiers, E.M. (1987) In *Cancer of the Liver, Esophagus and Nasopharynx* (Wagner, G. and Zhang, Y.H. eds.). Berlin: Springer, pp. 132–133. Papillomavirus infections in esophageal cancer.

Hollstein, M.C., Smits, A.M., Galiana, C., Yamasaki, H., Bos, J.L., Mandard, A., Partensky, C. and Montesano, R. (1988) *Cancer Res.* **48**, 5119–5123. Amplification of epidermal growth factor receptor gene but no evidence of *ras* mutations in primary human esophageal cancers.

Houldsworth, J., Cordon-Cardo, C., Ladanyi, M., Kelsen, D.P. and Chaganti, R.S.K. (1990) *Cancer Res.* **50**, 6417–6422. Gene amplification in gastric and esophageal adenocarcinomas.

Lipkin, M. (1988) *Cancer Res.* **48**, 235–245. Biomarkers of increased susceptibility to gastrointestinal cancer: new application to studies of cancer prevention in human subjects.

Negri, E., La Vecchia, C., Franceschi, S., D'Avanzo, B. and Parazzini, F. (1991) *Int. J. Cancer* **48**, 350–354. Vegetable and fruit consumption and cancer risk.

Ozawa, S., Ueda, M., Ando, N., Abe, O. and Shimizu, N. (1988) *Jpn. J. Cancer Res.* **79**, 1201–1207. Epidermal growth factor receptors in cancer tissues of esophagus, lung, pancreas, colorectum, breast and stomach.

Rodriguez, E., Rao, P.H., Ladanyi, M., Altorki, N., Albino, P., Kelsen, D.P., Jhanwar, S.C. and Chaganti, R.S.K. (1990) *Cancer Res.* **50**, 6410–6416. 11p13–15 is a specific region of chromosomal rearrangement in gastric and esophageal adenocarcinomas.

Rumsby, G., Carter, R.L. and Gusterson, B.A. (1990) *Br. J. Cancer* **61**, 365–368. Low incidence of *ras* oncogene activation in human squamous cell carcinomas.

Scaramauzzino, D., Stoner, G.D. and Goldblatt, P.J. (1986) *Proc. Am. Assoc. Cancer Res.* **27**, 69. Keratin protein expression in non-tumorigenic and tumorigenic rat esophageal epithelial cells.

Tsuda, T., Nakatani, H., Matsumura, T., Yoshida, K., Tahara, E., Nishihira, T., Sakamoto, H., Yoshida, T., Terada, M. and Sugimura, T. (1988) *Jpn. J. Cancer Res.* **79**, 584–588. Amplification of the *hst-1* gene in human esophageal carcinomas.

Tsuda, T., Tahara, E., Kajiyama, G., Sakamoto, H., Terada, M. and Sugimura, T. (1989) *Cancer Res.*, **49**, 5505–5508. High incidence of coamplification of *hst*-1 and *int*-2 genes in human esophageal carcinomas.

Umbenhauer, D., Wild, C.P., Montesano, R., Saffhill, R., Boyle, J.M., Huh, N., Kirstein, U., Thomale, J., Rajewsky, M.F. and Lu, S.H. (1985) *Int. J. Cancer* **36**, 661–665. O^6-Methyldeoxyguanosine in oesophageal DNA among individuals at high risk of oesophageal cancer.

van Rensburg, S.J. (1982) *S. Afr. Cancer Bull.* **26**, 153–159. Nutritional factors in human carcinogenesis.

Victor, T., Du Toit, R., Jordaan, A.M., Bester, A.J. and van Helden, P.D. (1990) *Cancer Res.* **50**, 4911–4914. No evidence for point mutations in codons 12, 13 and 61 of the *ras* gene in a high-incidence area for esophageal and gastric cancers.

Wang, Y., You, M., Reynolds, S.H., Stoner, G.D. and Anderson, M.W. (1990) *Cancer Res.* **50**, 1591–1595. Mutational activation of the cellular Harvey *ras* oncogene in rat esophageal papillomas induced by methylbenzylnitrosamine.

Wagata, K., Ishizaki, M., Imamura, Y., Shimada, M. and Tobe, T. (1991) *Cancer Res.* **51**, 2113–2117. Deletion of 17p and amplification of the *int*-2 gene in esophageal carcinomas.

Index